MW00723262

Transcultural Nursing Education Strategies

Priscilla Limbo Sagar, EdD, RN, ACNS-BC, CTN-A, is a professor of nursing at Mount Saint Mary College in Newburgh, New York. She received a BS in nursing from the Philippine Women's University; an MS in adult nursing, with a minor in education from Pace University; and an EdD in nursing education/professorial role from Teachers College, Columbia University.

She is board certified in adult health from the American Nurses Credentialing Center and has advanced certification in transcultural nursing from the Transcultural Nursing Certification Commission (TNCC). She is a Transcultural Nursing Society (TCNS) transcultural scholar and a member of the Nursing Hall of Fame at Columbia University. Dr. Sagar is a site evaluator for the Commission of Collegiate Nursing Education (CCNE). Her research interests include transcultural nursing (TCN); mentoring; and international nursing, partnerships, and collaborations. She serves as consultant in the areas of cultural diversity and promotion of cultural competence as well as in curriculum development, implementation, and evaluation. In addition, Dr. Sagar has facilitated several national and international conferences to disseminate TCN research and knowledge. She is a long time member of TCNS and has chaired the Eligibility and Credentialing Committee of the TNCC. Her other professional memberships include the Philippine Nurses Association of America and the Sigma Theta Tau Honor Society for Nursing.

Dr. Sagar also teaches as an adjunct faculty for University of Phoenix Online's School of Advanced Studies where she functions as a committee member in dissertations with cultural diversity and transcultural foci. Her publications include *Transcultural Nursing Theory and Models: Application in Nursing Education, Practice, and Administration* as well as contributions to *Giving Through Teaching: How Nurse Educators Are Changing the World* and the forthcoming third edition of *Culture Care Diversity and Universality: A Worldwide Theory of Nursing.*

Transcultural Nursing Education Strategies

Priscilla Limbo Sagar, EdD, RN, ACNS-BC, CTN-A

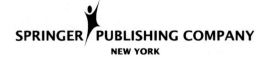

SPRINGER PUBLISHING COMPANY
NEW YORK

Copyright © 2014 Springer Publishing Company, LLC

All rights reserved.

No part of this publication may be reproduced, stored in a retrieval system, or transmitted in any form or by any means, electronic, mechanical, photocopying, recording, or otherwise, without the prior permission of Springer Publishing Company, LLC, or authorization through payment of the appropriate fees to the Copyright Clearance Center, Inc., 222 Rosewood Drive, Danvers, MA 01923, 978-750-8400, fax 978-646-8600, info@copyright.com or on the Web at www.copyright.com.

Springer Publishing Company, LLC
11 West 42nd Street
New York, NY 10036
www.springerpub.com

Acquisitions Editor: Margaret Zuccarini
Production Editor: Michael O'Connor
Composition: Newgen Imaging

ISBN: 978-0-8261-9593-7
e-book ISBN: 978-0-8261-9594-4

Instructors' Materials: Qualified instructors may request the ancillary package by emailing textbook@springerpub.com
Instructors' Ancillary Package: 978-0-8261-2754-9

14 15 16 17 18/ 5 4 3 2 1

The author and the publisher of this Work have made every effort to use sources believed to be reliable to provide information that is accurate and compatible with the standards generally accepted at the time of publication. The author and publisher shall not be liable for any special, consequential, or exemplary damages resulting, in whole or in part, from the readers' use of, or reliance on, the information contained in this book. The publisher has no responsibility for the persistence or accuracy of URLs for external or third-party Internet websites referred to in this publication and does not guarantee that any content on such websites is, or will remain, accurate or appropriate.

Library of Congress Cataloging-in-Publication Data
Priscilla Limbo Sagar, author.
  Transcultural nursing education strategies/Priscilla Limbo Sagar.
      p. ; cm.
  Includes bibliographical references and index.
  ISBN 978-0-8261-9593-7—ISBN 978-0-8261-9594-4 (e-book)
  I. Title.
  [DNLM: 1. Transcultural Nursing–methods. 2. Cultural Competency–education. 3. Education, Nursing–methods. WY 107]
  RT86.54
  610.73—dc23   2014000283

Special discounts on bulk quantities of our books are available to corporations, professional associations, pharmaceutical companies, health care organizations, and other qualifying groups. If you are interested in a custom book, including chapters from more than one of our titles, we can provide that service as well.

For details, please contact:
Special Sales Department, Springer Publishing Company, LLC
11 West 42nd Street, 15th Floor, New York, NY 10036–8002
Phone: 877-687-7476 or 212-431-4370; Fax: 212-941-7842
E-mail: sales@springerpub.com

Printed in the United States of America by Gasch Printing.

This book is dedicated to:

*My loving family; husband Drew Sagar for
his unconditional love and support; daughter Alexa and grandson Andrew Michael Cass;
parents Trinidad and Mercedes Limbo; sisters Virgenes, Soledad, and Cristina; brothers
Ruben, Marto, Juanito, Roberto, and Virgilio Limbo;
and all members of my extended family.*

*The late Dr. Madeline Leininger, founder and leader of transcultural nursing (TCN),
for her courageous and untiring effort for six decades in building
transcultural nursing knowledge, and her laborious work on behalf
of TCN in general. She was a mentor who continues to inspire my work.*

*Other pioneering transcultural nurses who contributed, are contributing,
and will contribute to the field of TCN. Because of Dr. Leininger and
these nurses, we have a wealth of knowledge for evidence-based practice
in transcultural nursing.*

*To mentoring; my past and current mentors; my mentees, and to
those they will mentor.*

*To the Philippine Women's University College of Nursing faculty for the
excellent nursing education that prepared me not only to be a nurse
and a leader, but also a writer, through opportunities to edit both the
College of Nursing and university papers.*

*To Professor Elisea de la Cruz,
for nurturing my love of writing and for demanding excellence.*

*To all nurses and student nurses; to take up the challenge and lead others
to bring TCN to all settings of nursing education, practice, administration,
and research. TCN is the water of necessity and the settings are what I called "the villages of the world" in my poem "Who Will Fetch the Water?"*

Who Will Fetch the Water [Today, Tomorrow, and in the Future]?
(To my fellow nurses)

1

The late foundress dug the well. That well is now a river . . .
I will fetch the water today.
And bring it to the villages.
We are 3,063,163* strong. We could lead the throng . . .
Will you be coming along?

2

Will they?
Staff nurses: guardians and caregivers.
Educators: opening the floodgates to minds.
Administrators: channeling flow through organizations.
Researchers: divining into new knowledge.

3

You, and I, and them. We are privileged.
We have strength in numbers. We have been constantly trusted.
Should we all fetch the water?

4

We are ready.
We are on clear vantage points.
If we bring water to all villages
Health for all may not just be a promise.

Priscilla Limbo Sagar

*United States Department of Health and Human Services, Health Resources Services Administration. (2010). *The registered nurse population: Initial findings from the 2008 national sample survey of registered nurses*. Retrieved February 7, 2014, from http://bhpr.hrsa.gov/healthworkforce/rnsurveys/rnsurveyfinal.pdf

Contents

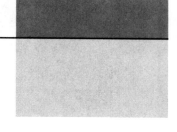

ADDITIONAL SYLLABI AVAILABLE IN DIGITAL ANCILLARY PRODUCT

Note: All Appendices in the book, in addition to the additional sample syllabi listed below, are part of a digital ancillary product provided in Word format and available to qualified instructors. This ancillary package can be requested by e-mailing textbook@springerpub.com.

AP-1. Sample Syllabus: Introduction to Nursing

AP-2. Sample Syllabus: Health History and Physical Assessment

AP-3. Sample Syllabus: Child-Rearing: Infancy to Adolescence

AP-4. Sample Syllabus: Nursing Research

AP-5. Sample Syllabus: Culturally Congruent Care: Pharmacology

AP-6. Sample Syllabus: Culturally Congruent Care of Older Adults

AP-7. Sample Syllabus: Mental Health and Psychiatric Nursing

AP-8. Sample Syllabus: Community Health Nursing

AP-9. Sample Syllabus: Professional Nursing Transition Course

AP-10. Sample Syllabus: Advanced Transcultural Nursing

Contributors

Mollie Bowman, BS, RN
Staff Nurse
Saint Luke's Cornwall Hospital
Newburgh, New York

Caroline Camuñas, EdD, RN
Adjunct Associate Professor
Health and Behavior Studies
Teachers College, Columbia University
New York, New York

Toni Ann Cervone, BS, RN
Staff Nurse
Sing Sing Correctional Facility
Psychiatric Crisis Unit
Ossining, New York

Julie Coon, EdD, RN
Director, School of Nursing
Ferris University
Big Rapids, Michigan

Ann D. Corcoran, DNP, RN-BC
Assistant Professor of Nursing
Mount Saint Mary College
Newburgh, New York

Debra A. Hrelic, PhD, RN-C
Professor of Nursing
Mount Saint Mary College
Newburgh, New York

Teresa V. Hurley, DHEd, RN
Associate Professor of Nursing
Mount Saint Mary College
Newburgh, New York

Barbara J. Joslyn, EdD, RN
Former Assistant Professor
Mount Saint Mary College
Newburgh, New York

Sheila O'Shea Melli, EdD, RN
Adjunct Associate Professor, Organization and
    Leadership
Teachers College, Columbia University
New York, New York

Nancy Spear Owen, MA, RN
Instructor of Nursing
Mount Saint Mary College
Newburgh, New York

Drew Y. Sagar, MS, RN, ANP-C
Nurse Practitioner
Axis Medical
Poughkeepsie, New York
Adjunct Faculty of Nursing
Mount Saint Mary College
Newburgh, New York

Priscilla Limbo Sagar, EdD, RN, ACNS-BC, CTN-A
Professor of Nursing
Mount Saint Mary College
Newburgh, New York

Elizabeth Simon, PhD, RN, ANP-BC
Director and Professor, School of Nursing
Nyack College
Nyack, New York

Foreword

Transcultural Nursing Education Strategies is Dr. Priscilla Limbo Sagar's most recent contribution to the body of knowledge in the fields of transcultural nursing and nursing education. This book, along with her previous work titled *Transcultural Nursing Theory and Models: Application in Nursing Education, Practice, and Administration,* make her among the world's foremost experts in transcultural nursing.

This is a much anticipated comprehensive compendium of evidence-based and best practices in transcultural nursing that contains exceptionally useful and helpful material for nurse educators in academic and staff development settings and for their students. Professional nurses are expected to plan, implement, and evaluate cultural competence and diversity initiatives within their respective organizational systems while simultaneously meeting state and national accreditation mandates and/or standards of care. Dr. Sagar provides a fresh, multidimensional, and multifaceted approach to transcultural nursing education strategies by including a wide array of transcultural conceptual and theoretical models, cultural assessment instruments, and key concepts and content found in toolkits used by the National League for Nursing and the American Association of Colleges of Nursing to integrate cultural competence and transcultural nursing concepts into undergraduate and graduate curricula. Among the purposes of the book is to teach cultural competence to nurses in clinical practice settings and students in undergraduate and master's academic nursing programs. Dr. Sagar addresses the culture care needs of individual patients across the life span, as well as families and groups from diverse cultures. Dr. Sagar's book provides a unique perspective on the subject matter because it includes so many different types of teaching strategies and pedagogical aids, such as role-playing exercises, case studies, modules, continuing education lesson plans, and course syllabi. The stand-alone modules developed for nursing courses typically found in school of nursing curricula are also suitable for staff development in the areas of cultural competence, diversity, and transcultural nursing.

Dr. Sagar has divided the text into seven major parts. Part I provides an overview of transcultural concepts, history, theory, and models; reviews research findings and the best available evidence for culturally competent nursing and health care; presents well-researched modules for teaching transcultural nursing concepts; and examines transcultural nursing concepts in the NCLEX-RN® examination. Part II integrates transcultural nursing into foundational and introductory nursing courses such as fundamentals of nursing, nursing skills, and health assessment courses. In Part III transcultural nursing concepts across the life span are introduced in courses with content related to childbearing, child-rearing, adolescent and adult health, and gerontological nursing. Part IV focuses on transcultural nursing concepts in specialty courses such as mental health and psychiatric nursing, pharmacology, nutrition, nursing research, and a professional nursing transition course. Of particular interest is the unique chapter on transcultural concepts in the simulation laboratory in which Dr. Sagar discusses the use of simulation to teach diversity and transcultural nursing knowledge and skills. In Part V the chapters focus on integrating transcultural concepts across undergraduate and graduate nursing programs and in faculty orientation. Part VI is dedicated to integrating transcultural concepts into staff development and includes transcultural modules for use when orienting new domestic and international nurses and other health care workers; annual online and face-to-face modules for yearly staff updates on transcultural nursing such as those required by the American Nurses Credentialing Center (ANCC) for magnet designation; preparing policies and procedures using evidence-based and best practices that are congruent with current mandates and accreditation standards; and preparing for accreditation by reviewing transcultural concepts in the mission, goals resources, curricula, and evaluation outcomes. In Part VII, Dr. Sagar's concluding chapter features the vision for the future of transcultural nursing, including transcultural concepts in consultation, mentoring, international partnerships and collaborations, and future trends for this increasingly vital specialty as the global society becomes increasingly interconnected while at the same time growing more multicultural.

In closing, I would like to express appreciation to Dr. Priscilla Sagar for sharing her extensive knowledge and years of experience as a scholar, teacher, and leader in the field of transcultural nursing in *Transcultural Nursing Education Strategies*. This text provides valuable information for undergraduate and graduate nursing students, nursing faculty, nurse educators in staff development settings, and all other professional nurses who strive to use transcultural nursing concepts to provide culturally competent care for individual patients, families, and groups from diverse cultural backgrounds. *Transcultural Nursing Education Strategies* provides readers with important, state-of-the-art, well-researched, and carefully documented, evidence-based, and best practices for delivering culturally competence care.

Margaret M. Andrews, PhD, RN, FAAN, CTN
Editor, *Online Journal of Cultural Competence in Nursing and Healthcare*
Director and Professor of Nursing
School of Health Professions and Studies
University of Michigan—Flint

Foreword

Our nation has seen a dramatic transformation in the demographic characteristics of its citizens and residents. From a historical beginning of a Eurocentric migrant population to our current highly diverse characteristics, this nation has evolved to include multiple communities representing the entire globe's population. Current statistics regarding birth rates provide evidence that the term *minority* is no longer relevant for the description of individuals from diverse ethnic or racial groups. Moreover, the diverse other cultural perspectives that are present in the United States, including gender, religion, sexual orientation, and others, mandate that our nation's nursing education programs prepare a professional nursing workforce capable of understanding and respecting this diversity as they seek to design and implement the highest quality care for the individuals for whom they are privileged to care.

Transcultural nursing is not a new concept; however, the extreme complexity of this nation's diversity will challenge nurse educators to develop resources, tools, curricula, and experiences that will shape the new or advancing professionals' perspectives and skills for providing appropriate and patient-centered care. The growing concerns related to the appropriateness of care, the need to be patient centered in that care, and the importance of health literacy in delivering good care mandates a strong focus on culture as a central element in the design of care. Patient-centered care can only occur when all clinicians have an appreciation for, and an understanding of, the cultural norms that will guide an individual's choices and behaviors in care experiences.

Transcultural Nursing Education Strategies is a valuable new resource to support efforts by both nurse educators and practicing nurses in their goals to provide high-quality care that is culturally appropriate. The wide array of content, including the strong theoretical model that frames this work and the tools for implementing these, creates a framework that will stand the test of time. Moreover, the text's appreciation and explication of the numerous issues affected by cultural norms and expectations gives the professional nurse a road map for engaging in culturally appropriate, patient-centered, and high-quality care. I am honored to be able to provide this Foreword for an enormously important piece of work that will assist us to do the right things for our nation's diverse population.

Geraldine (Polly) Bednash, PhD, RN, FAAN
Chief Executive Officer and Executive Director
American Association of Colleges of Nursing, Washington, DC

Foreword

Transcultural Nursing Education Strategies, written by Priscilla Limbo Sagar, EdD, RN, ACNS-BC, CTN-A, is a welcome resource for enhancing cultural competence for both individuals and organizations. While this book is derived from transcultural nursing theory, the content is applicable to other health care professionals and their educators.

Transcultural nursing is not an academic exercise. It is critical to the provision of competent care to diverse populations and central to the survival of health care organizations.

Dr. Sagar's first book, *Transcultural Nursing Theory and Models: Application in Nursing Education, Practice, and Administration,* focused on the review and application of six transcultural nursing models and provided assessment tools for nursing education, practice, and administration. This, her second ground-breaking book, provides course syllabi, lesson plans, modules, case studies, and role-plays based on Madeleine Leininger's Theory of Culture Care Diversity and Universality, conceptual models from Purnell, Campinha-Bacote, Choi, Giger and Davidhizar, Spector, and Jeffreys, and the Andrews and Boyle nursing assessment guide. Dr. Sagar makes valuable resources available to faculty teaching at all levels.

Dr. Sagar clearly addresses the imperative for integrating transcultural concepts into both academic and practice settings. She begins the book by providing an overview of transcultural concepts, history, theory, and models. Using an evidence-based approach, Dr. Sagar summarizes the evidence for integration of transcultural concepts into nursing education at all levels; identifies the challenges inherent in training for cultural competence; describes the tools available for measuring cultural competence among faculty, students, and staff; and explores the use of modules to effectively teach knowledge and skills.

In chapters focused on the academic setting, Dr. Sagar provides strategies for integrating transcultural nursing concepts into a variety of courses: introduction to nursing, nursing skills, health assessment and physical examination, childbearing and child-rearing, adult health, gerontology, mental health and psychiatric nursing, pharmacology, nutrition, nursing research, community health, professional nursing transition, and the simulation laboratory. Each chapter is filled with essential information and creative approaches for teaching cultural competence and the care of culturally diverse clients. Dr. Sagar addresses the various levels of academic preparation for nurses, including LPN/LVN, diploma, associate degree, baccalaureate degree, masters, and doctoral programs. She also provides an overview of transcultural nursing concepts for faculty members.

Arguably the greatest contribution of this book is the rigor with which Dr. Sagar approaches the rationale for and strategies to incorporate transcultural concepts into practice settings. Today's practicing nurses have been educated in a variety of settings, at a variety of times. Some graduated in the 1960s, before transcultural concepts were addressed in academic curricula. Others are international graduates. Dr. Sagar clearly addresses the compelling need for transcultural nursing in the practice setting, addressing both government and accreditation mandates. She provides essential tools, including education modules and policies, for practice settings.

This ambitious book is a must-read synthesis of the existing knowledge related to transcultural nursing education. Dr. Sagar has created a comprehensive collection that bridges both education and practice settings. Application of the concepts she presents will build cultural competence in individuals and in organizations, and will help to address the gap in quality that is so often seen with diverse patient populations. As a practice profession, meeting the health care needs of all people must be our ultimate goal. In this book, Dr. Sagar makes an exceptional contribution to transcultural health care and nursing and to the delivery of culturally competent care in all settings.

Patti Ludwig-Beymer, PhD, RN, CTN, NEA-BC, FAAN
Associate Editor
Journal of Transcultural Nursing
Vice President and Chief Nursing Officer
Edward Hospital and Health Services
Naperville, IL

Preface

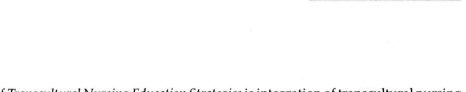

The focus of *Transcultural Nursing Education Strategies* is integration of transcultural nursing (TCN) in both academic and staff development settings. Much work went into highlighting TCN amid current trends, accreditation, professional standards, government mandates and guidelines, and an increasingly diverse nation and world.

In academia, the materials and strategies in this book can be applied to all levels of undergraduate and graduate nursing education. In staff development, concepts and materials are applicable for orientation, in-service, continuing education, competency programs, evidence-based practice, and research and scholarship programs as specified by the American Nurses Association and National Nursing Staff Development Organization. There are brief discussions about Leininger's Culture Care Theory and the models of Purnell, Jeffreys, Campinha-Bacote, Giger and Davidhizar, Choi, and Spector, and the assessment tools of Andrews and Boyle; the reader is encouraged to go back to these theories and models.

The American Association of Colleges of Nursing (AACN) uses Leininger, Purnell, Campinha-Bacote, Giger and Davidhizar, and Spector in its *Cultural Competency in Baccalaureate Nursing Education* (AACN, 2008). Recently, the AACN (2011) updated its *Toolkit for Cultural Competence in Master's and Doctoral Education* to include the Jeffreys Cultural Competence model. The National League for Nursing (2009) utilizes the Giger and Davidhizar model in its *Diversity Toolkit*.

This book is organized into seven parts dealing with specific integration of TCN concepts. **Part I** covers TCN in education, both in academia and in staff development settings. Discussion is provided in the integration of TCN in existing nursing courses, as modules into current courses, or as a separate course or courses in nursing programs. While many schools of nursing and allied health have made diversity and cultural competence a priority, there is no standard method for integration of these in to curricula or in to the National Council Licensing Examination (NCLEX) blueprint. Diversity and cultural competence integration on the NCLEX and as a requirement for licensure and registration of all nurses will contribute much to the culturally and linguistically appropriate care of all clients in health care.

Part II comprises the integration of TCN in foundation courses. Beginning a nursing program is significant, a milestone in a student's life. It is imperative to integrate TCN concepts very early on to emphasize the importance of culturally and linguistically congruent care and to thread it vertically and horizontally, from foundation to capstone courses.

Part III involves TCN integration in courses across the life span. Throughout the life span, every person's culture, values, and beliefs influence the lens used for viewing health, illness, health promotion, health-seeking behavior, and acceptance of therapeutic modalities. Care of clients, families, and significant others is emphasized.

Part IV contains integration of TCN in specialty area courses. Cultural attitudes, values, and beliefs vary among and within cultures. Strategies are illustrated in integration of TCN in specialty courses such as mental health and psychiatric nursing; pharmacology; nutrition; and research. Graduating students, preparing for and on the verge of their own professional nursing practice, aptly need a strong background in culturally and linguistically appropriate services (CLAS) in nursing classes and in clinical practicum.

Part V covers integration of TCN across nursing programs and in faculty orientation and mentoring. The faculty has a daunting task of preparing graduates to care for the complex needs of a diverse population with decreasing resources. Faculty themselves—already facing critical shortages—need formal preparation in TCN to be effective at this task.

Part VI encompasses integration of TCN in staff development and the role of the nursing professional development (NPD) specialist. Strategies in weaving TCN concepts are included for staff orientation, continuing competence development, preparation of policies and procedures, and credentialing. The last chapter covers recruitment and retention of foreign-educated nurses (FENs). An overview of development of nursing education in the Philippines is included to provide a starting point in understanding the Filipino nurse. Nurses from the Philippines have persistently outnumbered other FENs since developed countries began recruiting nurses from developing countries, triggering a nurse drain that now has reached critical proportions and health implications in sending countries.

Part VII, the concluding section, embraces vision in TCN. Six decades after Dr. Madeleine Leininger founded TCN, the authors look at TCN's history, development, and knowledge building; its increasing relevance in today's diverse society; and the implementation of CLAS and other guidelines, and envisioned the future of TCN.

CRITICAL THINKING EXERCISES

Critical thinking exercises (CTEs) are in every chapter. The authors anticipate that these CTEs may stimulate readers to reflect on and assess their own journey to cultural competence; to critically think and integrate TCN knowledge and skills when caring for clients, families, or significant others; and to be culturally sensitive when dealing with others from diverse cultures. While the questions are addressed to undergraduate and graduate students, faculty in academia, and faculty in staff development, the questions are applicable to other learners as well.

According to Rubenfeld and Scheffer (2006), critical thinking (CT) dates back to the Socratic method of providing questions with questions—with deeper questioning entailed for ideas known as fact. CT emerged as a focus for nursing education in the 1990s (Rubenfeld & Scheffer, 2006). The American Association of Colleges of Nursing ([AACN], 2008) and the National League for Nursing ([NLN], 2010) both require CT as program outcomes, emphasizing that all nursing programs should address CT in their respective nursing curricula.

EVIDENCE-BASED PRACTICE BOXES

Evidence-based practice (EBP) boxes are in every chapter in recognition of the continuing addition to the body of professional nursing knowledge for use in practice to improve health outcomes; to increase quality and access to health care; and to improve the cultural competence of health providers. These can be used as assignments in academic and staff development settings and may be helpful when planning access of research articles for use in academic or staff development purposes. A list of research studies in EBP boxes is available in Appendix 21.

The EBP boxes attempt to encourage all nurses to be consumers of research, to promote and undertake research that will improve health outcomes for all and not just the select few, and to recruit and retain diverse participants in research and evidence-based practice. The synopsis of each research study may be helpful in the decision to go further and access the original research articles as befits the learner's purpose. Viewing some of these research studies, hopefully, will lead to the pursuit of research studies where gaps in knowledge exist.

SELF-LEARNING MODULES

There are four stand-alone self-learning modules (SLMs) in this book: CLAS; posttraumatic stress disorder (PTSD) among women; hot and cold theory; and care of an Orthodox Jewish child with asthma. These can be used as learning tools to enhance the learner's cultural competence in academia and staff development. The enhanced CLAS standards, implemented since 2001, need to be threaded through all academic courses and staff development initiatives. Violence against women is prevalent in any culture. The use of hot and cold theory is common among many cultures and is gaining more prominence in Western cultures using complementary and alternative medicine (CAM).

UNFOLDING CASE SCENARIOS

Two unfolding case scenarios are contained in the book. One scenario involves a school nurse providing care to a culturally diverse individual, family, and school population. The second scenario deals with caring for a migrant worker with Chagas disease. Case scenarios are widely used in nursing education to promote critical thinking and clinical judgment.

Finally, all contributors wish that educators—both in academic and staff development settings—will find this book useful in enhancing the cultural competence of current health professionals and in the preparation of the next generation of nurses.

SAMPLE SYLLABI

Sample syllabi are provided in the Appendix section (Appendices 22–25) and in the electronic ancillary package. All sample syllabi are in Word format so they can easily be revised, tailored, or enhanced based on the curricular level or the user's need. Qualified instructors can access the ancillary package by emailing *textbook@springerpub.com*.

Priscilla Limbo Sagar

REFERENCES

American Association of Colleges of Nursing. (2008). *The essentials of baccalaureate education for professional nursing practice.* Washington, DC: Author.

National League for Nursing. (2010). *NLN education competencies model.* New York, NY: Author. Retrieved October 16, 2013, from www.nln.org/facultyprograms/competencies/pdf/comp_model_final.pdf

Rubenfeld, M. G., & Scheffer, B. K. (2006). *Critical thinking TACTICS for nurses: Tracking, assessing, and cultivating thinking to improve competency-based strategies.* Sudbury, MA: Jones & Bartlett.

Acknowledgments

There are so many individuals I would like to thank, without whom it would be impossible to complete the writing of my second book. My first book was *Transcultural Nursing Theory and Models: Application in Nursing Education, Practice, and Administration.*

- My family for their love, support, and patience despite my being a constant "absentee" from many family gatherings because of the attention and time I needed to spend on this book.
- Dr. Margaret M. Andrews, Dr. Geraldine (Polly) Bednash, and Dr. Patti Ludwig-Beymer, for their very generous Forewords. These Forewords sustained me, especially during times when I could hardly write as a result of some health issues. Dr. Andrews deserves special note for her constant support of my work and my personal and professional endeavors.
- All contributors to this book for enriching the content in their specialties, and for their patience in following through as I asked for yet another concept or further discussion that needed to be in subsequent chapters.
- My friends, too many to mention by name, for forgiving me for absences at gatherings and for my lapses in communication due to the many, many hours spent on this work.
- Dr. Larry Purnell, Dr. Marianne Jeffreys, Dr. Joyce Newman Giger, and Dr. Hesseung Choi for the generous reprint of their respective models.
- Oldways for the most generous reprint of three of their food pyramids: African American, Asian, and Hispanic.
- Margaret Zuccarini for her support, understanding, and consideration throughout this book. Allan Graubard for challenging me to produce a proposal and table of contents that crystallized my ideas concerning TCN and meld and interweave it with education, current national and global trends, and vision for the future of TCN. Chris Teja for his support and follow-up with details about this work. Michael O'Connor for his attention to details during the production of this book.
- The American Nurses Association and National Nursing Staff Development Organization for the permission to reprint their *Nursing Professional Development as a Specialist Practice Model.*
- All contributors from Mount Saint Mary College are grateful specifically to Fr. Kevin Mackin and many others who create a climate of faculty and staff scholarship, creativity, and productivity; Curtin Library Director Barbara Petruzzelli and her staff, especially Theresa Davis, Vivian Milczarski, Denise Garofalo, Derek Sanderson, and Mary Spear for their assistance in the use of library resources.

Transcultural Nursing Education Strategies

Nursing Education and Transcultural Nursing

Priscilla Limbo Sagar

KEY TERMS

Boyle and Andrews: Transcultural Nursing
  Assessment Guides
Campinha-Bacote: The Process of Cultural
  Competence in the Delivery of Healthcare
  Services and A Biblically Based Model of
  Cultural Competence in the Delivery of
  Healthcare Services: Seeing "Imago Dei"
Choi: Theory of Cultural Marginality

Giger and Davidhizar: Transcultural Assessment
  Model
Jeffreys: Cultural Competence and Confidence
  Model
Leininger: Cultural Care Theory
Purnell: Model for Cultural Competence
Spector: Heritage Assessment Model

LEARNING OBJECTIVES

At the completion of this chapter, the learner will be able to

1. Discuss the role of transcultural nursing (TCN) in nursing education, practice, administration, and research.
2. Compare and contrast TCN theory and models in terms of applicability at the learner's own setting.
3. Analyze the necessity of integrating TCN concepts in academic settings.
4. Examine the necessity of integrating TCN concepts in staff development settings.
5. Compare and contrast standards and guidelines for inclusion of diversity and cultural competence in nursing and allied health curricula.

OVERVIEW

The inclusion of cultural diversity in nursing curricula is not a new phenomenon. The curricular integration of cultural diversity in nursing started in 1917 when the National League for Nursing (NLN) Committee on Curriculum published a guide focusing on sociology and social issues in nursing (DeSantis & Lipson, 2007). In 1937, the NLN Committee further included the cultural background in the guide to understand the individual's reaction to being ill.

The first promotion of cultural competence integration of transcultural nursing (TCN) in academia dates back to 1965 through 1969, when Leininger not only developed the first TCN course and telecourses but also established the first PhD nurse–scientist program at the Colorado School of Nursing (Andrews & Boyle, 2012). The American Nurses Association ([ANA], 1991, 1995, 2003), American Association of Colleges of Nursing (AACN, 1998, 1999, 2008a, 2008b, 2011), and the NLN (2005, 2009a, 2009b) have all been consistently vocal in their commitment to cultural diversity and cultural competence in nursing practice, education, administration, and research. The Accreditation Commission for Education in Nursing ([ACEN], 2013), formerly the National League for Nursing Accreditation Commission (NLNAC), explicitly includes diversity among its standards under "curriculum."

Nurses are at the front line of health care, spending more time and working closely with clients more than any other health professionals. Globally, nurses provide 80% of health services (International Council for Nurses [ICN], 2007) to individuals and communities. It is not surprising that in the United States, consumers have rated nurses as the most trusted of health care professionals for 12 years in a row according to the Gallup survey of professionals (ANA, 2011). The National Partnership for Action (NPA) to End Health Disparities (Tomer, 2012) called upon nurses for identification and responsive solutions in eliminating health disparities. There are continuing disparities not only in health status but also in health access among African Americans, Hispanics, and Native Americans (AACN, 2008a, 2011; Sullivan Commission, 2004). To eliminate disparities, the U.S. Department of Health and Human Services (USDHHS) Office of Minority Health ([OMH], USDHHS & OMH, 2013) continue to refine the culturally and linguistically appropriate services (CLAS) that it initially published in 2000.

It is then imperative for nurse academicians to prepare nurses for this role by integrating health disparities and solutions in all nursing curricula preparing licensed practical, diploma, associate, baccalaureate, master's, and doctoral level nurses. National and global health disparities need to be included in discussions in all classes and in clinical practice in nursing and allied health care fields such as medicine, dentistry, physical therapy, pharmacy, and other professions. Policy development, an important key when working to eliminate health disparities (TCNS, 2010), must also be integrated. The Affordable Health Care Act, since its inception 2 years ago, has provided access to preventable care for 86 million people; its provision to extend parental coverage for children from age 21 to 26 further covered 2.5 million people (Tomer, 2012). While this would improve access, there remains the question of quality of care and elimination of factors that continue to show disparate results among African Americans, Hispanics, and Native Americans (Sullivan Commission, 2004).

Sagar (2012) emphasized the overlapping dynamic connections between the realms of nursing education, practice, and administration in health promotion and in the provision of equal, safe, and quality health care. The role of nurse professional development (NPD) specialist is vital in planning, implementing, and evaluating the ongoing professional development of staff nurses and colleagues. While this book concentrates on **staff**

development settings along with academia, the role of nursing administration leadership in supporting such endeavors to promote cultural competence at the individual and organizational levels could not be underestimated. Nor could we forget nurse researchers studying health disparities in access and quality of care; these are the guardians of the recruitment, ethical treatment, and retention of participants, and discovery of new knowledge in improving minority client health outcomes. Nurse educators in academic and staff development settings need to work closely and hand-in-hand to develop culturally and linguistically appropriate approaches to students, faculty, colleagues, clients and their families, and the community. This hand-in-hand collaboration is an example of what Brown and Doane (2007) referred to as the purposeful alignment of education and nursing practice wherein both of these realms benefit.

SOME TRANSCULTURAL THEORIES AND MODELS

Leininger: Culture Care Theory

Dr. Madeleine Leininger is widely accepted as the mother and founder of TCN (Ryan, 2011; Sagar, 2012). Leininger started the development of her *Culture Care Theory (CCT)* in the 1940s. Leininger's theory depiction is the *sunrise enabler* (Figure 1.1), a symbol of hope to generate new knowledge for nursing. The CCT—carefully refined in six decades—is applicable for individuals, families, groups, communities, and institutions, and has been used in nursing as well as health-related disciplines (Leininger, 1995a, 2002; Leininger & McFarland, 2006; McFarland & Leininger, 2002). Fanning into sunrays in Leininger's model are seven factors that influence individuals, families, and groups in health and illness: *technological; religious and philosophical; kinship and social; cultural values, beliefs, and ways of life; political and legal; economic;* and *educational* (Leininger, 1995, 2002, 2006). There are 11 theoretical assumptions from the major tenets of CCT; the essence of two of those assumptions center on (1) caring as the essence of nursing, and (2) diversities and commonalities existing between cultures (Leininger, 1995, 2002, 2006). Nursing care sits between—and could strategically and effectively bridge—generic folk care and professional care. At this vantage point, the nurse can be most influential and effective in the assessment, planning, implementation, and evaluation of culturally congruent care.

Leininger (1995, 2002, 2006) uses three action modes in the CCT for provision of holistic, culturally congruent care: *preservation or maintenance* for decisions that promote helpful and desirable values and beliefs; *accommodation and/or negotiation* when adapting care that fits the client's culture, values, and beliefs; and *repatterning and/or restructuring* as the nurse and client mutually modify or change nursing actions to promote better health outcomes. Globally and in the United States, Leininger's CCT is one of the most widely used frameworks in nursing education, practice, administration, and research.

Purnell: Purnell Model for Cultural Competence

Initially intended as a framework for clinical assessment, the *Purnell Model for Cultural Competence* ([PMCC], Figure 1.2) was developed in 1991 (Purnell, 2002). Foremost among the purposes of the PMCC is to serve as a framework whereby health care providers could "interrelate characteristics of culture to promote congruence and … delivery of consciously sensitive and competent healthcare" (Purnell, 2013, p. 15). The PMCC has 12 wedge-shaped

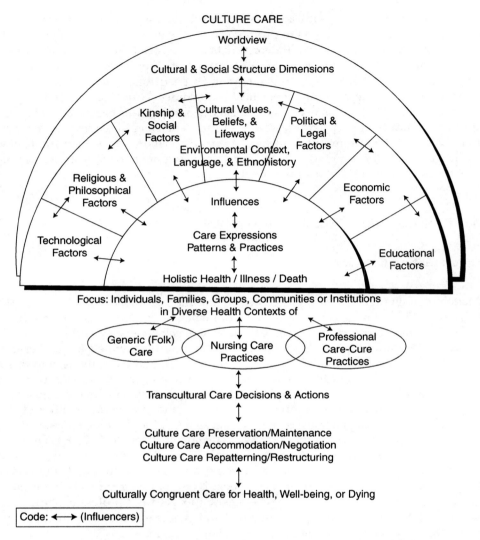

CULTURE CARE

FIGURE 1.1 Leininger's sunrise enabler to discover culture care. *Source:* Reprinted from Leininger, M. M., & McFarland, M. M. (2006). *Culture care diversity and universality: A worldwide nursing theory.* Burlington, MA: Jones & Bartlett. Reprinted with permission. www.jblearning.com

sections as an organizing framework surrounded by four rims that signify global society (outside rim), community (second rim), family (third rim), and individual (fourth rim; Purnell, 2002, 2007, 2008, 2013). The 12 domains could be used in their entirety or their concepts could be used selectively when applying the model.

The PMCC is one of the most widely used models in nursing curricula (Lipson & Desantis, 2007); its 12 domains could be threaded both into theoretical nursing courses as well as clinical components (Sagar, 2012). Notably, this model is not only widely used in nursing practice, administration, and research but also in other health-related fields and in international projects. The PMCC has been adopted as the framework of the Commission on Internationalization and Cultural Competence for the European Union project for the Bologna-Sorbonne-Salamanca World Health Organization declarations (Purnell, 2007).

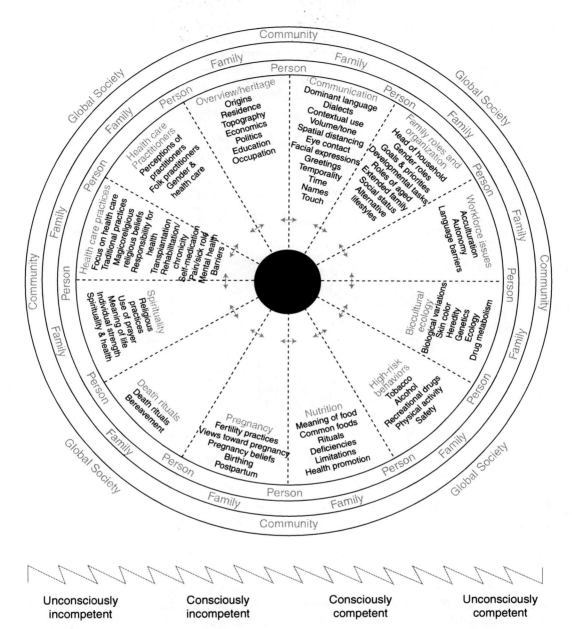

Unconsciously incompetent   Consciously incompetent   Consciously competent   Unconsciously competent

FIGURE 1.2 Purnell Model for Cultural Competence. *Source:* Purnell (2013). Reprinted with permission from Dr. Larry Purnell, PhD, RN, FAAN.

Jeffreys: Cultural Competence and Confidence Model

The *Cultural Competence and Confidence Model* (CCC; Figure 1.3) aims to connect concepts that predict learning of cultural competence and integrate "the construct of transcultural self-efficacy (TSE) (confidence)" (Jeffreys, 2010, p. 46). Jeffreys views cultural competence as a learning process in three dimensions: *cognitive, practical,* and *affective*; as mainly influenced by the transcultural self-efficacy (TSE); and directed toward culturally congruent care. According to Jeffreys (2010), the TSE is the "perceived confidence for performing or

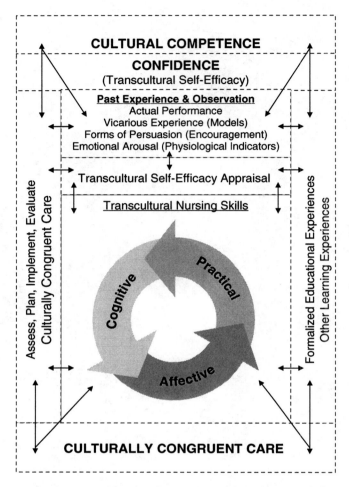

FIGURE 1.3   Jeffreys's Cultural Competence and Confidence Model (CCC).
Source: Jeffreys (2010). Reprinted with permission from Springer Publishing.

learning" (p. 46) TCN skills when working with clients whose culture is different from the nurse's own. In the course of time, formal education and other structured learning experiences could affect the three dimensions of TSE and the development of cultural competence which further leads to culturally congruent care (Jeffreys, 2010).

Jeffreys (2010) emphasized that the cognitive learning dimension includes knowledge and comprehension about cultural factors and its influence on professional care of culturally diverse clients throughout the life span. Jeffreys (2010) pointed out the similarity of the *practical learning dimension* and psychomotor domain; in the context of TCN, this refers to verbal and nonverbal communication skills when performing cultural assessment. The *affective learning dimension* involves "attitudes, values, and beliefs" (Jeffreys, 2010, p. 52); this dimension is of prime importance in professional value and attitude development. The CCC is highly applicable in nursing education, practice, administration, and research, as well as in other health-related disciplines.

Campinha-Bacote: The Process of Cultural Competence in the Delivery of Healthcare Services and A Biblically Based Model of Cultural Competence in the Delivery of Healthcare Services: Seeing "Imago Dei"

Campinha-Bacote (2007) developed the initial version of *The Process of Cultural Competence in the Delivery of Healthcare Services* (*PCCDHS*) in 1991. The PCCDHS was called *A Culturally Competent Model of Care* then, represented by four interrelated constructs of *cultural awareness, cultural knowledge, cultural skill,* and *cultural encounters* (Campinha-Bacote, 2007, 2011, p. 42). To keep up with development in TCN, to add to the four existing constructs, and to portray the interdependence of the constructs, she added a fifth construct of *cultural desire* in 1998 (Campinha-Bacote, 2011, 2012). It was then that Campinha-Bacote renamed her model to PCCDHS; its pictorial image denoted five Venn circles that overlap, mirroring interdependent relationships among constructs (Campinha-Bacote, 2011, 2012). Campinha-Bacote (2007) developed the *Inventory for Assessing the Process of Cultural Competence Among Healthcare Professionals—Revised* (*IAPCC-R*), a self-assessment tool that indicates level of cultural competence. To assess the cultural competence of student nurses, Campinha-Bacote also created the *IAPCC-Student Version* (*IAPCC-SV*).

In recognition of the key role of cultural desire in the journey to cultural competence, Campinha-Bacote (2011, 2012) further revised the PCCDHS in 2002. At this time, her model illustrated an erupting volcano, representing the desire for cultural competence. In 2010, based on review of literature and evidence-based studies utilizing the IAPCC-R (Campinha-Bacote, 2007), the PCCDHS further evolved to portray and "center on the construct of cultural encounters" (Campinha-Bacote, 2011, p. 43). In terms of cultural encounters, health care professionals must continuously interact with clients from diverse cultures to "validate and refine values and beliefs" (Campinha-Bacote, 2011, p. 43) in order to develop the other constructs of the PCCDHS. The evolution of her model is illustrated on the Transcultural Clinical Administrative Research and Education (C.A.R.E.) website at http://transculturalcare.net.

Campinha-Bacote (2007) also developed *A Biblically Based Model of Cultural Competence in the Delivery of Healthcare Services* (*BBMCCDHS*) from her own earlier work in 2007, from Leininger and McFarland in 2006, and from those of Kleinman (1980) and Chapman (2005), among others (both as cited by Campinha-Bacote in 2013). When using the BBMCCDHS, it is imperative that health care professionals see the image of God ("Imago Dei") in their clients and integrate love, caring, humility, compassion, and other virtues (Campinha-Bacote, 2013, para 1). In both the PCCDHS and BBMCCDHS, health care professionals must view themselves as becoming culturally competent rather than being culturally competent (Campinha-Bacote, 2011, 2013); both models are highly applicable in nursing education, practice, administration, and research. Notably, Campinha-Bacote's IAPCC-R and IAPCC-SV have been extensively used in nursing education and practice to measure the cultural competence of health care practitioners and students, respectively. The BBMCCDHS is also demonstrated on her C.A.R.E.) website at http://transculturalcare.net.

Giger and Davidhizar: Transcultural Assessment Model

There were few cultural assessment tools in 1988 when Giger and Davidhizar (2002, 2004, 2008) started the *Transcultural Assessment Model* (*TAM*) as a solution to students' need to provide care to culturally diverse clients. Giger and Davidhizar (2002, 2008) based the TAM on the groundbreaking work of Leininger as well as that of Spector; Orque, Bloch, and Monroy; and Hall.

The TAM espouses six cultural phenomena, namely *biological variations, environmental control, time, social orientation, space,* and *communication* (Dowd, Davidhizar, & Giger, 1998; Giger & Davidhizar, 2002, 2004, 2008, 2013, Figure 1.4). Each cultural phenomenon occurs in cultures, relates to each other, overlaps with one another, and varies in its utility and application (Dowd et al., 1998; Giger & Davidhizar, 2013). The TAM offers a functional and thorough assessment tool in planning culturally congruent care for clients (AACN, 2008; Giger & Davidhizar, 2013).

Spector: Heritage Traditions Model

Spector (2002, 2004a, 2004b, 2009) incorporated Giger and Davidhizar's six cultural phenomena of environmental control, biological variations, communication, social orientation, space, and time to form the *Health Traditions Model (HTM)* in 1993. The HTM first appeared in Potter and Perry's *Fundamentals in Nursing* textbook (Davidhizar & Giger, 1998; Giger & Davidhizar, 2008, 2013). Spector also refers to this model as *personal health traditions of a unique cultural being.*

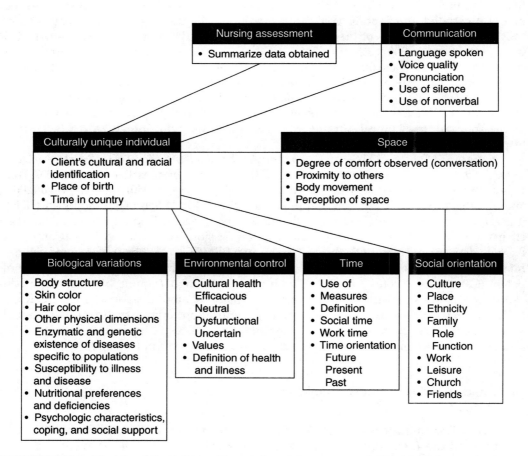

FIGURE 1.4 Giger and Davidhizar: Transcultural Assessment Model (TAM). *(continues)*
Source: Reprinted from Giger & Davidhizar (2008). Copyright Elsevier Mosby.

(continued)

CULTURALLY UNIQUE INDIVIDUAL
1. Place of birth
2. Cultural definition
   What is…
3. Race
   What is…
4. Length of time in country (if appropriate)

COMMUNICATION
1. Voice quality
   A. Strong, resonant
   B. Soft
   C. Average
   D. Shrill
2. Pronunciation and enunciation
   A. Clear
   B. Slurred
   C. Dialect (geographical)
3. Use of silence
   A. Infrequent
   B. Often
   C. Length
      (1) Brief
      (2) Moderate
      (3) Long
      (4) Not observed
4. Use of nonverbal
   A. Hand movement
   B. Eye movement
   C. Entire body movement
   D. Kinesics (gestures, expression, or stances)
5. Touch
   A. Startles or withdraws when touched
   B. Accepts touch without difficulty
   C. Touches others without difficulty
6. Ask these and similar questions:
   A. How do you get your point across to others?
   B. Do you like communicating with friends, family, and acquaintances?
   C. When asked a question, do you usually respond (in words or body movement, or both)?
   D. If you have something important to discuss with your family, how would you approach them?

SPACE
1. Degree of comfort
   A. Moves when space invaded
   B. Does not move when space invaded
2. Distance in conversations
   A. 0 to 18 inches
   B. 18 inches to 3 feet
   C. 3 feet or more
3. Definition of space
   A. Describe degree of comfort with closeness when talking with or standing near others
   B. How to objects (e.g., furniture) in the environment affect your sense of space?

4. Ask these and similar questions:
   A. When you talk with family members, how close do you stand?
   B. When you communicate with coworkers and other acquaintances, how close do you stand?
   C. If a stranger touches you, how do you react or feel?
   D. If a loved one touches you, how do you react or feel?
   E. Are you comfortable with the distance between us now?

SOCIAL ORGANIZATIONS
1. Normal state of health
   A. Poor
   B. Fair
   C. Good
   D. Excellent
2. Marital status
3. Number of children
4. Parents living or deceased?
5. Ask these and similar questions:
   A. How do you define social activities?
   B. What are some activities you enjoy?
   C. What are your hobbies, or what do you do when you have free time?
   D. Do you believe in a Supreme Being?
   E. How do you worship that Supreme Being?
   F. What is your function (what do you do) in your family unit/system?
   G. What is your role in your family unit/system (father, mother, child, advisor)?
   H. When you were a child, what or who influenced you most?
   I. What is/was your relationship with your siblings and parents?
   J. What does work mean to you?
   K. Describe your past, present, and future jobs.
   L. What are your political views?
   M. How have your political views influenced your attitude toward health and illness?

TIME
1. Orientation to time
   A. Past-oriented
   B. Present-oriented
   C. Future-oriented
2. View of time
   A. Social time
   B. Clock-oriented
3. Physiochemical reaction to time
   A. Sleeps at least 8 hours a night
   B. Goes to sleep and wakes on a consistent schedule
   C. Understands the importance of taking medication and other treatments on schedule

FIGURE 1.4 Giger and Davidhizar: Transcultural Assessment Model (TAM). *(continues)*
Source: Reprinted from Giger & Davidhizar (2008). Copyright Elsevier Mosby.

(continued)

4. Ask these and similar questions:
   A. What kind of timepiece do you wear daily?
   B. If you have an appointment at 2 pm, what time is acceptable to arrive?
   C. If a nurse tells you that you will receive a medication in "about a half hour," realistically, how much time will you allow before calling the nurses' station?

ENVIRONMENTAL CONTROL

1. Locus-of-control
   A. Internal locus-of-control (believes that the power to affect change lies within)
   B. External locus-of-control (believes that fate, luck, and chance have a great deal to do with how things turn out)
2. Value orientation
   A. Believes in supernatural forces
   B. Relies on magic, witchcraft, and prayer to affect change
   C. Does not believe in supernatural forces
   D. Does not rely on magic, witchcraft, or prayer to affect change
3. Ask these and similar questions:
   A. How often do you have visitors to your home?
   B. Is it acceptable to you for visitors to drop in unexpectedly?
   C. Name some ways your parents or other persons treated your illnesses when you were a child.
   D. Have you or someone else in your immediate surroundings ever used a home remedy that made you sick?
   E. What home remedies have you used that worked? Will you use them in the future?
   F. What is your definition of "good health"?
   G. What is your definition of illness or "poor health"?

BIOLOGICAL VARIATIONS

1. Conduct a complete physical assessment noting:
   A. Body structure (small, medium, or large frame)
   B. Skin color
   C. Unusual skin discolorations
   D. Hair color and distribution
   E. Other visible physical characteristics (e.g., keloids, chloasma)
   F. Weight
   G. Height
   H. Check lab work for variances in hemoglobin, hematocrit, and sickle cell phenomena if Black or Mediterranean
2. Ask these and similar questions:
   A. What diseases or illnesses are common in your family?
   B. Has anyone in your family been told that there is a possible genetic susceptibility for a particular disease?

C. Describe your family's typical behavior when a family member is ill.
D. How do you respond when you are angry?
E. Who (or what) usually helps you to cope during a difficult time?
F. What foods do you and your family like to eat?
G. Have you ever had any unusual cravings for:
   (1) White or red clay dirt?
   (2) Laundry starch?
H. When you were a child what types of foods did you eat?
I. What foods are family favorites or are considered traditional?

NURSING ASSESSMENT

1. Note whether the client has become culturally assimilated or observes own cultural practices.
2. Incorporate data into plan of nursing care:
   A. Encourage the client to discuss cultural differences; people from diverse cultures who hold different world views can enlighten nurses.
   B. Make efforts to accept and understand methods of communication.
   C. Respect the individual's personal need for space.
   D. Respect the rights of clients to honor and worship the Supreme Being of their choice.
   E. Identify a clerical or spiritual person to contact.
   F. Determine whether spiritual practices have implications for health, life, and well-being (e.g., Jehovah's Witnesses may refuse blood and blood derivatives; an Orthodox Jew may eat only kosher food high in sodium and may not drink milk when meat is served).
   G. Identify hobbies, especially when devising interventions for a short or extended convalescence or for rehabilitation.
   H. Honor time and value orientations and differences in these areas. Allay anxiety and apprehension if adherence to time is necessary.
   I. Provide privacy according to personal need and health status of the client (NOTE: the perception of and reaction to pain may be culturally related).
   J. Note cultural health practices:
      (1) Identify and encourage efficacious practices.
      (2) Identify and discourage dysfunctional practices.
      (3) Identify and determine whether neutral practices will have a long-term ill effect.
   K. Note food preferences:
      (1) Make as many adjustments in diet as health status and long-term benefits will allow and that dietary department can provide.
      (2) Note dietary practices that may have serious implications for the client.

FIGURE 1.4 Giger and Davidhizar: Transcultural Assessment Model (TAM).
Source: Reprinted from Giger & Davidhizar (2008). Copyright Elsevier Mosby.

Spector (2013) views health as "the balance of the person, both within one's being—physical, mental, and spiritual—and in the outside world" (p. 91). The physical, mental, and spiritual facets of health added to the *personal methods of maintaining health, protecting health,* and *restoring health* comprise the nine interrelated facets of health (Spector, 2013, p. 93). For example, to restore health, an individual may use cupping (physical), exorcism (mental), and meditation (spiritual).

Boyle and Andrews: Transcultural Nursing Assessment Guides

In 1989, the *Transcultural Concepts in Nursing Care* textbook was initially published from a collaboration between faculty and students at the University of Utah to clarify the application of transcultural nursing in clinical practice (Andrews & Boyle, 2012). Nursing schools preferring not to use a specific TCN model use the Andrews and Boyle textbook (Boyle, 2007; Lipson & Desantis, 2007).

Boyle and Andrews (2012a) developed the *Transcultural Nursing Assessment Guide for Individuals and Families (TCNGIF),* consisting of 12 major categories of cultural knowledge to guide cultural and physical assessment and development of culturally congruent care. The guide consists of *biocultural variations and cultural aspects of the incidence of disease; communication; cultural affiliations; cultural sanctions and restrictions; developmental considerations; economics; educational background; health-related beliefs and practices; kinship and social networks; nutrition; religion and spirituality;* and *values orientation* (Boyle & Andrews 2012a, pp. 451–455).

To foster systematicity, Boyle and Andrews (2012b) also devised the *Andrews/Boyle Transcultural Nursing Assessment Guide for Groups and Communities (TCNAGGC).* This guide has eight major categories: *family and kinship systems; social and life networks; political or government systems; language and traditions; worldviews, value orientations, and cultural norms; religious beliefs and practices; health beliefs and practices;* and *healthcare systems* (Boyle & Andrews, 2012b, pp. 456–458).

In recognition of the need to also strive for culturally competent organizations, Boyle, Andrews, and Ludwig-Beymer (2012) developed the *Andrews/Boyle Transcultural Nursing Assessment Guide for Health Care Organizations and Facilities.* The nine areas in this guide are *environmental context; language and ethnohistory; technology; religious/philosophical; social factors; cultural values; political/legal; economic;* and *education* (Boyle et al., 2012, pp. 459–461). The cultural competence of organizations rests in every individual health care provider; this, too, is a lifetime journey and commitment (Ludwig-Beymer, 2012).

Choi: Theory of Cultural Marginality

Choi (2008, 2013) developed the *Theory of Cultural Marginality (TCM)* to foster understanding of the unique experiences of immigrant persons who are living between two cultures. Choi called this complex living "straddling of cultures" (2008, p. 243). Choi is hopeful that TCM will assist health care providers and offer them directions for culturally congruent care of immigrants.

The three major concepts of the TCM are *marginal living, across-culture conflict recognition,* and *easing cultural tension* (Choi, 2008, 2013). Marginal living entails passivity and feelings of being in between two cultures—living and shaping new relationships in the midst of the old culture—simultaneously being in conflict and in promise (Figure 1.5). Feeling of passivity and being in between are primary attributes of marginal living (Park, 1928).

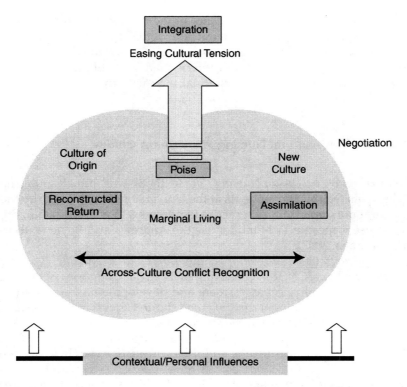

FIGURE 1.5 Theory of Cultural Marginality. *Source:* Choi (2013). Copyright Springer Publishing.

Across-culture conflict recognition signals the initial understanding of differences between contradiction in "cultural values, customs, behaviors, and norms" (Choi, 2008, p. 250). To resolve across-culture conflict, the individual resorts to adjustment responses.

Choi adapted Weisberger's (1992, as cited in Choi, 2013) four responses from his study on marginality among German Jews: *assimilation, reconstructed return, poise,* and *integration.* The process of assimilation entails absorption into the majority culture, striving hard to adopt its new language, customs, and ways of life. The pattern of *reconstructed return* happens when an individual chooses to return to one's own culture either due to conflicts with the new culture or as a consequence of longing for the old culture (Choi, 2001, 2008, 2013; Choi, Meninger, & Roberts, 2006). Overidentification with the old or new culture are common manifestations in reconstructed return. The characteristic pattern response of poise is its tentativeness; the cycle of emotional conflicts and struggle may return. The response pattern of *integration* signifies adjustment; the individual forges a third culture through the blending of the old and new cultures (Choi, 2008, 2013). Research among foreign nurses from India conducted by DiCicco-Bloom (2004) painfully reflects the marginality of individuals as "a foot here, a foot there, a foot nowhere" (p. 28).

To explore marginal living experiences of immigrant children in South Korea, Choi (2013) developed the 13-item *Cultural Marginality Scale (CMS)*. Choi adapted the CMS from the *Societal, Attitudinal, Familial, and Environmental Acculturative Stress Scale for Children (SAFE-C;* Chavez et al., 1997 as cited in Choi, 2013). Choi is currently conducting cognitive interviews with young children from age 10 to 13 years; this is in preparation for testing the brand new CMS.

HISTORY: TCN IN ACADEMIA

The NLN Committee on Curriculum initiated the integration of sociology and social issues in nursing in 1917 (Desantis & Lipson, 2007). Aimed at understanding individual reaction to illness, the NLN Committee further added the individual's cultural background in its guide in 1936 (Desantis & Lipson, 2007). The ANA (ANA, 1991, 1995, 2003), AACN (AACN, 1998, 1999, 2008, 2011), and NLN (NLN, 2005, 2009a, 2009b, 2011) have been steadfast in their commitment to address cultural diversity and promotion of cultural competence in all levels of nursing education. The AACN offers two vital premier documents for member schools: *Cultural Competency in Baccalaureate Nursing Education: End of Program Competencies for Baccalaureate Nursing Program Graduates and Faculty Toolkit for Integrating These Competencies Into Undergraduate Curriculum* (2008) and *Toolkit for Cultural Competence in Master's and Doctoral Nursing Education* (2009, 2011).

HISTORY: TCN IN STAFF DEVELOPMENT

Academia and practice are intertwined. It is imperative that a two-way feedback loop exist, mutually feeding and energizing each other. Practice ought to actively inform academia in terms of the latest practice innovations and the performance and areas of graduate preparation needed for an ever changing health care delivery system. Academia must actively inform practice of educational innovations and new knowledge generated in research. In so doing, we will dispel the ivory tower of academia and the muck of practice riddled with complex problems (Schon, 1987); instead, we will be fostering a powerful two-way feedback loop.

To serve as a forum for discussion of national issues by college and university providers of continuing education (CE), the initial national conference on nursing CE was held in 1969 (ANA and National Nursing Staff Development Organization [ANA & NNSDO, 2010]). While the Commission on Continuing Education was established by the ANA in 1972, the standards for CE in nursing were not published until 1974 (ANA & NNSDO, 2010). The NNSDO was established in 1989, the same year when the ANA Council on CE evolved into the Council of Continuing Education and Staff Development. ANCC, an ANA subsidiary, was founded in 1991 to implement the credentialing process including specialty nursing certification and CE accreditation (ANA & NNSDO, 2010). The NNSDO (ANA & NNSDO, 2010) works to advance the staff development practice specialty with an end goal of improving health care outcomes. Staff development, basing its standard on research, is essential to enhancing patient and organizational outcomes (ANA & NNSDO, 2010). The NNSDO published its third edition of *Core Curriculum for Nursing Staff Development* in 2009.

The ANA has consistently advocated for the inclusion of cultural diversity in all patient interactions (ANA, 1991, 1995, 2003). The ANA and The Joint Commission (TJC, 2010a, 2010b) mandate competency assessment. Competency skills are essential in staff development.

The model of nursing professional development specialist (NPD) practice (Figure 1.6) has seven areas surrounding evidence-based practice (EBP) and practice-based evidence (PBE): inservice, continuing education (CE), career development and role transition, research and scholarship, academic partnerships, orientation, and competency program (ANA & NNSDO, 2010). In its inservice area, TCN concepts may be offered for nurses in all shifts. CE offerings may be offered face-to-face or online in the forms of modules. The NPD specialist may also be helpful in supporting other nurses in career development, in role

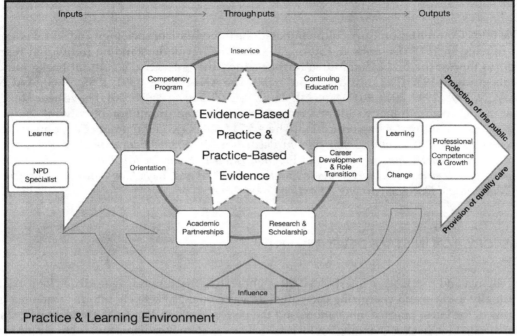

FIGURE 1.6   The model of nursing professional development specialist practice.
Source: American Nurses Association & National Nursing Staff Development
Organization (2010). Copyright ANA & NNSDO.

transition, and in succession planning. For example, the NPD specialist may guide other nurses in TCN certification, in planning to return to school for baccalaureate and graduate degree completion, or in mentoring other nurses for leadership roles. When partnering with academic institutions, collaborative TCN scholarship and research may be pursued in addition to diversity and cultural competence initiatives that would benefit all partners. The area of orientation presents a timely opportunity to offer TCN workshops and modules. During periodic competency evaluations, online and face-to-face TCN CE offerings may be required. Self-learning modules (SLMs) are another method of delivery for staff competency and to ensure organizational compliance with accreditation and government mandates and guidelines. Chapter 3 provides discussions and two examples of SLMs.

INTEGRATION OF TCN CONCEPTS

Although many advocate for the formal teaching of TCN concepts in nursing curricula, there are no standard curricular guidelines or mandates for content integration (Lipson & Desantis, 2007; Ryan, Carlton, & Ali, 2000; Sagar, 2012). Furthermore, there is a growing evidence that graduates of nursing programs are not prepared to care for increasingly diverse U.S. populations (Kardong-Edgreen & Campinha-Bacote, 2008).

Ryan et al. (2000) conducted a national survey of 610 National League for Nursing accredited schools. With a return of 36%, Ryan et al. (2000) indicated that 89 undergraduate and 27 graduate schools had formal courses in TCN. It is interesting to note that TCN concepts had varying degrees of inclusion: integrated in existing courses (197); modules in courses (135); and formal courses (89). Among the graduate schools in the survey, TCN concepts were integrated into existing courses (86); modules (56); and formal courses (27). Furthermore, Ryan et al. (2000) showed integration of TCN concepts in a wide variety of degree content and depth.

There has been increasing research about cultural competence in education. Among these researchers are Grant and Letzring (2003) on intensive review of cultural competence content, teaching strategies used by faculty, and tools used to measure cultural competence; Kardong-Edgreen (2007) on cultural competence of faculty; Kardong-Edgreen and Campinha-Bacote (2008) and Kardong-Edgreen et al. (2010) on cultural competence of graduating baccalaureate students; McFarland, Mixer, Lewis, and Easley (2006) on recruitment, engagement, and retention of diverse nursing students; and Mixer (2008, 2011) in the use of Leininger's CCT to explore faculty expressions, patterns, and practices in teaching culture care.

Kennedy, Fisher, Fontaine, and Martin-Holland (2008) modeled a School of Nursing's (SON) long-time commitment to diversity, as well as its ability to critically appraise its progress and proceed on its journey toward goal attainment. An intensive curricular evaluation was conducted by Kennedy et al. (2008) to appraise their university's initiatives for addressing diversity (EBP 1.1).

EBP 1.1

Kennedy et al. (2008) used a mixed method evaluation to examine the University of California at San Francisco (UCSF) School of Nursing's (SON) attainment of its goal of addressing diversity. UCSF has a long history of seeking diversity among its students, faculty, and staff. The SON established a Diversity in Action Committee (DIVA) in 1994; this volunteer group of faculty has mentored faculty and students to offer diversity programs.

The mixed method consisted of four steps: (1) content analysis of all SON syllabi; (2) comparison of content analysis to students' evaluation of diversity in their education; (3) survey of 2006 graduates; and (4) an analysis of responses from faculty to the findings (Kennedy et al., 2008). From an institutional database, codes developed by the DIVA committee were used to analyze 262 syllabi in the *first step*: basic nursing (11), masters (192), and doctoral (60) courses. Included in the concepts list were cross-cultural comparisons, disabilities, end of life, ethics, health/social policy, language barriers, power, and social determinants of health, among others. Each course received a diversity concept (DC) score. The final code, reflecting the analyst's evaluation of the integration of diversity (ID) throughout the syllabus, was given a *yes* or *no* score. The DC score for each syllabus ranged from 0 to 437; median was 6 with an interquartile range of 25. Thirty-six out of 262 (14%) courses received a *yes* for ID content in the syllabus.

(*continued*)

EBP 1.1 *(continued)*

In the *second step*, all SON students were requested to complete the online course evaluation of the 262 courses using a 4-point Likert-type scale. The researchers used Spearman's Rho to assess the association between the DC and ID scores with the students' evaluation average for the course. The mean for all course evaluation was 3.25, ranging from 1.7 to 4.0. The association between students' evaluation and the DC score was .196 two-tailed Spearman's Rho; $p < .05$ (Kennedy et al., 2008). The investigators' findings also included higher ID scores for basic nursing and doctoral courses than master of science (MS) courses; they attributed this to the assumption of some faculty that clinical placement in diverse settings will ensure skill development.

In the *third step*, 143 graduates were sent several e-mail invitations to complete an electronic survey. The survey contained questions about the graduate's perception of effectiveness of courses in addressing diversity in health care. Of the 31 (22%) respondents who completed the survey, 84% were MS and 16% were doctoral students. Twenty-six (26) out of 31 respondents provided qualitative data for the question that asked them to identify the three courses that best addressed diversity and the reasons for choosing those courses.

In the *fourth step*, when findings were presented to the faculty, the primary investigator deleted the actual name of courses so there was no identification of the faculty members. The strength, weakness, opportunity, threat (SWOT) analysis was revealing: 53 strengths, 57 weaknesses, 62 opportunities, and 55 threats. More than a third of the faculty admitted they did not possess the skills and preparation to tackle diversity in the classroom. More than half of the faculty had challenges to increasing diversity in course content. Faculty verbalized appreciation in discussing examples of creative integration of diversity in courses; this gave them ideas for their own courses in the future.

Kennedy et al. (2008) acknowledged the following limitations of this study: syllabi only represent a "one dimensional aspect of the course" (p. 369), some syllabi on the databases are abbreviated versions, and there was a low response rate from graduates (22%), hence only representing a small portion of students. While limited in this assessment, information was useful for the SON in continuing to work toward the goal of fostering a climate of inclusion and embracing diversity. This research clearly pointed to the ongoing commitment of an SON in addressing the principles of diversity and preparing graduates who are ready to care for the increasingly diverse U.S. population. The researchers pose a challenge to other schools to reflect how they evaluate their own diversity initiatives. As SONs integrate diversity in nursing curricula, they move toward the AACN (2009, 2011) goals of cultural competence.

Applications to Practice

■ Investigate your nursing program's mission and philosophy in terms of diversity and cultural competence. Is it congruent with the mission and philosophy of your parent institution?

(continued)

EBP 1.1 (continued)

■ Analyze the course you are taking/teaching. How are cultural concepts integrated?
■ If you were to replicate this study, how would you conduct it? What would you change in terms of conceptual framework, collection of data, and analysis of findings?

Source: Kennedy, Fisher, Fontaine, & Martin-Holland (2008).

APPLICATION: CASE STUDY 1.1

Sunrise School of Nursing (SSN) at Fidelity College has an enrollment of about 700 students: 450 in traditional baccalaureate, 100 in accelerated baccalaureate, 50 in RN-BS, and 100 in the masters program that prepares nurse educators and family nurse practitioners. Although faculty members at SSN integrate TCN concepts in the undergraduate program, there is no separate TCN course.

About 6 years ago, DS, a doctorally prepared faculty who also has certification in advanced transcultural nursing (CTN-A), proposed a 3-credit undergraduate TCN course along with the NUR 5040-Transcultural Nursing for the masters program. NUR 5040 had been running for 6 years; DS teaches this as a blended course. The entire faculty approved NUR 5040; it was then consequently approved by the FC Curriculum Committee and later the Faculty Senate.

Currently, DS's proposal for HLT 3000, the undergraduate TCN course, is with the divisional nursing committee. HLT 3000 will be an elective for students in nursing, premedicine, and physical therapy. The decision to create a 3-credit elective transcultural health care course will be in line with ANA, AACN, NLN, and JC guidelines for cultural diversity and promotion of cultural competence. While the faculty is in agreement that HLT 3000 is needed, the majority of the members believe that there is no current room for another 3-credit course in the 120-credit BS in Nursing curriculum that contains anatomy and physiology (8 CR); chemistry (8 CR); microbiology (4 CR); pathophysiology (3 CR); statistics (3 CR); computer literacy (3 CR); sociology (3 CR); psychology (6 CR); philosophy (6 CR); religion (3 CR); arts and letters (6 CR); English (6 CR); history (3 CR); and electives (6 CR), in addition to 52 CR from 14 NUR courses.

Case study 1.1 outlines the arduous task of adding a separate TCN course in a packed baccalaureate curriculum. Truly, the journey to cultural competence could be difficult and demanding, much like "scaling the mountain" (Campinha-Bacote, 2007, p. 7). In the end, perseverance, commitment, and passion for TCN could overcome resistance.

CRITICAL THINKING EXERCISES 1.1

Undergraduate Student
1. You often hear faculty at your school say that you need to be prepared to care for culturally diverse clients for your clinical rotations and when you graduate. Have you felt this readiness?
2. Do you think there is enough content of cultural diversity and promotion of cultural competence integrated in your classes (theory) and in clinical?
3. Would you be in favor of including a 3-credit TCN course in your current curriculum? If yes, which course would you be in favor of deleting from your BS in Nursing curriculum? Why?

Graduate Student
1. How many credits do you need to complete in your masters or doctoral program?
2. How many TCN courses do you need to complete in this program? Do all courses in the program integrate TCN concepts? Describe.
3. As a nurse leader, how would you meet the challenge of promoting cultural competence among staff and colleagues? Describe.
4. As an advanced practice nurse (APN), how do you plan to manage culturally and linguistically appropriate services to your clients? Explain.

Faculty in Academia
1. How many credits do you have in the BS in Nursing program at your school?
2. If you were to add a 3-credit TCN course, which current course would you delete? Why?
3. How do you critically appraise diversity in your curricula?
4. Analyze strategies that you could implement according to the enhanced CLAS standards. Describe.

Staff Development Educator
1. Do you require a yearly module in cultural diversity and promotion of cultural competence?
2. What follow-up activities that celebrate diversity do you have for the nurses and ancillary staff? How often are these activities held?
3. How long has it been since you attended a workshop/conference on cultural diversity and promotion of cultural competence? When are you planning to attend a workshop/conference on this topic?

SUMMARY

This chapter provides an overview of TCN along with some theories and models. These theories and models are highly applicable in academic and staff development settings. Academia has the gigantic task of preparing practitioners primed to care for the diverse clients and their families or significant others in today's complex health care system. Staff development picks up from program completion and licensure to maintain continuing competence among practitioners. There is a brief history of integration of transcultural concepts in academia and the formation of professional staff development to oversee continuing education and competence. Partnerships between academia and clinical affiliating institutions are strongly encouraged to enhance consistency and harmony in theoretical and practice expectations and to improve client care outcomes.

REFERENCES

Accreditation Commission for Education in Nursing. (2013). *ACEN standards and criteria: Baccalaureate.* Retrieved August 22, 2013, from www.acenursing.net/manuals/SC2013_BACCALAUREATE.pdf

American Association of Colleges of Nursing. (1998). *The essentials of baccalaureate education for professional nursing practice.* Washington, DC: Author.

American Association of Colleges of Nursing. (1999). *Nursing education's agenda for the 21st century.* Washington, DC: Author.

American Association of Colleges of Nursing. (2008a). *Cultural competency in baccalaureate nursing education.* Washington, DC: Author.

American Association of Colleges of Nursing. (2008b). *The essentials of baccalaureate education for professional nursing practice.* Washington, DC: Author.

American Association of Colleges of Nursing. (2011). *Toolkit for cultural competence in master's and doctoral nursing education.* Washington, DC: Author.

American Nurses Association. (1991). *Position statement on cultural diversity in nursing practice.* Kansas City, MO: Author.

American Nurses Association. (1995). *Nursing's social policy statement.* Washington, DC: Author.

American Nurses Association. (2003). *Nursing's social policy statement* (2nd ed.). Washington, DC: Nurses Books.

American Nurses Association. (2011). *Nurses keep top spot for honesty and ethics in poll ranking professions.* Retrieved August 7, 2013, from www.nursingworld.org/FunctionalMenuCategories/MediaResources/PressReleases/2011-R/Nurses-Keep-Top-Spot-in-Poll.pdf

American Nurses Association & National Nursing Staff Development Organization. (2010). *Nursing professional development: Scope and standards of practice.* Silver Spring, MD: Nursesbooks.org.

Andrews, M. M., & Boyle, J. S. (2012). *Transcultural concepts in nursing care* (6th ed.). Philadelphia, PA: Wolters Kluwer/Lippincott Williams & Wilkins.

Boyle, J. (2007). Commentary on "Current approaches to integrating elements of cultural competence in nursing education." *Journal of Transcultural Nursing, 18*(1), 21S–22S.

Boyle, J. S., & Andrews, M. M. (2012a). Andrews/Boyle transcultural nursing assessment guide for individuals and families. In M. M. Andrews & J. S. Boyle (Eds.), *Transcultural concepts in nursing care* (6th ed., pp. 451–455). Philadelphia, PA: Wolters Kluwer/Lippincott Williams & Wilkins.

Boyle, J. S., & Andrews, M. M. (2012b). Andrews/Boyle transcultural nursing assessment guide for groups and communities. In M. M. Andrews & J. S. Boyle (Eds.), *Transcultural concepts in nursing care* (6th ed., pp. 456–458). Philadelphia, PA: Wolters Kluwer/Lippincott Williams & Wilkins.

Boyle, J. S., Andrews, M. M., & Ludwig-Beymer, P. (2012). Andrews/Boyle transcultural nursing assessment guide for health care organizations and facilities. In M. M. Andrews & J. S. Boyle (Eds.), *Transcultural concepts in nursing care* (6th ed., pp. 459–461). Philadelphia, PA: Wolters Kluwer/Lippincott Williams & Wilkins.

Brown, H., & Doane, G. H. (2007). From filling a bucket to lighting a fire: Aligning nursing education and nursing practice. In L. E. Young & B. L. Paterson (Eds.), *Teaching nursing: Developing a student-centered learning environment* (pp. 97–118). Philadelphia, PA: Lippincott Williams & Wilkins.

Campinha-Bacote, J. (2007). *The process of cultural competence in the delivery of healthcare services: The journey continues.* Cincinnati, OH: Transcultural C.A.R.E. Resources.

Campinha-Bacote, J. (2011). Coming to know cultural competence: An evolutionary process. *International Journal for Human Caring, 15*(3), 42–48.

Campinha-Bacote, J. (2012). *The process of cultural competence in the delivery of healthcare services.* Retrieved September 17, 2013, from www.transculturalcare.net

Campinha-Bacote, J. (2013). *A biblically based model of cultural competence in the delivery of healthcare services: Seeing "Imago Dei."* Retrieved September 17, 2013, from www.transculturalcare.net

Choi, H. (2001). Cultural marginality: A concept analysis with implications for immigrant adolescents. *Issues in Comprehensive Pediatric Nursing, 24,* 193–206.

Choi, H. (2008). Theory of cultural marginality. In M. J. Smith & P. R. Liehr (Eds.), *Middle range theory for nursing* (3rd ed., pp. 243–259). New York, NY: Springer Publishing.

Choi, H. (2013). Theory of cultural marginality. In M. J. Smith & P. R. Liehr (Eds.), *Middle range theory for nursing* (3rd ed., pp. 289–307). New York, NY: Springer Publishing.

Choi, H., Meininger, J. C., & Roberts, R. E. (2006). Ethnic differences in adolescents' mental distress, social stress, and resources. *Adolescence, 41*(162), 263–283.

Davidhizar, R. E., & Giger, J. N. (1998). *Canadian transcultural nursing: Assessment and intervention.* St. Louis, MO: Mosby.

Desantis, L. A., & Lipson, J. G. (2007). Brief history of inclusion of content on culture in nursing education. *Journal of Transcultural Nursing, 18*(1), 7S–9S.

DiCicco-Bloom, B. (2004). The racial and gendered experiences of immigrant nurses from Kerala, India. *Journal of Transcultural Nursing, 15*(1), 26–33.

Dobbins, M., Ciliska, D., Estabrooks, C., & Hayward, S. (2005). Changing nursing practice in an organization. In A. DiCenso, G. Guyatt, & D. Ciliska (Eds.), *Evidence-based nursing: A guide to clinical practice* (pp. 172–200). St. Louis, MO: Elsevier Mosby.

Dowd, S. B., Giger, J. N., & Davidhizar, R. E. (1998). Use of Giger and Davidhizar's transcultural assessment model by health professions. *International Nursing Review, 45*(4), 119–122, 128.

Giger, J. N., & Davidhizar, R. E. (2002). The Giger and Davidhizar transcultural assessment model. *Journal of Transcultural Nursing, 13*(3), 185–188.

Giger, J. N., & Davidhizar, R. E. (2004). *Transcultural nursing: Assessment and intervention* (4th ed.). St. Louis, MO: Mosby Elsevier.

Giger, J. N., & Davidhizar, R. E. (2008). *Transcultural nursing: Assessment and intervention* (5th ed.). St. Louis, MO: Mosby Elsevier.

Giger, J. N., & Davidhizar, R. E. (2013). *Transcultural nursing: Assessment and intervention* (6th ed.). St. Louis, MO: Mosby Elsevier Health Science. Retrieved August 9, 2013, from pageburstls .elsevier.com/books/978–0-323–08379-9/Root/0

Grant, L. F., & Letzring, T. D. (2003). Status of cultural competence in nursing education: A literature review. *Journal of Multicultural Nursing & Health, 9*(2), 6–13. Retrieved December 26, 2012, from ProQuest Nursing & Allied Health Source.

International Council of Nurses. (2007). *Nurse retention and migration.* Retrieved July 11, 2013, from www.icn.ch/images/stories/documents/publications/position_statements/C06_Nurse_ Retention_Migration.pdf

Jeffreys, M. R. (2010). A model to guide cultural competence education. In M. R. Jeffreys, *Teaching cultural competence in nursing and health care* (2nd ed., pp. 45–59). New York, NY: Springer. Publishing.

Kardong-Edgreen, S. (2007). Cultural competence of baccalaureate nursing faculty. *Journal of Nursing Education, 46*(8), 360–366.

Kardong-Edgreen, S., & Campinha-Bacote, J. (2008). Cultural competency of graduating US Bachelor of Science nursing students. *Contemporary Nurse, 28*, 37–44.

Kardong-Edgreen, S., Cason, C. L., Walsh Brennan, A. M., Reifsnider, E., Hummel, F., Mancini, M., & Griffin, C. (2010). Cultural competency of graduating BSN students. *Nursing Education Perspectives, 31*(5), 278–285.

Kennedy, H. P., Fisher, L., Fontaine, D., & Martin-Holland, J. (2008). Evaluating diversity in nursing education. *Journal of Transcultural Nursing, 19*(4), 363–370. doi:10.1177/104.3659608322500

Leininger, M. M. (1995). Overview of Leininger's culture care theory. In M. M. Leininger (Ed.), *Transcultural nursing: Concepts, theories, research, and practice* (2nd ed., pp. 93–114). New York, NY: McGraw-Hill.

Leininger, M. M. (2002). Culture care theory: A major contribution to advance transcultural nursing knowledge and practices. *Journal of Transcultural Nursing, 13*(3), 189–192.

Leininger, M. M. (2006). Culture care diversity and universality and evolution of the ethnonursing method. In M. Leininger & M. McFarland (Eds.), *Culture care diversity and universality: A worldwide nursing theory* (pp. 1–41). Sudbury, MA: Jones & Bartlett.

Leininger, M. M., & McFarland, M. M. (2006). *Culture care diversity and universality: A worldwide nursing theory.* Sudbury, MA: Jones & Bartlett.

Lipson, J. G., & Desantis, L. A. (2007). Current approaches to integrating elements of cultural competence in nursing education. *Journal of Transcultural Nursing, 18*(1), 10S–20S.

Ludwig-Beymer, P. (2012). Creating culturally competent organizations. In M. M. Andrews & J. S. Boyle (Eds.), *Transcultural concepts in nursing care* (6th ed., pp. 211–242). Philadelphia, PA: Wolters Kluwer/Lippincott Williams & Wilkins.

McFarland, M. R., & Leininger, M. M. (2002). Transcultural nursing: Curricular concepts, principles, and teaching and learning activities for the 21st century. In M. M. Leininger & M. R. McFarland (Eds.), *Transcultural nursing: Concepts, theories, research, and practice* (3rd ed., pp. 527–561). New York, NY: McGraw-Hill.

McFarland, M., Mixer, S., Lewis, A. E., & Easley, C. (2006). Use of the culture care theory as a framework for the recruitment, engagement, and retention of culturally diverse nursing students in a traditionally European American baccalaureate nursing program. In M. M. Leininger & M. R. McFarland (Eds.), *Culture care diversity and universality: A worldwide nursing theory* (2nd ed., pp. 239–254). Sudbury, MA: Jones & Bartlett.

Mixer, S. (2011). Use of the culture care theory to discover nursing faculty care expressions, patterns, and practices related to teaching culture care. *Online Journal of Cultural Competence in Nursing and Healthcare, 1*(1), 3–14.

Mixer, S. J. (2008). Use of the culture care theory and ethnonursing method to discover how nursing faculty teach culture care. *Contemporary Nurse, 28,* 23–36.

National League for Nursing. (2005). *Core competencies of nurse educators with task statements.* New York, NY: Author. Retrieved January 26, 2013, from www.nln.org/aboutnln/core_competencies/cce_dial3.htm

National League for Nursing. (2009a). *A commitment to diversity in nursing and nursing education.* Retrieved August 22, 2013, from www.nln.org/aboutnln/reflection_dialogue/rfl _dial3.htm

National League for Nursing. (2009b). *Diversity toolkit.* Retrieved August 22, 2013, from www.nln.org/facultyprograms/Diversity_Toolkit/index.htm

Park, R. E. (1928). Human migration and the marginal man. *The American Journal of Sociology, 33,* 881–893.

Purnell, L. D. (2002). The Purnell model for cultural competence. *Journal of Transcultural Nursing, 13*(3), 193–196.

Purnell, L. D. (2007). Commentary on "Current approaches to integrating elements of cultural competence in nursing education." *Journal of Transcultural Nursing, 18*(1), 23S–24S.

Purnell, L. D. (2008). The Purnell model for cultural competence. In L. D. Purnell & B. J. Paulanka. *Transcultural health care: A culturally competent approach* (3rd ed., pp. 15–44). Philadelphia, PA: F. A. Davis.

Purnell, L. D. (2013). The Purnell model for cultural competence. In L. D. Purnell, *Transcultural health care: A culturally competent approach* (4th ed., pp. 15–44). Philadelphia, PA: F. A. Davis.

Ryan, M. (2011). A celebration of a life of commitment to transcultural nursing: Opening of the Madeleine M. Leininger Collection on Human Caring and Transcultural Nursing. *Journal of Transcultural Nursing, 22*(1), 97.

Ryan, M., Carlton, K. H., & Ali, N. (2000). Transcultural nursing concepts and experiences in nursing curricula. *Journal of Transcultural Nursing, 11*(4), 300–307.

Sagar, P. L. (2012). *Transcultural nursing theory and models: Application in nursing education, practice, and administration.* New York, NY: Springer Publishing.

Schon, D. A. (1987). *Educating the reflective practitioner.* San Franciso, CA: Jossey Bass.

Spector, R. E. (2002). Cultural diversity in health and illness. *Journal of Transcultural Nursing, 13*(3), 197–199.

Spector, R. E. (2004a). *Cultural diversity in health and illness* (6th ed.). Upper Saddle River, NJ: Pearson Education.

Spector, R. E. (2004b). *Cultural care guide to heritage assessment and health traditions* (3rd ed.). Upper Saddle River, NJ: Pearson Prentice Hall.

Spector, R. E. (2009). *Cultural diversity in health and illness* (7th ed.). Upper Saddle River, NJ: Pearson Education.

Spector, R. E. (2013). *Cultural diversity in health and illness* (8th ed.). Boston, MA: Pearson Education.

Sullivan Commission. (2004). *Missing persons: Minorities in the health professions: A report of the Sullivan Commission on diversity in the health care workforce.* Retrieved July 26, 2013, from health-equity.pitt.edu/40/1/Sullivan_Final_Report_000.pdf

TCNS Expert Panel on Global Nursing & Health. (2010). *Standards of practice for culturally competent nursing care.* Retrieved February 3, 2012, from www.tcns.org/TCNStandardsofPractice.html

The Joint Commission. (2010a). *Advancing effective communication, cultural competence, and patient- and family-centered care: A roadmap for hospitals.* Oakbrook Terrace, IL: Author.

The Joint Commission. (2010b). *Cultural and linguistic care in area hospitals.* Oakbrook Terrace, IL: Author.

Tomer, J. (2012). Health disparities: The beginning of the end. *Minority Nurse,* 20–23.

United States Department of Health and Human Services, Office of Minority Health. (2013). *Enhanced national CLAS standards.* Retrieved August 16, 2013, from https://www.thinkculturalhealth.hhs.gov/Content/clas.asp

Integrating Transcultural Nursing in Education: Academia and Staff Development

Priscilla Limbo Sagar

KEY TERMS

Academia
Accommodation/negotiation
Boyle and Andrews' Transcultural Assessment
    Guide for Individuals, Families, and Groups
Curriculum threads
Discussion questions
Eclectic approach
Evidence-based practice
Grading rubrics
Horizontal threads
Independent study

Journaling
Knowing-in-action
Mirror
Preservation/maintenance
Reflection-in-action
Reflection-on-action
Repatterning/restructuring
Self-learning modules
Staff development
Vertical threads

LEARNING OBJECTIVES

At the completion of this chapter, the learner will be able to

1. Analyze barriers and challenges in integrating diversity and cultural competence into nursing curricula.
2. Discuss strategies used to integrate transcultural nursing (TCN) in nursing education.
3. Demonstrate vertical and horizontal threading of concepts in nursing curricula.
4. Propose creative strategies to integrate TCN concepts in existing and proposed nursing curricula.
5. Compare and contrast tools for measuring students' and faculty's cultural competence.

OVERVIEW

The curricular integration of cultural diversity in nursing started in 1917 when the National League for Nursing (NLN) Committee on Curriculum published a guide focusing on sociology and social issues in nursing (DeSantis & Lipson, 2007). Twenty years later, in 1937, the NLN Committee added cultural background in order to understand individual response to illness. Almost 100 years later, we are still grappling with a more consistent, standardized inclusivity of diversity, and culturally congruent care not only in nursing but also in allied health professional curricula such as medicine, pharmacy, and dentistry.

In nursing alone, the nation's largest health care professionals with current membership at 3,163,063 (United States Department of Health and Human Services, Health Resources Services Administration, 2010), a huge difference could be made if diversity will be consistently integrated and standardized across all levels of curricula and included as required competence for registration and licensure. In addition to the power in number, Gallup polls show public trust for nurses among all health care professionals for 11 years in a row (American Nurses Association, 2012). As an initiative to expand the affordable health care coverage, Vice-President Biden capitalized on this trust as he exhorted all nurses—through a phone conference with nursing leaders and more than 5,000 nurses participating on September 26, 2013—to continue teaching and advocating for clients in this endeavor (Health Insurance Marketplace, 2013).

Meanwhile, the population of the United States has increasingly become more culturally and ethnically diverse. The minority populations, now at 37%, are projected to be the majority by the year 2060 at 57% (U.S. Census Bureau, 2012). Moreover, health care professionals do not mirror the diverse population that they serve—and will be less representative of these populations in the future; there is evidence that this is contributing to the disparities in health care access and quality among minority populations (Sullivan Commission, 2004; U.S. Commission on Civil Rights, 2010). The American Association of Colleges of Nursing ([AACN], 2008, 2011, 2012) and the NLN (2009a, 2009b) have been consistently supportive of the recruitment and retention of both minority students and faculty as well as the integration of diversity and cultural competence in nursing education.

Integration of TCN concepts has been the most common method of inclusion of cultural competency in nursing curricula (Kardong-Egren et al., 2010; Lipson & DeSantis, 2007). There is continuing evidence suggesting that there is a wide variation in content, depth, and level of integration (Ryan, Carlton, & Ali, 2000). Moreover, if there is integration of TCN concepts in the curricula, there is usually no conceptual framework used (Mixer, 2011). Furthermore, surveys point to lack of cultural competence and lack of formal preparation among faculty themselves. It is imperative that national surveys be replicated—ensuring representativeness of existing undergraduate and graduate schools of nursing throughout the United States—to explore preparation of graduates with the knowledge, skills, and competencies to care for culturally diverse clients (Sagar, 2012).

SOME STRATEGIES TO INTEGRATE TCN INTO THE CURRICULUM

An introspective, reflective look at one's undergraduate curriculum is the first step when planning integration of TCN concepts. The following strategies of TCN concept inclusion will be discussed: using theory or model, weaving-in as curricular threads, integrating guiding students in independent studies, into clinical experiences, adding concepts as modules, integrating **evidence-based practice**, creating a separate course or courses, and integrating into simulations. Various teaching strategies such as cultivating reflection, assigning reflective journals, creating and implementing grading rubrics, using role-plays, developing unfolding case scenarios, teaching literary works, and creating user-friendly websites are also discussed.

Using Conceptual Theory or Model

The use of theories or models may be a helpful guide when planning to integrate TCN concepts in the curricula or when embarking into curricular overhaul or revision. Agreeing on a theory or a model is in itself a daunting task, since individual faculty may have established preferences. Chapter 1 discusses a theory and several models in TCN.

Carefully examining the congruency between the university or college mission, philosophy, and goals may guide the selection of theory or model. Some schools or divisions of nursing prefer to adopt an **eclectic approach**—that is, adopting two or more theories and/or models—and using those to develop the school's mission, philosophy, and goals. When using several theories or models, the faculty need to analyze the blending of a group of concepts into a congruent, harmonious whole. Tables 2.1 and 2.2 illustrate curricular

TABLE 2.1   Old Curriculum at Sunrise University That Used the Medical Model

Fall Semester	Spring Semester
Year I BIO 101-Anatomy & Physiology I (4) CHM103-Biochemistry (4) NUR 1000-History of Nursing (1) ANT 101-Anthropology (3) PSY-General Psychology (3) <div align="right">15</div>	Year I BIO 102-Anatomy & Physiology II (4) BIO 200-Microbiology (4) NUR 100-Transcultural Health Care (3) PSY-Developmental Psychology (3) <div align="right">14</div>
Year II NUR 204-Nursing Assessment and Physical Examination (3) PHL 103-Intro to Philosophy (3) NUR 200-Mental Health Nursing (5) CIT 101- Computer Literacy (3) <div align="right">14</div>	Year II NUR 204-Foundations of Nursing Practice (4) MUS, LANG, THR, CMA (3) MTH 207-Statistical Concepts in Health Care (3) BIO 303-Pathopysiological Concepts (3) HIS 101- History and Culture (3) <div align="right">16</div>
Year III NUR 322-Nursing Care of Adults (8) REL 103-Culture and Religion (3) NUR 300-Pharmacology and Calculation (3) *Elective (3) <div align="right">17</div>	Year III NUR 323- Family I: Maternal and Newborn Care (5) NUR 324-Family II: Child Care (5) NUR 303- Nutrition and Culture (3) MUS, LANG, THR, CMA (3) <div align="right">16</div>
Year IV NUR 421-Promotion of Community Health (5) NUR 4000-Cultural Competence in Research and Evidence Based Practice (3) PHL 3500-Ethics in Healthcare (3) NUR 420-Special Topic in Nursing (3) <div align="right">14</div>	Year IV NUR 4500-Transition to Professional Nursing (8) NUR 4001-Leadership in Health Care (4) *Elective (3) <div align="right">15</div>

TABLE 2.2 Sample 120-Credit BS in Nursing Curriculum at Sunrise University Utilizing the Andrews and Boyle Transcultural Assessment for Individuals, Families, Groups, and Communities

Fall Semester	Spring Semester
Year I BIO 103-Anatomy & Physiology I (4) CHM 106-Biochemistry (4) NUR 1000-History of Nursing (1) ANT 101-Anthropology (3) PSY-General Psychology (3) 15	Year I BIO 104-Anatomy & Physiology II (4) BIO 202-Microbiological Concepts (4) NUR 100-Transcultural Health Care (3) PSY-Developmental Psychology (3) 14
Year II NUR 204-Cultural Competence in Health Assessment and Physical Examination (3) PHL 103-Intro to Philosophy (3) NUR 200-Multicultural Perspectives: Mental Health Nursing (5) CIT 101-Computer Literacy (3) 14	Year II NUR 204-Cultural Competence in the Performance of Nursing Skills (4) MUS, LANG, THR, CMA (3) MTH 207-Statistical Concepts in Health Care (3) BIO 303-Pathophysiological Concepts (3) HIS 101- History and Culture (3) 16
Year III NUR 302-Cultural Competence in Adult Health (8) REL 103-Culture and Religion (3) NUR 300-Multicultural Perspectives: Pharmacology (3) 14	Year III NUR 304-Cultural Competence in Maternal and Child Health (5) NUR 305-Multicultural Perspectives: Child Care (5) NUR 303- Nutrition and Culture (3) MUS, LANG, THR, CMA (3) 16
Year IV NUR 402-Cultural Competence in Community Health (5) NUR 4000-Cultural Competence in Research and Evidence-Based Practice (3) PHL 367-Ethics and Health Care (3) NUR 406-Multicultural Perspectives: Professional Nursing (3) *Elective (2) 16	Year IV NUR 405-Cultural Competence in Complex Health Settings (8) NUR 4001-Multicultural Perspectives: Leadership in Health Care (4) *Elective (3) 15

Sources: Developed from Boyle & Andrews (2012a, 2012b).

revision from a medical model curriculum to a curriculum that uses Boyle and Andrews's (2012a, 2012b) *Transcultural Assessment Guide for Individuals, Families, and Groups.*

Weaving TCN Concepts as Curricular Threads

When threading TCN concepts in the curriculum, it is of prime importance to first assess the program's conceptual framework, expected outcomes, and TCN content already in the curriculum. Based upon the conceptual framework and expected results of the program, essential elements that unify the curriculum are referred to as vertical and horizontal threads.

Vertical threads are content focused (Jeffreys, 2010) and allow the students to have both breadth and depth as they advance in the nursing program. Most nursing curricula are progressive; new concepts are introduced as the complexity of nursing interventions increases. For example, when integrating vertical threads about the recipient of care, communication, and professional role, the Culturally and Linguistically Appropriate Services (CLAS) standards (U.S. Department of Health and Human Services [USDHHS], Office of Minority Health [OMH], 2013) could be integrated. To illustrate further, CLAS could be introduced in nursing skills in caring for individuals, into childbearing and child-rearing courses to care for families, and into community health nursing to care for groups and communities.

Horizontal threads are essential elements of the framework and expected program results; these elements are introduced in the first level of the program. Consequently, horizontal threads gain in breadth when applied at various levels and in diverse care settings. If cultural diversity is a horizontal **curriculum thread** that adopts Leininger's CCT (2006), her three-action and decision modes of **preservation and/or maintenance, accommodation and/or negotiation**, and **repatterning and/or restructuring** will be introduced in the first nursing course and consistently applied in the care of childbearing and child-rearing families; care of adults; care of individuals, groups, and communities; and care of clients in mental health and illnesses. In this way, the concept of the three-action and decision modes of Leininger's CCT theory is woven throughout the curriculum. The creative weaving-in of concepts creates a "durable fabric that provides long-lasting learning" (Jeffreys, 2010, p. 125) and achievement of program outcomes.

Integrating TCN Concepts Into Clinical Experiences

Clinical experiences are worth two or more times the academic credit hours than to the theory portion of nursing courses; integration of TCN concepts in clinical experiences is vital in achieving outcomes for culturally congruent care. The theoretical or didactic portion of the curriculum only partially contributes to the knowledge, skills (Emerson, 2007), and attitudes of the future practitioner.

Pre- and postconferences as well as individual conferences with students are excellent opportunities to discuss culturally congruent care of all clients. Planned learning activities such as the invitation of a guest speaker for postconference represent this kind of integration. The faculty member may invite a certified transcultural nurse (CTN) if one is employed at the hospital, the **staff development** educator, a leader of migrant workers, or someone from the neighborhood health clinic or a homeless shelter. Assigning a student to include culturally congruent interventions in his or her plan of care is an approach to ensure integration of TCN concepts in the clinical area. Using transcultural theories and models such as Purnell, Jeffreys, Campinha-Bacote, Giger and Davidhizar, and Spector in developing course assessment tools and nursing care plans for clients is another way of including this content in the clinical component of nursing courses.

Adding Concepts as Self-Learning Modules

Self-learning modules (SLMs), stand-alone learning packages offering a variety of uses for both nurse educators and learners (Alvir, 1975), are easier to add to existing courses when revisions to make way for TCN content or development of a separate TCN course are not yet possible. In some literature, SLMs are also referred to as self-learning packets (SLPs), independent studies (Aucoin, 1998), or individualized learning packets (ILPs; Rowles & Briggs, 2005). Some advantages of using SLMs are independence in learning, flexibility of time, enhancement of classroom and discussion methods (Rowles & Brigham, 2005), and the adaptability of offering hard copies of the packages or posting them on the institution's intranet or web-based server. Disadvantages in using SLMs on the learner's part may be procrastination or inability to complete the module on time; in addition, SLMs are time consuming and expensive to prepare and revise on the educator's part (Rowles & Brigham, 2005).

This book contains four modules—*Module 3.1: Culturally and Linguistically Appropriate Services (CLAS) Standards*, and *Module 3.2: Generic Folk Practices: Theory of Hot and Cold*, Chapter 3; *Self-Learning Module 10.1: An Orthodox Jewish Child With Asthma*, Chapter 10; and *Self-Learning Module 13.1: Posttraumatic Stress Disorder (PTSD) in Women*, Chapter 13. Any or a combination of these modules could be used as assignments for learners. See Chapter 3 for more information about SLMs.

Online modules, mostly offered with continuing education credits (CEs), are widely available; some are offered without any cost. Nurse educators must choose online courses that encourage independent learning, self-reflection, and self-evaluation (Nielsen, 2011). Completion of required modules may be rewarded with incentives such as placing them in a newsletter, or applying them toward annual required competence.

Integrating Research and Evidence-Based Practice

There has been heightened focus on using research and EBP in health care (Polit & Beck, 2010). Even if a school of nursing does not have a separate TCN course, integrating research and EBP could easily be integrated in an existing course. The nurse educator's creativity in this process is displayed by using research and EBP related to diversity and cultural competence. There is a time lag of 8 to 15 years between the generation of new knowledge and its utilization in the practice setting and in the development of policy (Dobbins, Ciliska, Estabrook, & Hayward, 2005). It is imperative that we reduce this time lag and adopt research evidence to improve teaching and learning and to foster cultural competence among our students, faculty, and colleagues.

African Americans, Hispanics, and Native Americans are underrepresented among health care professionals such as nurses, physicians, dentists, and psychologists (Sullivan Commission, 2004). Asians, in addition to these groups, are also underrepresented among nurse educators (AACN, 2010, 2011; NLN, 2009a, 2010). Both the AACN (2008, 2009, 2011) and the NLN (2009) developed faculty toolkits that include evidence-based, best practices to guide educators in assessment, integration, and evaluation of diversity content in the nation's nursing curricula. In addition, many advocates feel there's a need to transform nursing education and foster a climate of inclusivity, offering evidence-based practices such as mentoring (Davis-Dick, 2009; Vance, 2002, 2011) and recruitment and retention

(Jeffreys, 2010; McFarland, Mixer, Lewis, & Easley, 2006) to increase minority success in nursing. Many more voices have joined in—sounding distinct calls— and are challenging all of us to look, listen, feel, and reflect on the many intentional and unintentional practices of exclusivity.

Guiding Students in Independent Studies

An **independent study** (IS), a nonrequired, focused study of a specific area pursued by a student and guided by a faculty member, provides an avenue for nursing students or those in allied health to pursue areas of interest in health care that are not otherwise covered or only covered minimally in the curriculum. When a student is interested in pursuing an IS with a faculty mentor, the student must submit clear, specific, and measurable objectives. In general, three to four objectives are enough for a 1-credit IS; this is equivalent to 15 hours of supervised work. In Appendix 1, the student aimed to explore Filipino Americans' (FAs) folk and folk-healing practices and Filipino nurse migration to the United States in a 1-credit IS. The student's reflections throughout the 10-week semester as she was learning more about FAs are shown in Box 2.1.

BOX 2.1 A SENIOR STUDENT'S REFLECTIONS: INDEPENDENT STUDY

Independent Study: NUR 497- Filipino Americans and Filipino Nurse Migration to the United States

Mollie Bowman, BS, RN
Staff Nurse, Saint Luke's Cornwall Hospital, Newburgh, New York

I am truly enjoying my independent study on Filipino Americans. My future sister-in-law is Filipino and I always wanted to learn more about her culture. I am grateful that I now have the opportunity to do a literature search about Filipino Americans and their role in nursing. I think it is vital to learn about other cultures, especially the Filipino culture because they make up a large percentage of nurses in the United States. I think all nursing students should take a transcultural nursing class during their college years and I think it should be offered in hospitals for the nursing staff. A transcultural nursing class will help students and nursing staff to better care for their patients of different cultures.

I have learned so much about the migration and acculturation process. I did not know that one of the largest immigrant populations to the United States is from the Philippines. I also did not know that many of the nurses are recruited to the United States and trained here. I found it very interesting that many of the newly recruited Filipino nurses start on the evening and night shifts at the hospitals. The poor working conditions and the economic hardship intrigued me to find out more information about the country. I heard about the poor areas of the country but it was an eye opener reading about it. I would like to learn more about the country and what the government is doing to help support the hospitals in the Philippines.

I think it is interesting that Filipino nurses migrate to the United States to find nursing jobs. I know that there is a nursing shortage and that these nurses are

---

(continued)

BOX 2.1 A SENIOR STUDENT'S REFLECTIONS: INDEPENDENT STUDY *(continued)*

helping to fill the void. Nurses from other countries such as the Philippines create diversity in the work place. Diversity is needed in hospitals to help the staff and the patients. I have come across many patients from different cultures and countries. I think it is comforting to have a nurse who is from the same culture as you are and who understands your values and customs. I always enjoy working with nurses from other cultures because I learn about their cultures and they learn about mine. It is always important to be helpful to these nurses because if they do not feel welcomed they may not accomplish all they want to in the nursing profession and it may impact the nursing care given to their patients.

Acculturation takes time and effort, especially from a country like the Philippines because its culture is much different than the American culture. According to literature, the Filipino nurses succeed in the acculturation process better than immigrants from other countries. Before writing this paper, I never knew how much acculturation and job satisfaction went hand in hand. It now makes much more sense than when I began writing this paper. Job satisfaction is extremely important in any field of work and I am interested to learn about the factors that create higher job satisfaction.

Learning about the folk and healing practices are always interesting because it is much different than the way of life in the United States and the way I was raised. I respect their values and customs very much. I found it very hard to find literature on the Filipino folk practices and I used one solid source that I could find. The hot and cold theory is always very interesting to read about; I also found the herbal medicines fascinating. It amazes me how herbs can be used for so many different ailments. I would have liked to learn more about the roots of these folk healing practices and how long they have been practiced.

I am looking forward to finding more information about folk practices in the Filipino culture. I did not find many articles about them and I am curious to see if I can search out more information about herbal medicines. I am enjoying this independent study and I know it will help me immensely in my future nursing career.

Journal 2: In my last journal, I wrote about my findings and what I thought was very interesting about my independent study. I have learned so much about the Filipino culture throughout this independent study. I think the topics I chose were very interesting but were somewhat broad. If I had to write another paper, I would have liked to search other topics and would have narrowed my search.

In addition, I would have liked to learn more about the perspective of American nurses toward their Filipino coworkers. I wrote a paper about the acculturation process and the job satisfaction of Filipino nurses in the United States. If I had to write another paper for an independent study, I would include American nurses and how they feel when nurses from other countries such as the Philippines come to work with them. It would be interesting to hear their point of view during the time they worked with them and when they trained these nurses on the floors.

(continued)

BOX 2.1 A SENIOR STUDENT'S REFLECTIONS: INDEPENDENT
STUDY (continued)

Everyone has his or her own perceptions about other cultures and it would be interesting to see if these perceptions changed or remained the same during the training
process.

Another area of interest for me is the statistics of nurses coming from the
Philippines from when they first immigrated until now. I did not use many statistics in this independent study but in the future I would like to include this. I
think the statistics are striking and would interest the readers even more. I did not
find many statistics for this paper so I would have to use other search engines and
other books.

When I first began getting my ideas together for the independent study, I was
going to interview my future sister-in-law about the Filipino lifestyle and her
experience growing up in a family with Filipino nurses. I would have liked to hear
her perspective and I still plan on asking her even though I will not add it into my
paper. When her family comes to the United States from the Philippines this sum-
mer I also plan on talking to them. I think I am very fortunate to have written a
paper on this culture and to have members of this culture easily available to speak
to and ask questions.

As I mentioned earlier, if I had to write another independent study, I would have
liked to personally interview American nurses about their perspectives. I would
like to create five to ten questions to ask the nurses. I would start with basic questions such as:

■ How long have you been a nurse?
■ What are your thoughts before, during, and after working with the Filipino
  nurses?
■ Was this your first time working with a nurse from a different culture?
■ What did you learn from working with a nurse from a different culture?
  Discuss.
■ Would you work with a nurse from a different culture again in the future?
  Discuss.

I think it would be very interesting to interview a nurse who has worked with
nurses from other cultures and to get feedback about this process. I could possibly
make a chart or graph of their answers to go along with my paper. That would
also be very helpful if I had to present my findings.

As I come to the end of writing a paper for my independent study, I am looking
back on what I have learned and what I am taking away from this one-credit
course. When I began this course, I thought the Filipino culture would be similar to other cultures I have learned about in the past and I was very wrong. The
Filipino culture is very unique and intriguing. I am fortunate to have taken this
independent study and included it in my workload this semester. It has not only
taught me how to care for Filipino Americans but also how to be culturally sensitive to other people.

Creating a Separate TCN Course

The creation of a separate course could take time, depending on the receptivity of other faculty members to examine the existing curriculum. When instituting a 3-credit TCN course, there will be a need to remove a 3-credit course from the current curriculum. This course deletion will necessitate careful assessment of curriculum content by reviewing content maps, level objectives, and course syllabi. Following divisional or departmental consensus, the course may need approval from the college-wide or university-wide curriculum committee and later the faculty senate or a similar body.

This author's undergraduate TCN course was rejected 6 years ago primarily due to an already overcrowded baccalaureate curriculum at the same time that the master's level TCN course received divisional approval. It took 6 years before this author was able to resubmit a proposal for a 3-credit transcultural health care course, which finally obtained approval in March 2013 to be initially offered in spring 2014. Persistence and perseverance are indeed imperative when initiating change. See Chapter 3 for further discussions regarding a separate TCN course for students in nursing and allied health.

Integrating Into Simulation

The evolution from Mrs. Chase—an adult-sized mannequin used for demonstration of basic nursing skills at the Hartford Hospital Training School for Nurses (Decker et al., 2011)—to the prevailing use of simulation in nursing schools has been an amazing example of paradigm shift to keep up with the changing times. The use of simulation has likewise flourished tremendously in the training of allied health professionals such as physicians, dentists, and those in the military. In the early 1960s, Laerdal, a plastic toy manufacturer, introduced Resusci Annie for mouth-to-mouth resuscitation (Cooper & Taqueti, 2004). Since then, the medical simulation industry has grown by leaps and bounds. For more information about simulation, see Chapter 19. Whether planning for high- or low-fidelity mannequin acquisition, some careful preparation has to be done.

Tarnow and Butcher (2005) strongly advocated for lifelike laboratory simulation experiences; they argued that the more lifelike the LRC, the better it is to portray the behaviors anticipated in nurse–client interactions. Currently, in many schools of nursing, the LRC reflects acute and chronic management of clients and are furnished accordingly, resembling actual client settings. The technology seems to attract prospective students and their parents. Cultural and ethnic diversities in actual client settings need to be reflected in these LRCs. Box 19.1, Chapter 19 will help faculty reflect on the diversity score for their LRC. The maximum possible score is 20 points, indicating an LRC that resembles actual client settings. This proposed evaluation tool may be adapted to the ethnocultural groups prevalent in a particular community.

TEACHING AND LEARNING STRATEGIES

Some teaching and learning strategies include journaling, role-plays, unfolding scenarios, literary works, **discussion-questions**, course website, and grading rubrics.

For online classes, discussion questions (DQs), both in individual and in group format, are quite effective in engaging student learning. In blended classes, it is amazing to observe the "blossoming" of a quiet student while participating or facilitating DQs.

Cultivating and Fostering Reflection

Schon (1983, 1987) expanded on Dewey's (1933) work on reflection as part of personal growth and discerned two kinds of reflective thinking: reflection-in-action and reflection-on-action. Schon (1983) referred to **reflection-in-action,** or thinking while absorbed in the action, as "thinking on our feet" (p. 54). This entails using our experiences, coming in touch with our feelings, and listening to assumptions being used (Cohen, 2005). **Reflection-on-action,** or thinking after doing the action, gives us opportunities to explore why we performed the way we did.

Although primarily used in sports, coaching may enable reflection-in-action in educating professionals (Schon, 1987) and is exemplified by the evolving role of educators from being "sages on a stage" to "facilitators on the side." Faculty could use coaching to foster reflection among students when caring for diverse clients, groups, and communities such as those with different ethnic backgrounds, cultural values and beliefs, socioeconomic status, or sexual orientation. The coach, acting as role model, mirrors reflective practice.

Shellenbarger, Palmer, Labant, and Kuzneski (2005) emphasized the need for nurse educators to engage in reflection. Educators are unable to teach what they themselves do not practice. To foster reflective practice, Shellenbarger et al. (2005) proposed a reflection map for reflecting alone and for reflecting with colleagues during a course or program.

Assigning Reflective Journals

Journaling is a form of writing, recording, and guiding thinking and reflection. When started in the initial nursing course and nurtured in succeeding courses, journaling refines critical thinking; sustains interest; and promotes alternate, creative approaches for client care. Journaling gives students opportunities for critical reflection regarding their learning experiences (Yonge & Myrick, 2005) and for engaging in introspection (Schuessler, Wilder, & Byrd, 2012). The faculty member needs to provide carefully constructed questions as a guide for student thinking and reflection. Journaling may be an effective tool to use when embarking on a journey toward cultural competence. The beginning of this journey is the exploration of one's cultural values and beliefs (CVBs) regarding other individuals of different race, ethnicity, gender, sexual orientation, social and economic status, and with differing CVBs (Emerson, 2007; Jeffreys, 2010). Schuessler et al. (2012) utilized journaling as a teaching method to develop cultural humility (Review the synopsis of this study in EBP 17.1).

Journaling may entail substantial writing time on the student's part; it also requires significant time for instructor's reading and giving of feedback (Yonge & Myrick, 2005). In light of this, journaling as an assignment deserves weight in terms of grading. Some faculty may believe in ungraded journals whereas other faculty may opt for assigning grades. Continuing on with the impact of journaling as an assignment, Yonge and Myrick also reminded educators about student and teacher expectations, ethical aspects, and keeping the journaling as a teaching–learning tool and not a forum for unwarranted and unsolicited revelations from students.

When journals are required assignments in clinical, assigning grades may be a decision of the whole faculty and conveys to the student the importance of journaling at the programmatic level (Emerson, 2007). As with any assignments, grading rubrics are helpful for both faculty and students. Students are guided to hone critical thinking and clinical judgment while given the opportunity to optimize their grades by adhering to the grading rubrics. Rubrics also help faculty eliminate bias in grading.

Creating and Implementing Grading Rubrics

Carnegie Mellon University (2013) describes **grading rubrics** as a scoring tool that has explicit expectations for student performance for a specific assignment. When designing rubrics, it is essential for the nurse educator to analyze the objectives for the assignment (Starnes-Vottero, 2011). Rubrics are advantageous to both students and instructors. The students have a clear description of the type of work expected at various levels of mastery as well as the exact weight of the portions of the assignment. Students can gauge the level of effort necessary to achieve criteria or measures for performance (Starnes-Vottero, 2011) and could easily refer to these guides as they develop the assignment. Grading rubrics are tools that assist students to attain maximum grades for assignments or projects.

Rubrics provide consistency and bias reduction in instructor grading, whether dealing with a single instructor or multiple instructors for bigger classes or laboratory sections. The use of rubrics can reduce the need for writing lengthy comments when grading; instructors may instead refer or circle portion of the rubrics as part of the feedback and add brief comments as needed (Carnegie, 2013). Rubrics may be used in formative evaluation of student strength and areas for growth; in addition, referrals could be made early to available campus and online resources for remediation. See Appendix 2 for a sample grading rubric for a transcultural nursing assignment.

Using Role Plays

In **role playing**, individuals enact the role of others while observers analyze and interpret (Billings & Halstead, 2005). Role playing may enhance cultural awareness and give students the opportunity to use their creativity in fostering culturally appropriate care (Shearer & Davidhizar, 2003). The nurse educator's focus in role playing includes developing objectives for the experience; providing guidelines for the different roles and timeframe; monitoring the process and intervening as necessary; and facilitating analysis and debriefing (Rowles & Brigham, 2005; Shearer & Davidhizar, 2003).

Debriefing, the planned feedback at the end of the role play or simulation, provides an opportunity for participants to analyze their actions, address emotional reactions to the role play, and receive constructive comments (Decker, Gore, & Feken, 2011). It also needs to include learning outcomes, application to practice, further learning needed, and changes necessary to improve client care (Gaberson & Oermann, 1999).

Role plays may be used in all levels of students from licensed practical, associate, baccalaureate, master's, and doctoral programs. It is important for nurse educators to allow for maximal student creativity. Debriefing is an important part of role plays. (An example, Sample Role Play Scenario 6.1, is in Chapter 6.)

Developing Unfolding Case Study or Scenario

Case study, or case scenario, is an application of theoretical content to "real life, simulated life, or both" (Rowles & Brigham, 2005, p. 298) and could be used both as an instructional tool or as an assessment activity (Starnes-Vottero, 2011). An unfolding case scenario uses a basic scenario that unfolds into different scenarios.

It takes time, creativity, and patience to develop unfolding case scenarios, but the potential for developing critical thinking is tremendous. The availability of published case scenarios should be considered (Rowles & Brigham, 2005).

BOX 2.2   REFLECTION WORKSHEET: LITERARY WORK ASSIGNMENT WITH SELECTED CATEGORIES FROM BOYLE AND ANDREWS's TCNAGIF

Sunrise University School of Nursing

NUR 222-Nursing Care of Adult

Student name: _____   Literary work: _____

1. Compare and contrast your culture and that of the people in the novel.

2. Identify the values of people from this culture and explain each.

3. Describe the role of the family in health and illness.

    3.1   Healing practices

    3.2   Gender issues

4. Discuss the pattern of communication.

    4.1   Barriers to effective communication

    4.2   Facilitators for effective communication

5. Examine your biases and prejudices about people from this culture. Have your views changed after reading this novel? Explain.

Sources: Boyle & Andrews (2012a), and Boyle & Andrews (2012b).

Teaching Through Literary Works

The use of literary works in nursing education is limitless; it is not limited by available patients in the clinical setting. When assigning works, one important guideline is a direction to pick a different culture from the student's own (Halloran, 2009). One other approach is to assign one literary work for all students, or divide students into groups—either by self-selection or by random assignment. However the faculty decides on student assignment, there needs to be some guidelines or a set of questions to steer each student's reflections. Box 2.2 provides an example of such guidelines. This assignment is applicable to any undergraduate program in nursing or allied health and may be modified by faculty according to perceived student needs.

Creating User-Friendly Course Website

In addition to being a repository for the course, the course website—whether using Moodle, blackboard, Web CT, or other learning platforms—presents wonderful opportunities to link to government, private organization, or other school websites offering cultural diversity guidelines, standards, programs, and other resources. Actual websites or videos may be embedded within the course website; these would offer easier access whether for courses in academic settings or for staff development courses offered on the intranet. These online resources will enhance learning, foster networking, and fuel more curiosity for cultural competence.

Some strategies for integration of TCN concepts at different levels of nursing education are summarized in Table 2.3. In many instances, existing courses could accommodate essential TCN concepts. Possible evaluation methods are also provided.

TABLE 2.3 Strategies: Integration of TCN Concepts at Different Levels of Nursing Education

Existing Courses	Level	Concepts to Integrate	Evaluation Methods
Nursing Care of Adults, Other Integrated Courses With Mental Health, Family Nursing, Pharmacology, and Nutrition	Licensed Practical Nursing	Biocultural Variations, Andrews & Boyle, 2013; Biological Variations, Giger & Davidhizar, 2008; Biocultural Ecology, Purnell, 2013	NCLEX-PN®-type questions, assessment tools
Medical–Surgical Nursing, Child-bearing and Rearing, Mental Health	Associate Degree/ Diploma	Biocultural Variations, Andrews & Boyle, 2013; Biological Variations, Giger & Davidhizar, 2008; Biocultural Ecology, Purnell, 2013	NCLEX-RN®-type questions, assessment tools, pharmacology, and nutrition assignments
Caring for Adults, Child-bearing, Child-Rearing, Pharmacology, Nutrition, Mental Health, Complex Health, Nursing Research, Community Health	Baccalaureate	Biocultural Variations, Andrews & Boyle, 2013; Biological Variations, Giger & Davidhizar, 2008; Biocultural Ecology, Purnell, 2013	Assessment tools, care plans, NCLEX-RN®-type questions, pharmacology and nutrition assignments
Adult Health, Older Adult Health, Advanced Physical Assessment, Advanced Pharmacology, Advanced Nursing Research	Master's	Biocultural Variations, Andrews & Boyle, 2013; Biological Variations, Giger & Davidhizar, 2008; Ethnonursing method, Leininger, 2006; Biocultural Ecology, Purnell, 2013	Assessment tools, paper, classroom presentation, advanced pharmacology assignments
Doctoral Level Courses in Individual, Family, Group, and Population Health; Research-focused Doctoral	Doctoral	Biocultural Variations, Andrews & Boyle, 2013; Biological Variations, Giger & Davidhizar, 2008; Ethnonursing Method, Leininger, 2006; Biocultural Ecology, Purnell, 2013; Mixed-method research about persistent disparities in health care quality and access among minorities	Assessment and grading rubrics, certification examination, dissertation

Sources: Adapted from Boyle & Andrews (2012a); Giger & Davidhizar (2008); Leininger (2006); and Purnell (2013).

Tools for Measuring Cultural Competence

Several tools are available for measuring cultural competence among students, faculty, other health professionals, clinical settings and organizations, and patients. A few of the available tools are mentioned here. The *Inventory for Assessing the Process of Cultural Competence Among Healthcare Professionals*—Revised (*IAPCC-R*; Campinha-Bacote, 2007) is a self-assessment tool that indicates level of cultural competence. Campinha-Bacote also developed the *IAPCC-Student Version* (*IAPCC-SV*), specific to assessing the cultural competence of student nurses, and the *Inventory for Assessing Biblical Worldview of Cultural Competence Among Healthcare Professionals* (*IABWCC*) for use with her Biblically Based Model of Cultural Competence (Campinha-Bacote, 2005).

Another tool, the *Transcultural Self-Efficacy Tool* (*TSET*), was developed by Jeffreys (2010) in 1994. The TSET had undergone multiple reliability and validity tests and has been used with nursing students, physicians, and allied health care providers (Jeffreys, 2010). The *Cultural Competence Clinical Evaluation Tool* (*CCCET*) was adapted from the TSET with a revised rating scale and directions to allow the student/learner's self-evaluation (Jeffreys, 2010). Other modified versions of the CCCET are *Student Version* (SV), *Teacher Version* (TV), *Employee Version* (EV), and *Agency Evaluator Version* (AEV). In addition, Jeffreys developed the *Clinical Setting Assessment Tool-Diversity and Disparity* (*CSAT-DD*) for data collection of diverse client populations (Part I) and clinical problems aimed at the 28 *Healthy People 2010* focus areas (Part II; Jeffreys, 2010).

The Consumer Assessment of Healthcare Providers and Systems (CAHPS), a public–private program led by the Agency for Healthcare Research and Quality (AHRQ), has designed a survey to measure cultural competence from the patients' perspectives. The CAHPS, aiming beyond patient satisfaction, hopes to obtain patient reports of their experiences with health care services with the use of valid and reliable measures (Clancy, Brach, & Abrams, 2012; Weech-Maldonado et al., 2012). CAHPS cultural competency domains focus on doctor communication, health promotion, alternative medicine, shared decision making, and access to interpreter services. CAHPS has evolved into a family of surveys such as the Clinician/Group CAHPS with Item Set I, CAHPS Cultural Competence Item Set, and CAHPS Item Set for Addressing Health Literacy. The CAHPS Hospital Survey has CAHPS Item Set for Addressing Health Literacy (Clancy et al., 2012, p. S1). These are evidence of continuing efforts to implement culturally and linguistically appropriate services (CLAS). Considering that nurses are at the bedside for 24 hours a day, it is imperative to adapt CAHPS to survey patients' experiences with nurses (see EBP 2.1).

EBP 2.1

Mixer (2011) performed an ethnonursing study to explore nursing faculty practices when teaching baccalaureate students provision of culturally congruent care. This study used Leininger's Culture Care Theory (2006) and the sunrise enabler and ethnonursing method as framework. The ethnonursing method embraces the essence of discovery from the people's way of knowing. Leininger (2006) depicted *key informants* (KIs) as bearers of the most knowledge regarding the domain of inquiry, whereas *general informants* (GIs) may not be as knowledgeable. However, GIs offer reflective data, hence allowing the researcher to focus on similarities and differences.

(continued)

EBP 2.1 (continued)

There were a total of 27 participants in this study. The 10 KIs from rural and urban universities were all tenured faculty while the 17 GIs were on tenure track, adjunct, and/or clinical nursing faculty. Participants' ages ranged from 25 to 71 years with an average age of 52 years for KIs and 41 years for GIs. Average years in teaching and experience were significantly higher, respectively, for KIs (21, 30) than for GIs (4, 16). Only eight faculty had some TCN education; none of the faculty took or taught formal cultural immersion nursing courses. A lone informant had taught a TCN course. Of the 27 participants, seven spoke a language other than English, four had lived outside of the United States, and seven had been involved in nursing work outside of the United States. The researcher received approval from the University of Colorado Institutional Review Board (IRB). All participants signed written consent.

Using the four phases of ethnonursing data analysis, the researcher inferred four universal themes: 1) "faculty care is embedded in religious values, beliefs, and practices; 2) faculty taught students without an organizing conceptual framework; 3) faculty provided generic and professional care to students; and 4) care is essential for faculty health and well-being…" (Mixer, 2011, pp. 8–10).

This study shows the application of the CCT in nursing education, substantiating the six constructs discovered by Leininger and others: "respect, praying with, listening, collective care, reciprocal care, and surveillance care" (Mixer, 2011 p. 11). The researcher suggested similar faculty research focusing on faculty generic and professional care in allied disciplines.

Applications to Practice

■ Reflect on your faculty roles in teaching, service, and scholarship. Do you see caring behaviors toward students and other faculty members that are similar to the findings in this study? Explain.

■ Analyze the course you are taking/teaching. How are cultural concepts integrated? Is there a conceptual framework used? If yes, which one theory or model is utilized?

■ If you were to replicate this study, how would you conduct it? What would you change in terms of conceptual framework, sampling, and analysis of findings?

Source: Mixer (2011).

CRITICAL THINKING EXERCISES 2.1

Undergraduate Student
1. Are there enough clients in your school's affiliating hospitals and agencies whose culture are different from your own?
2. How many cultural encounters with culturally diverse clients do you usually have in a semester? Do you think those times are enough in your preparation to care for culturally diverse clients in your role as a graduate nurse?
3. How are cultural diversity and promotion of cultural competence content integrated in your classes (theory) and in clinical? Describe one that is the most interesting, fun, and applicable.

Graduate Student
1. In your clinical practice, do you encounter clients whose ethnic, cultural, and/or gender orientation are different from your own?
2. Are you comfortable in your encounters with the above clients?
3. Would you be able to practice culturally congruent care in your future roles in **academia** and/or advance practice nursing (APN)?

Faculty in Academia
1. How do you integrate TCN concepts in the courses that you teach?
2. Do you use a theory or model to apply those concepts? If no, which theory or model would you prefer to use? Why?
3. How do you critically appraise your own learning needs regarding diversity and promotion of cultural competence?
4. What is your first step in acquiring knowledge skills regarding cultural competence? Do you have support from the SON in this step? Describe.

Staff Development Educator
1. Do you require continuing education (CE) in cultural diversity and promotion of cultural competence among nurses and ancillary staff?
2. What activities that celebrate diversity do you have for everyone in your institution? How often are these activities held?
3. How do you critically appraise your own learning needs regarding diversity and promotion of cultural competence? What is your first step in acquiring knowledge and skills regarding cultural competence? Do you have support from the department of nursing to undergo this step? Describe.

SUMMARY

Nursing education is grappling with the challenge of preparing graduates to provide culturally and linguistically congruent care to an increasingly diverse population. Accreditation and government mandates and guidelines are useful tools when planning integration of concepts. This chapter reviewed various methods of integrating TCN concepts in nursing and allied health curricula such as using theories or models, weaving-in as curricular threads, adding concepts as modules, integrating into clinical experience, developing a separate course, guiding students in independent studies, and integrating in simulations. Various teaching strategies were likewise discussed.

REFERENCES

Alvir, H. P. (1975). *The module: A tool in nursing education.* Albany, NY: New York State Education Department.

American Association of Colleges of Nursing. (2008). *Cultural competency in baccalaureate nursing education.* Washington, DC: Author.

American Association of Colleges of Nursing. (2011). *Toolkit for cultural competence in master's and doctoral nursing education.* Washington, DC: Author.

American Association of Colleges of Nursing. (2012). *Fact sheet: Creating a more highly qualified nursing workforce.* Retrieved July 30, 2013, from www.aacn.nche.edu/media-relations/ NursingWorkforce.pdf

American Nurses Association. (2012). *Nurses earn highest ranking ever, remain most ethical of professions in poll.* Retrieved September 1, 2013, from www.nursingworld.org/ FunctionalMenuCategories/MediaResources/PressReleases/Nurses-Remain-Most-Ethical-of-Professions-in-Poll.pdf

Aucoin, J. W. (1998). Program planning: Solving the problem. In K. J. Kelly-Thomas (Ed.), *Clinical and nursing staff development: Current competence, future focus* (2nd ed., pp. 213–239). Philadelphia, PA: J. B. Lippincott.

Boyle, J. S., & Andrews, M. M. (2012a). Andrew/Boyle transcultural nursing assessment guide for individuals and families. In M. M. Andrews & J. S. Boyle (Eds.), *Transcultural concepts in nursing care* (6th ed., pp. 451–455). Philadelphia, PA: Wolters Kluwer/Lippincott Williams & Wilkins.

Boyle, J. S., & Andrews, M. M. (2012b). Andrews/Boyle transcultural nursing assessment guide for groups and communities. In M. M. Andrews & J. S. Boyle (Eds.), *Transcultural concepts in nursing care* (6th ed., pp. 456–458). Philadelphia, PA: Wolters Kluwer/Lippincott Williams & Wilkins.

Campinha-Bacote, J. (2005). *A Biblically based model of cultural competence in the delivery of healthcare services.* Cincinnati, OH: Transcultural C.A.R.E. Associates.

Campinha-Bacote, J. (2007). *The process of cultural competence in the delivery of healthcare services: The journey continues.* Cincinnati, OH: Transcultural C.A.R.E. Associates.

Carnegie Mellon University. (2013). *Grading and performance rubrics.* Retrieved March 29, 2013, from www.cmu.edu/teaching/designteach/teach/rubrics.html

Clancy, C., Brach, C., & Abrams, M. (2012). Assessing patient experiences of providers' cultural competence and health literacy practices: CAHPS item sets. *Medical Care, 50*(9), S1-S2. Retrieved July 25, 2013, from www.lwww-medicalcare.com

Cohen, J. A. (2005). The mirror as metaphor for the reflective practitioner. In M. H. Oermann (Ed.) & K. T. Heinrich (Associate Ed.), *Annual review of nursing education: Strategies for teaching, assessment, and program planning* (pp. 313–330). New York, NY: Springer Publishing.

Cooper, J. B., & Taqueti, V. R. (2004). A brief history of the development of mannequin simulators for clinical education and training. *Quality and Safety in Health Care, 13*(Suppl1), i11-i18. doi:10.1136/qshc.2004.009886. Retrieved May 20, 2013, from www.ncbi.nlm.nih.gov/pmc/ articles/PMC1765785/pdf/v013p00i11.pdf

Davis-Dick, L. R. (2009). It takes a village to raise a nurse. In S. D. Bosher & M. D. Pharris (Eds.), *Transforming nursing education: The culturally inclusive environment.* (pp. 345–361). New York, NY: Springer Publishing.

Decker, S., Gore, T., & Feken, C. (2011). Simulation. In T. J. Bristol & J. Zerwekh, *Essentials for e-learning for nurse educators* (pp. 277–294). Philadelphia, PA: F. A. Davis.

Desantis, L. A., & Lipson, J. G. (2007). Brief history of inclusion of content on culture in nursing education. *Journal of Transcultural Nursing, 18*(1), 7S–9S.

Dobbins, M., Ciliska, D., Estabrooks, C., & Hayward. (2005). Changing nursing practice in an organization. In A. DiCenso, G. Guyatt, & D. Ciliska (Eds.), *Evidence-based nursing: A guide to clinical practice* (pp. 172–200). St. Louis, MO: Elsevier Mosby.

Emerson, R. J. (2007). *Nursing education in the clinical setting.* St. Louis, MO: Elsevier Mosby.

Gaberson, K. B., & Oermann, M. H. (1999). *Clinical teaching strategies in nursing.* New York, NY: Springer Publishing.

Giger, J. N., & Davidhizar, R. E. (2008). *Transcultural nursing: Assessment and intervention* (5th ed.). St. Louis, MO: Mosby Elsevier.

Halloran, L. (2009). Teaching transcultural nursing through literature. *Journal of Nursing Education,* 48(9), 523–528.

Health Insurance Marketplace. (2013). *The marketplace: The health insurance marketplace is the new way to get coverage that meets your needs.* Retrieved September 26, 2013, from www.healthcare.gov/marketplace/individual

Jeffreys, M. R. (2010). Academic settings: General overview, inquiry, action, and innovation. In M. R. Jeffreys, *Teaching cultural competence in nursing and health care* (2nd ed., pp. 117–181). New York, NY: Springer Publishing.

Kardong- Edgren, S., Cason, C. L., Walsh Brennan, A. M., Reifsnider, E., Hummel, F., Mancini, M., & Griffin, C. (2010). Cultural competency of graduating BSN nursing students. *Nursing Education Perspectives, 31*(5), 278–285.

Leininger, M. M. (2006). Culture care diversity and universality theory and evolution of the ethno-nursing method. In M. M. Leininger & M. R. McFarland (Eds.), *Culture care diversity and universality: A worldwide nursing theory* (2nd ed., pp. 1–41). Sudbury, MA: Jones and Bartlett.

Lipson, J. G., & Desantis, L. A. (2007). Current approaches to integrating elements of cultural competence in nursing education. *Journal of Transcultural Nursing, 18*(1), 10S–20S.

McFarland, M., Mixer, S., Lewis, A. E., & Easley, C. (2006). Use of the culture care theory as a framework for the recruitment, engagement, and retention of culturally diverse nursing students in a traditionally European American baccalaureate nursing program. In M. M. Leininger & M. R. McFarland (Eds.), *Culture care diversity and universality: A worldwide nursing theory* (2nd ed., pp. 239–254). Sudbury, MA: Jones & Bartlett.

Mixer, S. (2011). Use of the Culture Care Theory to discover nursing faculty care expressions, patterns, and practices related to teaching culture care. *Online Journal of Cultural Competence in Nursing and Healthcare, 1*(1), 3–14.

National League for Nursing. (2009a). *A commitment to diversity in nursing and nursing education.* Retrieved August 22, 2013, from www.nln.org/aboutnln/refl ection_dialogue/rfl _dial3.htm

National League for Nursing. (2009b). *Diversity toolkit.* Retrieved August 22, 2013, from www. nln.org/facultyprograms/Diversity_Toolkit/index.htm

Nielsen, P. A. Z. (2011). Instructional design for e-learning in nursing education. In T. J. Bristol & J. Zerwekh, *Essentials for e-learning for nurse educators* (pp. 25–54). Philadelphia, PA: F. A. Davis.

Polit, D. F., & Beck, C. T. (2010). *Essentials of nursing research: Appraising evidence for nursing practice* (7th ed.). Philadelphia, PA: Wolters Kluwer Lippincott Williams & Wilkins.

Purnell, L. D. (2013). The Purnell model for cultural competence. In L. D. Purnell, *Transcultural health care: A culturally competent approach* (4th ed., pp. 15–44). Philadelphia, PA: F. A. Davis.

Rowles, C. J., & Brigham, C. (2005). Strategies to promote critical thinking and active learning. In D. Billings & J. Halstead (Eds.), *Teaching nursing: A guide for faculty* (2nd ed., pp. 283–315). St. Louis, MO: Elsevier/Saunders.

Ryan, M., Carlton, K. H., & Ali, N. (2000). Transcultural nursing concepts and experiences in nursing curricula. *Journal of Transcultural Nursing, 11*(4), 300–307.

Sagar, P. L. (2012). *Transcultural nursing theory and models: Application in nursing education, practice, and administration.* New York, NY: Springer Publishing.

Shearer, R. G., & Davidhizar, R. (2003). Using role play to develop cultural competence. *Journal of Nursing Education, 42*(6), 273–276.

Shellenbarger, T., Palmer, E. A., Labant, A. L., & Kuzneski, J. L. (2005). Use of faculty reflection to improve teaching. In M. H. Oermann (Ed.) & K. T. Heinrich (Associate Ed.), *Annual review of nursing education: Strategies for teaching, assessment, and program planning* (pp. 343–357). New York, NY: Springer Publishing.

Schon, D. A. (1983). *The reflective practitioner: How professionals think in action.* New York, NY: Basic Books.

Schon, D. A. (1987). *Educating the reflective practitioner.* San Francisco, CA: Jossey Bass.

Schuessler, J. B., Wilder, B., & Byrd, L. W. (2012). Reflective journaling and development of cultural humility in students. *Nursing Education Perspectives, 33*(2), 96–99.

Starnes-Vottero, B. (2011). E-learning assessment. In T. J. Bristol & J. Zerwekh (Eds.), *Essentials for e-learning for nurse educators* (pp. 165–179). Philadelphia, F. A. Davis.

Sullivan Commission. (2004). *Missing persons: Minorities in the health professions: A report of the Sullivan Commission on diversity in the health care workforce.* Retrieved July 26, 2013, from http://health-equity.pitt.edu/40/1/Sullivan_Final_Report_000.pdf

U.S. Census Bureau. (2012). *U.S. Census Bureau projections show a slower growing, older, more diverse nation a half century from now.* Retrieved August 3, 2013, from www.census.gov/newsroom/releases/archives/population/cb12–243.html

U.S. Commission on Civil Rights. (2010). *Healthcare disparities: A briefing before the United States Commission on Civil Rights.* Retrieved July 26, 2013, from www.usccr.gov/pubs/Healthcare-Disparities.pdf

U.S. Department of Health and Human Services, & Office of Minority Health. (2013). *Enhanced national CLAS standards.* Retrieved August 16, 2013, from www.thinkculturalhealth.hhs.gov/Content/clas.asp

U.S. Department of Health and Human Services, Health Resources and Services Administration. (2010). *The registered nurse population: Initial findings from the 2008 National sample survey of registered nurses.* Retrieved February 7, 2014 fromhttp://bhpr.hrsa.gov/healthworkforce/rnsurveys/rnsurveyfinal.pdf

Vance, C. (2002). Leader as mentor. *Nursing Leadership Forum, 7*(2), 83–90.

Vance, C. (2011). *Fast facts for career success in nursing: Making the most of mentoring in a nutshell.* New York, NY: Springer Publishing.

Weech-Maldonado, R., Carle, A., Weidmer, B., Hurtado, M., Ngo-Metzger, Q., & Hays, R. D. (2012). The Consumer Assessment of Healthcare Providers and Systems (CAHPS) Cultural Competence (CC) item set. *Medical Care, 50*(9), S2, S22-S31. Retrieved July 25, 2013, from www.lwww-medicalcare.com

Yonge, O., & Myrick, F. (2005). Shadows and corners: The other side of journaling. In M. H. Oermann (Ed.) & K. T. Heinrich (Associate Ed.), *Annual review of nursing education: Strategies for teaching, assessment, and program planning* (pp. 331–341). New York, NY: Springer Publishing.

Transcultural Nursing in Modules: Academic and Staff Development Settings

Priscilla Limbo Sagar

Computer-based learning
Continuing education credits
Culturally and linguistically appropriate services
Interpreter
Medical interpreter

Module
Self-learning modules
Self-learning packets
Theory of hot and cold
Translator

At the completion of this chapter, the learner will be able to

1. Discuss the use of modules in teaching transcultural nursing in academia.
2. Illustrate the use of TCN modules in staff development settings.
3. Analyze the best format to offer self-learning modules (SLMs) in a setting.
4. Evaluate the use of continuing education credits for SLMs.

OVERVIEW

Modules are all inclusive, self-contained packets that learners can complete at their own time and without an instructor. The stand-alone learning format offers a variety of uses for both teachers and learners (Alvir, 1975). In some books, modules are also referred to as **self-learning packets** (SLPs) or independent studies (Aucoin, 1998) that can be utilized for a class, as a supplement, as part of remedial learning (Rowles & Brigham, 2005), or when learners are unable to attend traditional education sessions (Nichols & Davis, 2009). The definition of modules includes independent sections of a curriculum or shorter section of a syllabus. The use of modules has evolved over the years. Copies of reading resources and audiovisual aids should be a part of the packet or easily accessible online. In many institutions, modules can utilize **computer-based learning** (CBL). CBL is considered any learning that utilizes a computer "as a focal point of delivery" (Avillion, Holstschneider, & Puetz, 2010). As technology further advances, many learners use personal digital assistants (PDAs) and smartphones to access resources. SLMs have many potential uses in academic as well as staff development settings.

Nursing professional development (NPD) itself has undergone major evolution. More than ever, the effects of technology, globalization, and evidence-based practice (EBP) have required new expertise in the NPD specialist (ANA & NNSDO, 2010). Technological advances have changed the modality and delivery of educational resources. Globalization has brought about new regulations, guidelines, and standards to ensure quality and integrity of programs in education. EBP has become the rule rather than the exception. Despite all these, the goal of nursing professional development is still to increase "the knowledge, skills, and attitudes of nurses in their pursuit for professional career goals" (American Nurses Association & National Nursing Staff Development Organization, 2010, p. 2). In this high-demand environment, there is preference for continuing education available during convenient times and in easily accessible formats for learners instead of the face-to-face traditional classrooms. **Self-learning modules** (SLMs) are popular means to acquire **continuing education credits** (CEs) for professional development, maintenance of certification, and enhancement of professional marketability.

While the benefits and advantages of SLMs are many, there are also some disadvantages: learner procrastination and inability to complete in a timely manner; expensive preparation and updates in terms of time and money; and preference of some learners for face-to-face classes (Rowles & Brigham, 2005). When offering new modules or SLPs, a pilot test for at least 10 learners should be conducted to ensure that ample time is provided for completion. Commercial providers of CE have increased in the last decades; this may be an alternative way for staff development instead of preparing their own SLMs. Staff members, in collaboration with human resources, need to develop a policy for compensation of hours for mandated learning activities including successful completion of SLMs. Paying staff nurses for mandatory CE is a huge incentive for pursuing nurse professional development. Offering staff development in a blended format—half online and half face-to-face—may strike the desired balance, retaining what learners prefer in both methods.

For the sake of brevity, this author will refer to this learning tool as SLMs. Whether offered in hard copy version, online on the facility intranet, or on the Internet, modules must be easily accessible to the staff. The formats of SLMs in this book show some variations to illustrate that any institution can modify their offerings to learners based on their specific needs.

The module template in this book is conveniently divided into pretest, overview, objectives, content, learning resources, learning activities, self-assessment, and posttests. A generic module evaluation form to aid in future revision and enhancement of the SLM is in Appendix 3. Although developed in similar template, the four SLMs presented in this book may vary in depth. Users are encouraged to adapt them according to learner needs and to enhance the content of the modules for their own purposes in academic or staff development settings. See Module 3.1: *Culturally and Linguistically Appropriate Services* (CLAS) *Standards* and Module 3.2: *Generic Folk Practices: Theory of Hot and Cold* in this chapter; Self-Learning Module 10.1: *An Orthodox Jewish Child With Asthma* in Chapter 10, and Self-Learning Module 13.1: *Posttraumatic Stress Disorder* (PTSD) *in Women* in Chapter 13.

Integration of TCN Concepts

Many transcultural concepts can be integrated in academia and staff development in modular format, especially during times when formal curricular revisions are not yet possible.

Four were selected for SLMs in this book: culturally and linguistically appropriate services (CLAS) standards (USDHHS, OMH, 2011, 2013), theory of hot and cold, asthma in an Orthodox Jewish child, and posttraumatic stress disorders (PTSD) in women. The U.S. population is getting more diverse; the need for culturally and linguistically appropriate care is now governed by mandates and guidelines to eliminate disparate quality and access to care. Box 3.1 contains the new enhanced CLAS standards. Generic folk or traditional care is pervasive in any culture. One example of generic folk care pertains to the theory of hot and cold; this theory is very old and is prevalent throughout the globe, with both similarities and differences in peoples' beliefs and practice. Understanding these diverse practices will assist health care professionals in providing culturally congruent care. The global violence against women must be eliminated. The PTSD SLM in Chapter 13 is a tool for health care professionals to assess, plan, implement, and evaluate clients with PTSD and make appropriate community referrals.

BOX 3.1   THE NEW ENHANCED CULTURALLY AND LINGUISTICALLY APPROPRIATE SERVICES (CLAS) STANDARDS

National Standards for Culturally and Linguistically Appropriate Services (CLAS) in Health and Health Care

The national **culturally and linguistically appropriate services** CLAS standards are intended to advance health equity, improve quality, and help eliminate health care disparities by establishing a blueprint for health and health care organizations to:

PRINCIPAL STANDARD

1. Provide effective, equitable, understandable, and respectful quality care and services that are responsive to diverse cultural health beliefs and practices, preferred languages, health literacy, and other communication needs.

GOVERNANCE, LEADERSHIP, AND WORKFORCE

2. Advance and sustain organizational governance and leadership that promotes CLAS and health equity through policy, practices, and allocated resources.
3. Recruit, promote, and support a culturally and linguistically diverse governance, leadership, and workforce that are responsive to the population in the service area.
4. Educate and train governance, leadership, and workforce in culturally and linguistically appropriate policies and practices on an ongoing basis.

COMMUNICATION AND LANGUAGE ASSISTANCE

5. Offer language assistance to individuals who have limited English proficiency and/or other communication needs, at no cost to them, to facilitate timely access to all health care and services.
6. Inform all individuals of the availability of language assistance services clearly and in their preferred language, verbally and in writing.
7. Ensure the competence of individuals providing language assistance, recognizing that the use of untrained individuals and/or minors as interpreters should be avoided.
8. Provide easy-to-understand print and multimedia materials and signage in the languages commonly used by the populations in the service area.

(continued)

BOX 3.1 THE NEW ENHANCED CULTURALLY AND LINGUISTICALLY APPROPRIATE SERVICES (CLAS) STANDARDS (continued)

ENGAGEMENT, CONTINUOUS IMPROVEMENT, AND ACCOUNTABILITY

9. Establish culturally and linguistically appropriate goals, policies, and management accountability, and infuse them throughout the organization's planning and operations.
10. Conduct ongoing assessments of the organization's CLAS-related activities and integrate CLAS-related measures into measurement and continuous quality improvement activities.
11. Collect and maintain accurate and reliable demographic data to monitor and evaluate the impact of CLAS on health equity and outcomes and to inform service delivery.
12. Conduct regular assessments of community health assets and needs and use the results to plan and implement services that respond to the cultural and linguistic diversity of populations in the service area.
13. Partner with the community to design, implement, and evaluate policies, practices, and services to ensure cultural and linguistic appropriateness.
14. Create conflict and grievance resolution processes that are culturally and linguistically appropriate to identify, prevent, and resolve conflicts or complaints.
15. Communicate the organization's progress in implementing and sustaining CLAS to all stakeholders, constituents, and the general public.

Source: Reprinted with permission from the United States Department of Health and Human Services, Office of Minority Health. (2013).

MODULE 3.1 CULTURALLY AND LINGUISTICALLY APPROPRIATE SERVICES (CLAS) STANDARDS

Take Pretest (Appendix 4)

OVERVIEW

This module focuses on the enhanced CLAS standards and their role in equitable health care, elimination of health disparities, and serving as a blueprint for all organizations and agencies (USDHHS, OMH, 2011, 2013). The standards are divided into the *Principal Standard* (Standard 1); *Governance, Leadership, and Workforce* (Standard 2, 3, 4); *Communication and Language Assistance* (Standards 5, 6, 7, 8); *Engagement, Continuous Improvement, and Accountability* (Standards 9–15) (USDHHS, OMH, 2013). The CLAS standards were first published in 2000. Standards 5–8 are mandates for all institutions receiving federal funding.

The learner is encouraged to critically reflect the work setting applications and compliance activities of these standards. As part of this module, the learner will analyze the vital importance of language when navigating the health care system.

Disparities in health care access and quality have been documented in the United States (Agency for Healthcare Research and Quality [AHRQ], 2012; Sullivan Commission, 2004). Providing culturally and linguistically appropriate services (CLAS) is one strategy to facilitate the elimination of health inequities (USDHHS,

(continued)

OMH, 2013). Health professionals can assist in generating positive health outcomes for diverse populations through culturally and linguistically appropriate care. It is imperative that health equity be a top priority since "dignity and quality of care are rights of all and not the privileges of a few" (USDHHS, OMH, 2013, para 3).

OBJECTIVES

At the completion of this module, the learner will:

1. Compare and contrast mandates and guidelines among the CLAS standards.
2. Discuss important applications or compliance activities for CLAS standards at his or her own work setting.
3. Apply concepts of language, communication patterns, and health literacy factors when caring for clients.
4. Analyze the importance of language when navigating the health care system.

CONTENT

History

The Office of Minority Health (OMH) of the U.S. Department of Health and Human Services developed the CLAS standards in 2000. In 2010, the OMH began a campaign to enhance the CLAS standards (USDHHS, OMH, 2013). There were 14 standards during its publication in 2000; the enhanced CLAS contains 15 standards.

Language Services

Language services such as translation and interpretation—in demand in this rapidly diversifying nation—are becoming profitable enterprises and may be an alternative employment for those interested in the health care industry Association of Language Companies (ALC, 2013).

The language industry has grown at around 7.4% annually, largely ahead of total growth in the U.S. economy; it currently provides more than 200,000 full-time jobs and $15 billion in direct economic activity (ALC, 2013). The ALC emphasizes that the language services industry, as well as the enterprises and government agencies it supports, is contingent upon the American educational system to supply proficient, culturally educated professionals in over 200 languages. Many institutions, including medical centers, are currently offering medical translation and interpretation training. Cultural diversity and promotion of cultural competence is usually part of this training.

National Board of Certification for Medical Interpreters (NBCMI)

The National Board of Certification for Medical Interpreters (NBCMI, 2013), an independent division of the International Medical Interpreters Association (IMIA), aims to promote better health care outcomes, patient safety, and improved patient/

(continued)

provider communication. NBCMI seeks advancement of standards and quality of medical interpretation through a nationally established and accredited certification for **medical interpreters** (MIs). The NBCMI recently began offering certification examinations until December 31, 2013, for those who have been employed as MIs for at least a year. The development of the certification exam started in 2009. The certification examination consists of a written and an oral portion. After December 31, 2013, only MIs who have completed a minimum of 40 hours of training will be eligible to sit for the certification examination (NBCMI).

The Joint Commission (TJC)

The Joint Commission (TJC, 2010a, 2010b), an accreditor of more than 20,000 health care institutions and programs, requires diversity and cultural competence among its standards. TJC (2010b) studied 14 Florida area hospitals for 1) availability of cultural and linguistic resources and 2) staff awareness and use of such services. While all the hospitals had resources and tools to meet clients' cultural and linguistic needs, the staff were not always aware of services, did not use services, and frequently used someone accompanying the patient for interpretations (TJC, 2010b).

Learning Resources

1. U.S. Department of Health and Human Services, Office of Minority Health. (2011). *National partnership for action to end health disparities.* Retrieved August 18, 2013, from http://minorityhealth.hhs.gov/npa
2. U.S. Department of Health and Human Services, Office of Minority Health. (2013). *Enhanced national CLAS standards.* Retrieved August 16, 2013, from https://www.thinkculturalhealth.hhs.gov/Content/clas.asp
3. Agency for Healthcare Research and Quality. (2012). *National healthcare disparities report, 2012.* Retrieved June 1, 2013, from www.ahrq.gov/research/findings/nhqrdr/nhdr12/nhdr12_prov.pdf
4. Sullivan Commission. (2004). *Missing persons: Minorities in the health professions: A report of the Sullivan Commission on diversity in the health care workforce.* Retrieved July 26, 2013, from http://health-equity.pitt.edu/40/1/Sullivan_Final_Report_000.pdf
5. Association of Language Companies. (2013). *The language industry and careers in the 21st century: A response to the Today Show.* Retrieved July 25, 2013, from www.alcus.org/news/careers_pr.cfm
6. National Board of Certification for Medical Interpreters. (2013). *Certified medical interpreter candidate handbook.* Retrieved August 19, 2013, from https://www.certifiedmedicalinterpreters.org/sites/default/files/national-board-candidate-handbook-2013.pdf
7. The Joint Commission. (2010a). *Advancing effective communication, cultural competence, and patient- and family-centered care: A roadmap for hospitals.* Oakbrook Terrace, IL: Author.
8. The Joint Commission. (2010b). *Cultural and linguistic care in area hospitals.* Oakbrook Terrace, IL: Author.

(continued)

MODULE 3.1   CULTURALLY AND LINGUISTICALLY APPROPRIATE SERVICES (CLAS) STANDARDS   (continued)

Learning Activities*

1. Critically reflect work setting applications and compliance activities of these standards.
2. Review an assessment tool used in your own work setting. Analyze this tool for integration of CLAS standards.
3. If you have the responsibility of revising your assessment tool, what would you add? Discuss.

Self-Assessment*

1. Were you aware of the difference between an **interpreter** and a **translator** prior to taking this module?
2. Did you know that MI is a possible career in health care?
3. Recall incidents when you were caring for clients who were unable to speak English or had limited English proficiency (LEP). Prior to learning the CLAS standards, who did you use as an interpreter?
4. View the assessment tool used in your own work setting. Were you conscious of the integration of TCN principles before taking this module?

Take Posttest (Appendix 5; the key to pretest and posttest is available in Appendix 6.)

Lesson Evaluation: Complete Module Evaluation Form (Appendix 3)

---

*If a module has an online component or is offered totally online, these may be used as discussion questions (DQs).

MODULE 3.2   GENERIC FOLK PRACTICES: THEORY OF HOT AND COLD

Take Pretest (Appendix 7)

OVERVIEW

This module focuses on the **theory of hot and cold**, the belief in harmony and balance that originated from the Greek concept of the four body humors: yellow bile, black bile, phlegm, and blood (Andrews, 2012). In healthy individuals, there is a balance of these humors. To restore balance during illness or disharmony, these two opposing forces—referred to as *yin* (female aspect, negative, dark, and empty) and *yang* (male, positive, full, warm) (Andrews, 2012)—need to be adjusted to restore body functioning (Mattson, 2013).

THEORY OF HOT AND COLD

Categorization of illnesses or disharmony and the corresponding remedies differ from culture to culture (Purnell, 2013). According to Spector (2013), among the Puerto Ricans, the theory has a third element: hot (*caliente*), cold (*frio*), cool (*fresco*);

(continued)

MODULE 3.2 GENERIC FOLK PRACTICES: THEORY OF HOT AND COLD *(continued)*

illnesses deemed cold are treated with hot remedies, diseases classified as hot are treated with cool or cold remedies.

Medications, herbs, foods, and beverages are considered hot or cold not because of their physical temperature but for their effects. Illnesses and disharmony are also classified as either hot or cold; the treatment, therefore, entails the subtraction or addition of a remedy that is opposite in effect. For example, if childbirth is deemed a hot condition, then the postpartum woman may avoid cold drinks; cool air; cool, uncooked fruits and vegetables; and showers—since most of the heat had already been lost during the birthing process (Lauderdale, 2012; Mattson, 2013). In some Asian cultures, postpartum perineal administration of steam from hot stones made fragrant by the addition of herbs and flowers are used for weeks. Health care providers, knowing that iron is considered hot, will be better able to negotiate approval when providing health education to pregnant or lactating Puerto Rican women (Purnell, 2013) or women from other cultural groups who have similar beliefs about hot and cold theory.

The nurse's knowledge about hot and cold theory is beneficial when planning, implementing, and evaluating patient education. Clients, families, and communities may be more receptive to health promotion from knowledgeable and respectful transcultural nurses and other health care providers who incorporate generic folk practices in nursing care across the life span.

OBJECTIVES
At the completion of this module, the learner will

1. Explain the theory of hot and cold.
2. Describe some classifications of hot and cold remedies and illnesses and corresponding practices in diverse cultures.
3. Discuss important applications of the theory of hot and cold in patient teaching activities at your own work setting.
4. Analyze the importance of awareness and respect for generic folk practices when caring for culturally diverse clients, families, and communities.

CONTENT
  I. Theory of hot and cold
     Origin
     Four humors
 II. Meanings in different cultures
     The concept of balance and harmony
III. Some classification of hot and cold illnesses or disharmony
     Among Asians
     Among Hispanics
IV. Some classifications of hot and cold remedies
     Among Asians
     Among Hispanics

(continued)

MODULE 3.2   GENERIC FOLK PRACTICES: THEORY OF HOT AND COLD   (continued)

V. Application to patient education
   Labor and delivery

Learning Resources

READINGS

1. Andrews, M. (2012). The influence of cultural and health belief systems on health care practices. In M. M. Andrews & J. S. Boyle (Eds.), *Transcultural concepts in nursing care* (6th ed., pp. 73–88). Philadelphia, PA: Wolters Kluwer/ Lippincott Williams & Wilkins.
2. Lauderdale, J. (2012). Transcultural perspectives in childbearing. In M. M. Andrews & J. S. Boyle (Eds.), *Transcultural concepts in nursing care* (6th ed., pp. 91–122). Philadelphia, PA: Wolters Kluwer/Lippincott Williams & Wilkins.
3. Mattson, S. (2013). People of Vietnamese heritage. In L. D. Purnell (Ed.), *Transcultural health care: A culturally competent approach* (4th ed., pp. 479–480). Philadelphia, PA: F. A. Davis.
4. Purnell, L. D. (2013). People of Puerto Rican heritage. In L. D. Purnell (Ed.), *Transcultural health care: A culturally competent approach.* (4th ed., (pp. 407–425). Philadelphia, PA: F. A. Davis.
5. Spector, R. E. (2013). *Cultural diversity in health and illness* (8th ed.). Boston, MA: Pearson.

Learning Activities*

1. Critically reflect work setting applications of the knowledge gained from this module.
2. Review a patient education tool in your own work setting. Analyze this tool for integration of the theory of hot and cold.
3. If you have the responsibility of revising your assessment tool, what would you add in order to assess client's generic health care practices? Discuss.

Self-Assessment*

1. Were you aware of the theory of hot and cold prior to taking this module?
2. Recall incidents when you were caring for clients who were trying to tell you about the hot and cold theory.
3. View an assessment tool used in your own work setting. Were you conscious of the integration of TCN principles before taking this module?

Take Posttest (Appendix 8; the key to pretest and posttest is available in Appendix 9.)

Lesson Evaluation: Complete Module Evaluation (Appendix 3)

---

*If a module has an online component or is offered totally online, these may be used as discussion questions (DQs).

CRITICAL THINKING EXERCISES 3.1

Undergraduate Student
1. How many SLMs with continuing education (CE) credits have you taken? Do you like them? Why?
2. Do you think there is enough content of cultural diversity and promotion of cultural competence integrated in your classes (theory) and in clinical?
3. Would you be in favor of taking SLMs with CE credits that are equivalent to a 3-credit TCN course in your current curriculum? Why?

Graduate Student
1. Are mandatory SLMs used in your graduate program? If they are used, are they for replacement of a face-to-face class or classes? Explain.
2. How are your SLMs similar to or different than the examples in this book? Compare and contrast.
3. Are you in favor of online SLMs? Explain.

Faculty in Academia
1. Are you in favor of using self-learning modules in academia?
2. If you are in favor of SLMs, how would you use those in your course? Why?
3. How do you critically appraise SLMs for use in academic settings?
4. Have you developed SLMs before? Is your SLM with the examples in this book? Describe.

Staff Development Educator
1. Do you require yearly modules with CE credits in cultural diversity and promotion of cultural competence?
2. Do you develop SLMs with CEs for your institution? If yes, how many have you developed? How often is the SLM used by staff?
3. If you do not develop SLMs, do you require the staff to use online modules with CEs? Which ones do you use? Why?
4. Do you reimburse staff for their time to complete required CE? How many hours are eligible for reimbursement?

SUMMARY

Modules have been around for many years and have been tapped in nursing education and in staff development. SLMs have evolved from hard copies in binders to intranet and web-based educational offerings that promote self-learning and convenience for the learner. Four SLMs that present TCN concepts such as CLAS, theory of hot and cold, asthma in an Orthodox Jewish child, and managing care of women with PTSD are offered in this book. These SLMs have not been all inclusive; users are encouraged to enhance these for their own unique needs.

REFERENCES

Agency for Healthcare Research and Quality. (2012). *National healthcare disparities report, 2012.* Retrieved June 1, 2013, from www.ahrq.gov/research/findings/nhqrdr/nhdr12/nhdr12_prov.pdf

Alvir, H. P. (1975). *The module: A tool in nursing education.* Albany, NY: New York State Education Department.

American Nurses Association (ANA) & National Nursing Staff Development Organization (NNSDO). (2010). *Nursing professional development: Scope and standards of practice.* Silver Spring, MD: Nursesbooks.org.

Andrews, M. (2012). The influence of cultural and health belief systems on health care practices. In M. M. Andrews & J. S. Boyle (Eds.), *Transcultural concepts in nursing care* (6th ed., pp. 73–88). Philadelphia, PA: Wolters Kluwer/Lippincott Williams & Wilkins.

Association of Language Companies. (2012). *ALC in partnership with MSP wins gold in the convention promotion package category in Association TRENDS 2012 All-Media Contest.* Retrieved July 25, 2013, from www.alcus.org/news/pr_121212.cfm

Association of Language Companies. (2013). *The language industry and careers in the 21st century: A response to the Today Show.* Retrieved July 25, 2013, from www.alcus.org/news/careers_pr.cfm

Aucoin, J. W. (1998). Program planning: Solving the problem. In K. J. Kelly-Thomas (Eds.), *Clinical and nursing staff development: Current competence, future focus* (2nd ed., pp. 213–239). Philadelphia, PA: J. B. Lippincott.

Avillion, A., Holstschneider, M. E., & Puetz, L. R. (2010). *Innovation in nursing staff development: Teaching strategies to enhance learner's outcomes.* Marblehead, MA: HCPro.

Lauderdale, J. (2012). Transcultural perspectives in childbearing. In M. M. Andrews & J. S. Boyle (Eds.), *Transcultural concepts in nursing care* (6th ed., pp. 91–122). Philadelphia, PA: Wolters Kluwer/Lippincott Williams & Wilkins.

Mattson, S. (2013). People of Vietnamese heritage. In L. D. Purnell (Ed.), *Transcultural health care: A culturally competent approach* (4th ed., pp. 479–480). Philadelphia, PA: F. A. Davis.

National Board of Certification for Medical Interpreters. (2013). *Certified medical interpreter candidate handbook.* Retrieved August 19, 2013, from https://www.certifiedmedicalinterpreters.org/sites/default/files/national-board-candidate-handbook-2013.pdf

Nichols, B. L., & Davis, C. R. (2009). *The official guide for foreign educated nurses: What you need to know about nursing and health care in the United States.* New York, NY: Springer Publishing.

Purnell, L. D. (2013). People of Puerto Rican heritage. In L. D. Purnell (Ed.), *Transcultural health care: A culturally competent approach* (4th ed., pp. 407–425). Philadelphia, PA: FA Davis.

Rowles, C. J., & Brigham, C. (2005). Strategies to promote critical thinking and active learning. In D. M. Billings & J. A. Halstead (Eds.), *Teaching in nursing: A guide for faculty* (2nd ed., pp. 283–315). St. Louis, MO: Elsevier Saunders.

Spector, R. E. (2013). *Cultural diversity in health and illness* (8th ed.). Boston, MA: Pearson.

Sullivan Commission. (2004). *Missing persons: Minorities in the health professions: A report of the Sullivan Commission on diversity in the health care workforce.* Retrieved July 26, 2013, from http://health-equity.pitt.edu/40/1/Sullivan_Final_Report_000.pdf

The Joint Commission. (2010a). *Advancing effective communication, cultural competence, and patient- and family-centered care: A roadmap for hospitals.* Oakbrook Terrace, IL: Author.

The Joint Commission. (2010b). *Cultural and linguistic care in area hospitals.* Oakbrook Terrace, IL: Author.

U.S. Department of Health and Human Services, Office of Minority Health. (2011). *National partnership for action to end health disparities.* Retrieved August 18, 2013, from http://minorityhealth.hhs.gov/npa

U.S. Department of Health and Human Services, Office of Minority Health. (2013). *Enhanced national CLAS standards.* Retrieved August 16, 2013, from https://www.thinkculturalhealth.hhs.gov/Content/clas.asp

Transcultural Nursing as a Separate Course in Nursing Programs

Priscilla Limbo Sagar

Corequisite course
Ethnocentric
Ethnorelative

Prerequisite course
Seamless articulation
Separate transcultural health care course

At the completion of this chapter, the learner will be able to

1. Discuss strategies in developing a separate transcultural health care course for nursing and allied health students in a baccalaureate nursing program.
2. Analyze the modules for inclusion in separate transcultural health care courses.
3. Develop grading criteria for separate transcultural health care courses.
4. Apply Leininger's Culture Care Theory and other models when planning integration of transcultural concepts in nursing courses.
5. Plan on evaluating transcultural health care courses in terms of enrollment and suggestions from students.

OVERVIEW

Many schools still do not have a **separate transcultural health care course**—that is, any stand-alone course whose focus is transcultural nursing (TCN)—in the curricula. Generally, nursing curricula are laden and crowded with courses in biological and psychosocial sciences; statistics; computer literacy; and 3- to 6-credit courses in arts and letters in addition to nursing classes. A baccalaureate in nursing curricula generally requires 120 credits; the associate degree involves 65 to 68 credits. Formal linkage between a baccalaureate and associate degree program, or a two-plus-two (2+2) program, collaboration with schools, may make it smoother to integrate TCN concepts. A separate course may take the place of 3 of the 3 to 6 credits of electives.

The overcrowding of nursing curricula and faculty reluctance have been the main reasons for incorporating TCN in nursing curricula (Leininger, 1995; McFarland & Leininger, 2002). Many schools do not have a separate TCN course or courses. In light of this, the most common approach to inclusion of TCN content is to integrate it in all nursing and health classes (Sagar, 2012). It is imperative that TCN be integrated in nursing and allied health curricula to prepare culturally competent practitioners. Offering a separate course or courses in the baccalaureate program ensures that the content is delivered and not just in a "hit or miss approach" (Boyle, 2007, p. 21S).

Staff development textbooks now contain at least a section or chapter in TCN (Ullrich & Haffer, 2009). The enhanced culturally and linguistically appropriate services (CLAS) standards (United States Department of Health and Human Services, Office of Minority Health, 2013) must be in institutional policies and procedures. Modifications for culturally diverse clients and their families must be added to existing policies and when planning new ones. In staff development settings, instead of a separate course, TCN workshops, continuing education, and online modules can be very effective in ensuring staff orientation and their continuing competence.

Separate TCN Course

There are few baccalaureate programs that offer a separate course in TCN; however, many curricula integrate TCN concepts (Sagar, 2012). Ryan, Carlton, and Ali (2000) surveyed 610 baccalaureate and master's programs; of these, 43% of baccalaureate and 26% of master's had formal courses in TCN. Among those reporting formal courses, 87% of schools with baccalaureate programs have one course and 13% have several courses. Among master's programs in this study, 86% have one course while 14% offer several TCN courses (Ryan et al., 2000). Integration of TCN concepts in nursing curricula with wide sampling is among the priority areas of future research in nursing education.

When developing a separate TCN course in the baccalaureate program, the American Association of Colleges of Nursing ([AACN], 2008) document titled *Cultural Competency in Baccalaureate Nursing Education* and National League for Nursing's *Diversity Toolkit* (NLN, 2009) both offer invaluable resources. The Commission on Collegiate Nursing Education ([CCNE], 2013) does not specify diversity but requires adherence to professional nursing standards and guidelines and "the needs and expectations of the community of interest" (p. 12). For Accreditation Commission for Education in Nursing (ACEN, 2013) accredited schools, the need for inclusion of diversity in nursing programs is specified under its standard on "curriculum."

In some schools, there is a protocol for development of new courses from the school of nursing (SON), or department or division level, to the college-wide curriculum committee and to a faculty senate or similar body. At the SON level, it is important to develop a matrix to see TCN concept integration in other courses and find out where gaps in knowledge, skills, and competencies exist as specified by the AACN or the NLN.

Planning an Interprofessional Health Care Course

When planning an interprofessional health care course, the focus of diversity and cultural competence is broader than in a nursing-focused course. The Institute of Medicine ([IOM], 2010) advocates for interprofessional education. When members of the interprofessional health team have opportunities to collaborate and work together as students, they may work as a team much better. Muñoz, DoBroka, and Mohammad (2009) piloted an interprofessional course among students in nursing, education, and social work (EBP 4.1).

EBP 4.1

Muñoz, DoBroka, and Mohammad (2009), all from Capital University (CU) in Ohio, utilized a multidisciplinary teaching model to develop a pilot course in cultural competence for students in nursing, education, and social work. The course is consistent with CU's mission of leadership and service in a progressively diverse society.

The authors received funding from the Intercultural Communication Institute in Portland, Oregon. CD, the education faculty member, obtained certification in using the Intercultural Development Inventory (IDI), a 60-item valid tool to measure intercultural sensitivity (Muñoz et al., 2009). The other faculty (CCM, nursing, and CM, social work) are "voices from nonwestern cultures" (p. 497) and experts who are published in their respective fields.

Muñoz et al. (2009) used Campinha-Bacote's model (2003) featuring five components of the process of cultural competence, namely: cultural awareness, cultural knowledge, cultural skill, cultural encounters, and cultural desire. These five constructs provided the structure for content in the course. The researchers further incorporated Bennett's developmental model of intercultural sensitivity ([DMIS], Bennett, 1993, as cited by Muñoz et al., 2009). The six stages of Bennett's DMIS are 1) denial of difference, 2) defense against difference, 3) minimization of difference, 4) acceptance of difference, 5) adaptation to difference, and 6) integration of difference (Bennett, 1993, as cited by Muñoz et al., 2009, p. 498). Stages 1, 2, and 3 of Bennett's DMIS are termed **ethnocentric**; students use their own culture as a frame of reference. Stages 4, 5, and 6 are characterized as **ethnorelative**; students manifested a desire to learn about others and to interact with them (Muñoz et al., 2009).

The number of actual participants was not specified in the article. The "small" sample consisted of junior and senior students in nursing, education, and social work at CU who registered for the pilot course. The students were required to write five reflection papers during the entire course; the students focused on linking theory and practice and on weekly cultural encounters and readings as they applied Bennett's (1993) DMIS and Campinha-Bacote's (2003) five processes of cultural competence.

The interprofessional course was designed for 7 weeks. The course was scheduled in the early evening for 2 hours per week. On week 2, although the researchers knew from training that one semester is needed to move students from ethnocentrism to ethnorelativism, they administered the IDI (Hammer & Bennett, 2002, as cited by Muñoz et al., 2009) to assess the students' developing cultural sensitivity.

(continued)

EBP 4.1 *(continued)*

Findings indicate that the respondents 1) demonstrated understanding of Campinha Bacote's (2003) five components of the process of cultural competence; 2) verbalized more preparedness to care for culturally diverse clients in their professions; and 3) demonstrated assessment of their own growth along Bennett's DMIS (Muñoz et al., 2009). Muñoz et al. cited challenges encountered in piloting this course such as the lack of time to measure the students' process of movement from ethnocentrism to ethnorelativism. According to the authors, support from university administration is necessary for an interprofessional course. The course, likewise, needs support from advisors. It was a challenge to recruit students since the course was an elective; students in allied health already had very full course schedules. It was also challenging to find outside speakers for a small fee or an honorarium. The course provided an opportunity to gain knowledge of culturally competent services and provided practice in intercultural collaborations.

Applications to Practice

- Investigate your nursing program mission and philosophy in terms of diversity and cultural competence. Is it congruent with the mission and philosophy of your parent institution?
- Analyze the TCN course you are taking/teaching. Is this an elective or a required course in your program? Discuss.
- If you were to pilot a similar course, how would you conduct it? What would you change in terms of conceptual framework, sampling, and analysis of findings?

Source: Muñoz DoBroka & Mohammad (2009).

MODULAR CONTENTS: HLT 3000-TRANSCULTURAL HEALTH CARE (3 CREDITS) OFFERING IN A 15-WEEK SEMESTER

Module 1	Basic Concepts: Health, Cultural Diversity	Weeks 1–2
Module 2	Culture, Healers, Rituals of Healing, and Institutions of Health	Weeks 3–4
Module 3	Cultural Assessments Relevant to Health Care	Weeks 5–6
Module 4	Guidelines, Requirements, and Perspectives on Accreditation	Weeks 7–8
Module 5	Using Evidence-Based Practice (EBP) in Health Promotion	Weeks 9–10
Module 6	Creating a Culturally Competent Organization	Weeks 11–12
Module 7	Journey to Cultural Competence	Weeks 13–14

Deciding on Requisite Courses

Prerequisite courses are courses that students need to take prior to a certain course. **Corequisite courses** are courses that need to be taken along with, or in conjunction with, a course. Usually in a college or university, the requisite course proposal is first presented to the divisional committees, then to the college-wide curriculum committee, and later to a college-wide committee that makes the final decision. At Mount Saint Mary College, this faculty committee is called the Faculty Senate. Through the governance committee structure, the faculty makes a decision to accept or reject proposals. Determining course prerequisites depends upon how many other TCN courses are in the curriculum, how TCN is threaded in the curriculum, and the SON program outcomes. This may vary from department to department in a school.

Planning Course Assignments and Evaluation

When selecting course assignments, the faculty needs to examine CCNE or ACEN accreditation standards and guidelines in terms of program outcomes. Course assignments and evaluation need to be in congruence with the program outcomes. As an example, a SON program outcome includes "attainment of cultural competence" and "service to the underserved population" among its graduates.

In HLT 3000, one of the course assignments can be an interview of a person from a different culture; this assignment is aimed at fostering increasing awareness of differences and similarities among people of diverse cultures. Another project might be a group visit to a homeless shelter, a neighborhood health clinic, or a department of health clinic to see how people navigate the health care system and access available resources. The assignments in general education and professional courses must build on each other to prepare professionals to care for clients in a complex health delivery system.

Offering the Interprofessional Course for the First Time

When offering the interprofessional course for the first time, it is important to make several announcements to faculty and students, to offer it with wide access by students, and schedule it at a convenient time wherein students from different programs may be able to fit the course in their schedule. Muñoz et al. (2009) used an invitational approach for their interprofessional course and had a small group of students.

At its initial offering in spring 2014, HLT 3000 is scheduled to meet 2 days a week from 5:15 to 6:40 in the early evening. Students in the accelerated program usually start at 6:45 in the evening while students in the traditional program generally take courses in the morning and early afternoon. Since HLT 3000 is an elective, the invitational approach is also helpful.

Theory Application: Cultural Care Theory in a Faculty Workshop

Seamless articulation—usually a SON and area community colleges (CCs)—is one of the strategies used to alleviate the nursing shortage. Students who complete 2 years with an

CRITICAL THINKING EXERCISES 4.1

Undergraduate Student
1. Do you have a separate course for diversity and cultural competence? Is this a required course for your program? Explain.
2. What are the corequisite and prerequisite courses for the above course?
3. Which among the course assignments did you like? Which ones help in preparing you to work with diverse populations? Why?

Graduate Student
1. How many separate TCN courses do you have in the graduate program?
2. Are these all required courses? Are there any elective TCN courses in the program?
3. Are these TCN courses, both required and elective, preparing you for your role as an advanced practice nurse (APN)? As an educator? As an administrator?

Faculty in Academia
1. Have you developed a separate TCN or transcultural health care course? Describe the development steps before offering the course.
2. Prior to adding a 3-credit TCN course, which course did you delete? Why?
3. Have you had time to evaluate your TCN course? Have you revised anything as a result of student feedback? Describe.

Staff Development Educator
1. Have you developed a TCN course or module for staff development? If not, what do you require your staff to complete annually for cultural diversity and promotion of cultural competence?
2. Is the requirement developed by staff development or was it purchased for staff training? Describe.
3. Do you have institutional subscription to journals on cultural diversity and promotion of cultural competence? Are these subscriptions part of memberships in organizations that foster cultural competence? Explain.

associate degree in nursing (ADN) will be admitted directly to an affiliate SON. This articulation may be called a 2+2 program. As preparation for a separate course, a 2+2 from an associate degree and baccalaureate school can plan a collaboration of curricular synchrony. For example, if an SON utilizes Leininger's (2006) Cultural Care Theory in its curricula, and the SON anticipates admitting associate degree graduates to their Registered Nurse to Bachelor of Science in Nursing (RN–BS) program, faculty from the SON and community college (CC) need to collaboratively develop an application of the CCT in planning care for clients across the life span in all CC nursing courses.

The lesson plan in Appendix 10 illustrates a joint workshop planned for faculty at a SON and the CC that is investigating avenues to incorporate Leininger's CCT in its nursing program. The CC faculty also requested to see other models in TCN as points of comparison prior to selecting the CCT.

SUMMARY

Most nursing curricula are already packed with courses. The addition of a new course presents problems of what course to delete or integrate in other current courses. However difficult, faculty must assess the current integration of TCN concepts and the SON compliance with accreditation, as well as government mandates and guidelines.

Integration of TCN concepts, if planned and coordinated between two programs of nursing, will proceed more smoothly. This will help prepare practitioners who are ready to provide care for culturally diverse clients and their families or significant other. Nursing education is entrusted with the noble task of preparing graduates to care for the nation's increasingly diverse population. Staff development's task is to continue that quest for lifelong learning, motivation for continuing education, and maintenance of continued competence.

REFERENCES

Accreditation Commission for Education in Nursing (ACEN). (2013). *ACEN standards and criteria: Baccalaureate*. Retrieved August 22, 2013, from www.acenursing.net/manuals/SC2013_BACCALAUREATE.pdf

American Association of Colleges of Nursing (AACN). (2008). *Cultural competency in baccalaureate nursing education*. Washington, DC: Author.

Boyle, J. S. (2007). Commentary on "current approaches to integrating elements of cultural competence in nursing education." *Journal of Transcultural Nursing, 18*(1), 21S–22S.

Commission on Collegiate Nursing Education (CCNE). (2013). *Standards for accreditation of baccalaureate and graduate nursing programs*. Retrieved September 20, 2013, from www.aacn.nche.edu/ccne-accreditation/Standards-Amended-2013.pdf

Institute of Medicine (IOM). (2010, October 5). *The future of nursing: Leading change, advancing health*. Washington, DC: National Academies Press.

Leininger, M. M. (1995). Teaching transcultural nursing in undergraduate and graduate nursing programs. In M. Leininger (Ed.), *Transcultural nursing: Concepts, theories, research, and practice* (2nd ed., pp. 605–625). New York, NY: McGraw-Hill.

Leininger, M. M. (2006). Culture care diversity and universality theory and evolution of the ethnonursing method. In M. M. Leininger & M. R. McFarland (Eds.), *Culture care diversity and universality: A worldwide nursing theory* (2nd ed., pp. 1–41). Sudbury, MA: Jones & Bartlett.

McFarland, M. R., & Leininger, M. M. (2002). Transcultural nursing: Curricular concepts, principles, and teaching and learning activities for the 21st century. In M. M. Leininger & M. R. McFarland (Eds.), *Transcultural nursing: Concepts, theories, research, and practice* (3rd ed., pp. 527–561). New York, NY: McGraw-Hill.

Muñoz, C. C., DoBroka, C. C., & Mohammad, S. (2009). Development of a multidisciplinary course in cultural competence for nursing and human service professions. *Journal of Nursing Education, 48*(9), 495–503.

National League for Nursing (NLN). (2009). *Diversity toolkit*. Retrieved August 22, 2013, from www.nln.org/facultyprograms/Diversity_Toolkit/index.htm

Rew, L., Baker, H., Cookston, J., Khosropour, S., & Martinez, S. (2003). Measuring cultural awareness in nursing students. *Journal of Nursing Education, 42*(6), 249–257.

Ryan, M., Carlton, K. H., & Ali, N. (2000). Transcultural nursing concepts and experiences in nursing curricula. *Journal of Transcultural Nursing, 11*(4), 300–307.

Sagar, P. L. (2012). *Transcultural nursing theory and models: Application in nursing education, practice, and administration*. New York, NY: Springer Publishing.

Ullrich, S., & Haffer, A. (2009). *Precepting in nursing: Developing an effective workforce*. Sudbury, MA: Jones & Bartlett.

United States Department of Health and Human Services (USDHHS), Office of Minority Health (OMH). (2013). *Enhanced national CLAS standards*. Retrieved August 16, 2013, from https://www.thinkculturalhealth.hhs.gov/Content/clas.asp

Integrating TCN Concepts in the National Council Licensing Examination

Priscilla Limbo Sagar

KEY TERMS

Blueprint
Content bias
Cultural bias
English as an additional language

English as a second language
Linguistic bias
NCLEX-PN®
NCLEX RN®

LEARNING OBJECTIVES

At the completion of this chapter, the learner will be able to

1. Discuss the importance of integration of transcultural (TCN) concepts in the NCLEX-PN.
2. Illustrate strategies of integration of TCN concepts in the NCLEX-RN.
3. Analyze potential language, cultural, and content bias in NCLEX-type questions.
4. Develop NCLEX-type questions using guidelines for both examinations.
5. Devise strategies to increase success in the NCLEX.

OVERVIEW

The National Council of State Boards of Nursing (NCSBN) owns and develops the National Council Licensure Examination (NCLEX) for entry level licensure in the United States and its territories (Woo & Dragan, 2012). Graduates of a practical nursing program must take and successfully pass the NCLEX for practical nurses (LPNs), or **NCLEX-PN,** for licensure and work as LPNs or licensed vocational nurses (LVNs). Graduates of diploma, associate, and baccalaureate programs take the NCLEX for registered nurses (RNs), or **NCLEX-RN**.

There are varying degrees of cultural diversity and competence in the NCLEX-PN and NCLEX-RN.

The goal of the NCLEX is to determine the candidate's adequacy of knowledge, skills, and ability to practice safe and effective care at an entry level (Woo & Dragan, 2012). Woo and Dragan further reiterated that all NCLEX items undergo analyses to ensure that the examination only evaluates content related to nursing and not unrelated concepts such as gender or ethnicity.

The current NCLEX-RN **blueprint** does not have a specific cultural diversity area in its four major categories of client needs, namely: safe effective care environment; health promotion and maintenance; psychosocial integrity; and physiological integrity. "Cultural awareness/cultural influences on health" is listed under psychosocial integrity (NCSBN, 2013a, p. 7). Cultural diversity and promotion of culturally competent care need to be more implicitly integrated in each of those four major categories of client needs. Full integration of specific TCN topics in the licensing examinations will be a compelling incentive for nursing schools to thread this concept into nursing curricula—and preferably with a separate course or courses dedicated to diversity and culturally congruent care (Sagar, 2012). Whether for programmatic or for licensure purposes, this integration needs to be discussed among various stakeholders such as education, accreditation, state boards, and consumers.

INTEGRATION OF TCN CONCEPTS ON THE NCLEX

Eliminating Bias

Nursing programs depend mainly on NCLEX-style examinations for evaluating students. Although there are testing supports available such as Assessment Technologies Incorporated (ATI, 2013) and Health Education Systems Incorporated (Elsevier HESI, 2013), faculty members of nursing schools, for the most part, develop their own course exams. The testing itself usually consists of multiple choice; the answer calls for four options with only one correct answer. In the last few years, NCLEX questions have included item questions in alternate formats such as filling in blanks, graph interpretation, or prioritization ordering (Dudas, 2011; NCSBN, 2013a, 2013b). However, **English as a second language** (ESL) students generally have difficulties with multiple choice exams (Bosher, 2009) from cultural or linguistic bias.

Linguistic bias occurs when the language content of the test is awkward and difficult to understand; **cultural bias** pertains to content that is not easily understood by all cultural groups (Dudas, 2011). **Content bias** refers to bias toward an ethnic focal group. For example, if "drinking warm tea before bedtime" is one of the options to answer an item, a Hispanic test taker may pick this option because drinking warm tea prior to bedtime is perceived as appropriate in Hispanic cultures (Woo & Dragan, 2012).

Mandates, Guidelines, Accreditation Standards

Government mandates and guidelines regarding culturally and linguistically appropriate services (CLAS) have been in effect since 2001 (United States Department of Health and Human Services [USDHHS], Office of Minority Health [OMH], 2013). The enhanced CLAS standards is a vital document that needs to be threaded in nursing and allied health curriculum and must be in the core of staff development orientation, continuing education, and evidence-based practice (EBP).

The American Nurses Association ([ANA], 1991) is a strong proponent of inclusion of diversity in the care of all clients. Both the American Association of Colleges of Nursing ([AACN], 2008a, 2008b, 2011) and the National League for Nursing ([NLN], 2009a, 2009b) are strong advocates for inclusion of TCN content in nursing education, as exemplified by their respective curricular essentials and faculty toolkits. When this content is included among the standards of their corresponding accrediting bodies, the Commission on Collegiate Nursing Education (CCNE) and the Accreditation Commission for Education in Nursing ([ACEN], formerly the National League for Nursing [NLNAC]), schools of nursing will be more likely to integrate TCN.

CCNE (2013) is implicit in the inclusion of diversity and cultural competence, as inferred in the use of its standards and guidelines. CCNE Standard 3 affirms, "The curriculum is developed in accordance with the program's mission, goals, and expected student outcomes." CCNE (2013) further states, "The curriculum reflects professional nursing standards and guidelines and the needs and expectations of the community of interest" (p. 11). ACEN's (2013) Standard 4.5 for baccalaureate curriculum is more explicit; it specifically states, "The curriculum includes cultural, ethnic, and socially diverse concepts and may also include experiences from regional, national, or global perspectives" (p. 4).

This would be similar to the way that The Joint Commission (TJC, 2011) addresses diversity and cultural competence in accredited institutions. TJC (2011) particularly expects accredited institutions to collect data of a client's race and ethnicity. TJC (2010a, 2010b) issued new and revised standards in 2010 for client-focused communication as part of a program to promote effective communication, enhance cultural competence, and uphold client and family-centered interventions. In addition, TJC designed these standards not only to expand client safety and quality of care but also to motivate hospitals to embrace practices promoting improved communication and client engagement.

With the continued and consistent implementation of these accreditation and government mandates, the various State Boards of Nursing (SBON) may be able to incorporate diversity and cultural competence among the required content for licensure. Additionally, these concepts need to be a prerequisite for initial registration and licensure—similar to reports of child and adult abuse and infection control that have to be verified by school program inclusion—and for renewal of registration and licensure. Schools of nursing will have to attest compliance with diversity and cultural competence content. This SBON mandate will make it imperative and standardized to include TCN concepts in all nursing curricula.

STRATEGIES TO REMOVE BARRIERS TO SUCCESS ON THE NCLEX

ESL students generally have difficulties with multiple choice exams (Bosher, 2009), especially with test items containing cultural or linguistic bias. Strategies have been proposed to improve testing for those graduates who speak English as a second language (ESL) or **English as an additional language (EAL)**. For consistency, this author will refer to these students as ESL.

Dudas (2011) also referred to students speaking EAL; this group poses challenges to faculty with their unique cultural and linguistic needs along with the need for success in program completion and in passing the NCLEX. While some ESL students are born in the United States, they have different views and perspectives about time, personal space, communication, environmental control, and social organization (Giger & Davidhizar, 2008, 2013) compared to mainstream U.S. culture.

Bosher (2009) recommended the following in order to remove language as a barrier to succeeding on multiple choice examinations: (1) training for faculty; (2) working with ESL experts to reduce language load; and (3) exercising care in wording test items. In terms of study groups, Bosher (2009) suggested fostering study groups that are diverse in race, culture, and language; encouraging students to use institutional resources such as the learning center; and offering study groups that are faculty-led. Another suggestion that Bosher offered is allowing ESL students one-and-a-half time (1.5) when taking exams and permitting them to take the exam at the learning center instead of in the classroom with the rest of the students. Educators are familiar with distractions during testing, such as faster test takers completing the exam in half the time or less; this could distract others taking the exam.

Passing Rate on the NCLEX

To alleviate the nursing shortage, developed countries such as the United States, United Kingdom, Canada, Australia, and others recruit nurses from developing countries such as the Philippines, India, Korea, and Nigeria. The massive exodus—nurse drain from developing countries—of RNs creates imbalance in health care since many of the sending countries are likewise experiencing marked nurse shortages. Chapter 27 includes more discussion about FEN.

Between 2000, 2004, and 2008, graduates of non-U.S. schools increased from 3.8% to 5.6%; corresponding countries of origin for these nurses are the Philippines (48.7%), Canada (11.5%), India (9.3%), United Kingdom (5.8%), Korea (2.6%), Nigeria (2.0%), other (17.3%), and U.S. territories (2.8%) [USDHHS, Health Resources and Services Administration (HRSA; Health Resources and Services Administration, 2010)]. The passing rate on the NCLEX-RN is much lower for FEN than for those educated in the United States (Figure 5.1). As an example, from January 2012 to March 2012, the average passing rate for U.S.-educated candidates from associate, diploma, and baccalaureate programs was 91.2% for first-time takers; in comparison, candidates from foreign nursing schools had a 37.2% success rate for first-time takers (NCSBN, 2012). A similar pattern was observed from October 2012 to December 2012, as shown in Figure 5.1.

Among FEN in the United States, few are from Mexico; Mexico is not among the five sending countries (NCSBN, 2012). The passing rate for Mexican nurses in the NCLEX-RN is 22%, much lower than among other FENs (Lujan & Little, 2010). The following program, with Mexico-educated nurses, is highly applicable to other group of FENs.

Programs for Recruitment, Retention, and NCLEX Success

Mexico NCLEX-RN Success Program. The goal of the 16-week Mexico NCLEX-RN Success Program (MNSP) is to alleviate the nursing shortage by tapping culturally and linguistically consistent resources, especially for underserved communities along the U.S.–Mexican border (Lujan & Little, 2010). The program aims to help underemployed Mexico-educated nurses who may have migrated to the United States due to the high unemployment rate in Mexico and are working in retail, housekeeping, and dietary departments in the United States. who may have. The inclusion criteria for the MNSP are diploma from a nursing program in Mexico; minimum of 6 months nursing experience; minimum score of 560 on the Test of English as a Foreign Language (TOEFL); and completion of a 75-question NCLEX-type multiple choice exam. From 30 applicants, the project directors admit 20 participants.

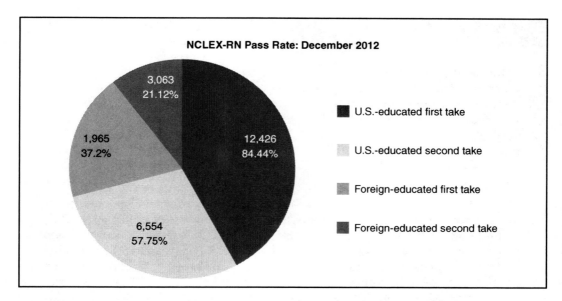

FIGURE 5.1 Comparison of NCLEX-RN Pass Rate Between U.S.- and Foreign-Educated Nurses, October to December 2012. *Source:* Developed from National Council of State Boards of Nursing (2012).

Intensive NCLEX preparation includes (1) thorough analysis of multiple choice NCLEX-type questions, as well as translating key verbs on test items; (2) case study presentations to colleagues; (3) video segments and role playing about U.S. authority and gender roles; and (4) verbal short answer tests. Except to clarify questions, English is used throughout the program; this provides opportunities for students to practice their skills in communicating in English (Lujan & Little). Through systematic preparation, 5 of 10 (50%) participants in the study successfully passed the NCLEX-RN at first take. From observation, Lujan and Little (2010) concluded that simulation with high-fidelity mannequins is effective in program sessions and is an ideal strategy for future participants (p. 706).

Opportunities for Professional Education in Nursing (OPEN). Project Open is a 3-year federally funded project for culturally diverse and financially disadvantaged students (McFarland, Mixer, Lewis, & Easley, 2006). Applying Leininger's Cultural Care Theory (CCT), McFarland et al. (2006) focused on the recruitment, engagement, and retention of students. Out of 200 Project Open students, 12 participants provided qualitative evaluation: seven European Americans, six African Americans, and one Asian American. There was an equal number of participants from rural and urban areas; five were males and seven were females.

Resources for students in Project Open consisted of (1) college success course; (2) peer tutoring and study groups; (3) prenursing course, *Nursing Connections for the Future*; and (4) other resources such as writing, studying, test taking, networking, and professional socializations, among others (McFarland et al., 2006). Notably, the project integrated TCN concepts in curriculum, preparing graduates to provide culturally congruent care for individuals, families, and groups.

Another funded project, affirming at-risk minorities for success (ARMS), also involves minority and educationally disadvantaged students (Sutherland, Hamilton, & Goodman, 2007). Sutherland et al. (2007) evaluated outcomes based on interventions to increase retention, graduation, and passing rate on the NCLEX-RN among 64 students. EBP 5.1 has a summary of this study.

EBP 5.1

Sutherland et al. (2007) evaluated 64 minority and educationally disadvantaged student outcomes based on interventions to increase retention, graduation, and passing rate on the NCLEX-RN in this ARMS program. The program was federally funded under the U.S. Department of Health and Human Services Basic Nurse Education and Practice Program grant. Inclusion criteria in this study were ethnic or minority background, first generation in college, rural community residence, and grade of C or presently failing in a nursing course.

The 64 students who were invited to participate in the 3-year study at a university in the south-central region of the United States were Whites (42%), Hispanics (42%), Asian Pacific Islanders (8%), and African Americans (8%). Other indices of group diversity included: single, widowed, or divorced (77%); married and had children (13%); unmarried with children younger than 12 years of age (3%); and unmarried with children over 12 years of age (5%) (Sutherland et al., 2007). The researchers used 265 non-ARMS students from the college of nursing database. The participants provided consent and the university institutional review board approved the study.

Interventions for students in the ARMS program consisted of advising and mentoring from faculty; tutoring from White and Hispanic practicing nurses; participating in Seminars in Success; and providing personal laptop, computer, and Internet access with accompanying NCLEX-RN Review 3000 (Springhouse, 2000). The faculty mentors met with students at least twice per semester. In addition to mentoring, the faculty encouraged students to utilize university resources such as the learning center, financial aid, and counseling. Tutors provided individual and group sessions preferred by students; sessions focused on taking notes, interpreting charts and tables, integrating clinical, and answering practice questions. The Seminars in Success, conducted by a Hispanic licensed professional counselor and consultant, involved test taking, anxiety reduction, relaxation, and positive imagery techniques.

The results indicated that interventions affected graduation (rate = 98%—one student dropped out because of pregnancy), increased grades in the leadership and management course, and "eliminated the effect of ethnicity on the NCLEX-RN" (Sutherland et al., 2007, p. 347). Increasing ethnic diversity among health care providers improved health care services to an increasingly diverse population (Sutherland et al., 2007). The chief limitation of this study was sample size, as it included relatively small percentages of African American and Asian American participants.

Applications to Practice

■ Do you have a recruitment, retention, and success program at your school? Discuss the interventions associated with this program.

(continued)

> **EBP 5.1** *(continued)*
>
> ■ Have you examined success rates in program completion in your school? Is there a difference in graduation and NCLEX rates between Whites and minority students? Discuss.
> ■ If you were to replicate this study, how would you conduct it? What would you change in terms of conceptual framework, sampling, and analysis of findings?
>
> _____
>
> *Source*: Springhouse (2000).

CRITICAL THINKING EXERCISES 5.1

Undergraduate Student
1. How would you rate the support services at your school in terms of preparing for the NCLEX? Is there a peer tutoring program? Is this helpful in your success of passing exams in your nursing classes?
2. Do you think there are enough content NCLEX-type questions included in the testing of all your nursing courses? Are the exams reviewed in class?
3. Is there a retention program at your school? Describe the components of this program.
4. Do you feel prepared to take the NCLEX after your program completion? Why?

Graduate Student
1. If your entry to practice is at the master's level, do you feel prepared to take the NCLEX exams upon graduating from your program?
2. Are NCLEX-type questions used enough in nursing courses? Explain.
3. Have you worked—as preceptor or mentor—with graduate nurses waiting to take or retake the NCLEX?
4. What kind of support or encouragement have you given graduate nurses preparing to take the NCLEX? Describe.

Faculty in Academia
1. Do you develop your own NCLEX-type examinations? How often do you revise these exams?
2. In addition to the NCLEX blueprint and its updates, are your revisions based upon student feedback? Describe.
3. Do you use a commercial testing program as an adjunct to teaching and to improve your graduates passing in the NCLEX? If yes, describe the components of this system.
4. How do you select peer tutors for your program? Are students paid for tutoring?

(continued)

> ## CRITICAL THINKING EXERCISES 5.1 *(continued)*
>
> **Staff Development Educator**
> 1. Do you provide support services such as onsite NCLEX review for your graduate nurses hired prior to passing the exams?
> 2. If you hire foreign-educated nurses (FENs), do you have ESL classes to enhance communication as well as help them prepare for the NCLEX? Describe the program that you have.
> 3. Do you use mentoring and precepting at your institution? How are preceptors and mentors assigned? What incentives do you offer mentors and preceptors? Why?
> 4. Do you reach out to professional nursing organizations for mentoring of your new nurses? Describe your collaboration with professional nursing organizations.

Ensuring Continuing Cultural Competence

There are varied entry programs in nursing with different lengths and number of credits required. The completion of cultural diversity and promotion of cultural competence modules post graduation or program completion may be another way to initially ensure the inclusion of this content for graduates from programs that are yet unable to place this on the curriculum.

Continuing education (CE) mandates are another way to ensure that practicing professionals continue to update their knowledge, skills, and awareness about culturally and linguistically congruent care. Presently, a total of 21 states require CE for renewal of licensure; the requirements vary from state to state. For example, nurses practicing in California are mandated 30 CE every 2 years; in comparison, nurses in Nebraska are only required 20 CE every 2 years (California State Board of Nursing, 2013; Nebraska Department of Health and Human Services, 2011; O'Shea & Smith, 2002). Another way to assure that each nurse has continuing competence is to make this a requirement for registration and licensure.

SUMMARY

Candidates for RN and LPN practice in the United States must take the NCLEX-RN and NCLEX-PN, respectively. This chapter examines the standards, mandates, and guidelines regarding diversity and cultural competence. While many schools of nursing and allied health have made diversity and cultural competence a priority, there is no standard method for inclusion of these in curricula or in integration in the NCLEX blueprint. Diversity and cultural competence integration on the NCLEX and as a requirement for licensure and registration of all nurses will contribute much to the culturally and linguistically appropriate care for all clients in health care.

REFERENCES

Accreditation Commission for Education in Nursing. (2013). *ACEN standards and criteria: Baccalaureate.* Retrieved August 22, 2013, from www.acenursing.net/manuals/SC2013_BACCALAUREATE.pdf

American Association of Colleges of Nursing. (2008a). *The essentials of baccalaureate education for professional nursing practice.* Washington, DC: Author.

American Association of Colleges of Nursing. (2008b). *Cultural competency in baccalaureate nursing education.* Washington, DC: Author.

American Association of Colleges of Nursing. (2011). *Toolkit for cultural competence in masters and doctoral nursing education.* Washington, DC: Author.

American Nurses Association. (1991). *Position statement on cultural diversity in nursing practice.* Kansas City, MO: Author.

Assessment Technologies Incorporated. (2013). *About ATI nursing education.* Retrieved August 22, 2013, from https://www.atitesting.com/About.aspx

Bosher, S. D. (2009). Removing language as a barrier to success on multiple-choice nursing exams. In S. D. Bosher & M. D. Pharris (Eds.), *Transforming nursing education: The culturally inclusive environment* (pp. 259–284). New York, NY: Springer Publishing.

California State Board of Nursing. (2013). *Continuing education for license renewal.* Retrieved August 22, 2013, from www.rn.ca.gov/licensees/ce-renewal.shtml#acceptable

Commission on Collegiate Nursing Education. (2013). *Standards for accreditation of baccalaureate and graduate nursing programs.* Retrieved August 22, 2013, from www.aacn.nche.edu/ccne-accreditation/Standards-Amended-2013.pdf

Dudas, K. (2011). Strategies to improve NCLEX® style testing in students who speak English as an additional language. *The Online Journal of Cultural Competence in Nursing and Healthcare, 1*(2), 14–23.

Elsevier HESI. (2013). *Elsevier HESI assessment.* Retrieved August 22, 2013, from https://hesifaculty-access.elsevier.com/index.aspx

Giger, J. N., & Davidhizar, R. E. (2008). *Transcultural nursing: Assessment and intervention* (5th ed.). St. Louis, MO: Mosby Elsevier.

Giger, J. N., & Davidhizar, R. E. (2013). *Transcultural nursing: Assessment and intervention* (6th ed.). St. Louis, MO: Elsevier Mosby.

Lujan, J., & Little, K. (2010). Preparing underemployed Latino US nurses through the Mexico NCLEX-RN Success Program. *Journal of Nursing Education, 49*(12), 704–707.

McFarland, M., Mixer, S., Lewis, A. E., & Easley, C. (2006). Use of the culture care theory as a framework for the recruitment, engagement, and retention of culturally diverse nursing students in a traditionally European American baccalaureate nursing program. In M. M. Leininger & M. R. McFarland (Eds.), *Culture care diversity and universality: A worldwide nursing theory* (2nd ed., pp. 239–254). Sudbury, MA: Jones & Bartlett.

National Council of State Boards of Nursing. (2012). *Number of candidates taking NCLEX examination and percent passing by type of candidates.* Retrieved August 20, 2013, from https://www.ncsbn.org/Table_of_Pass_Rates_2012.pdf

National Council of State Boards of Nursing. (2013a). *2013 NCLEX-RN® detailed test plan item writer/item reviewer/nurse educator version (2012).* Retrieved April 5, 2013, from https://www.ncsbn.org/2013_NCLEX_RN_Detailed_Test_Plan_Educator.pdf

National Council of State Boards of Nursing. (2013b). *2013 NCLEX-RN® detailed test plan candidate version.* Retrieved April 5, 2013, from https://www.ncsbn.org/2013_NCLEX_RN_Detailed_Test_Plan_Candidate.pdf

National League for Nursing. (2009a). *A commitment to diversity in nursing and nursing education.* Retrieved August 22, 2013, from www.nln.org/aboutnln/reflection_dialogue/rfl_dial3.htm

National League for Nursing. (2009b). *Diversity toolkit.* Retrieved August 22, 2013, from www.nln.org/facultyprograms/Diversity_Toolkit/index.htm

Nebraska Department of Health and Human Services. (2011). *Registered nurse/licensed practical nurse renewal information.* Accessed August 22, 2013, from http://dhhs.ne.gov/publichealth/Pages/crl_nursing_rn-lpn_renewal.aspx

O'Shea, K. L., & Smith, L. (2002). The mandatories. In K. L. O'Shea (Ed.), *Staff development nursing secrets* (pp. 185–195). Philadelphia, PA: Hanley & Belfus.

Sagar, P. L. (2012). *Transcultural nursing theory and models: Application in nursing education, practice, and administration.* New York, NY: Springer Publishing.

Springhouse. (2000). NCLEX review 3000 [Software]. Baltimore, MD: Author.

Sutherland, J. A., Hamilton, M. J., & Goodman, N. (2007). Affirming at-risk minorities for success (ARMS): Retention, graduation, and success on the NCLEX-RN®. *Journal of Nursing Education, 46*(8), 347–353.

The Joint Commission. (2010a). *Advancing effective communication, cultural competence, and patient- and family-centered care: A roadmap for hospitals.* Oakbrook Terrace, IL: Author.

The Joint Commission. (2010b). *Cultural and linguistic care in area hospitals.* Oakbrook Terrace, IL: Author.

The Joint Commission. (2011). *Use of technology urged to combat racial, ethnic disparities in health care.* Retrieved September 26, 2013, from www.pwrnewmedia.com/2011/joint_commission/jqps/#

U.S. Department of Health and Human Services, Health Resources Services Administration. (2010). *The registered nurse population: Initial findings from the 2008 National Sample Survey of registered nurses.* Retrieved March 9, 2013, from http://bhpr.hrsa.gov/healthworkforce/rnsurveys/rnsurveyfinal.pdf

U.S. Department of Health and Human Services, Office of Minority Health. (2013). *Enhanced national CLAS standards.* Retrieved August 16, 2013, from https://www.thinkculturalhealth.hhs.gov/Content/clas.asp

Woo, A., & Dragan, M. (2012). *Ensuring validity of NCLEX with differential item functioning analysis.* Retrieved April 5, 2013, from https://www.ncsbn.org/Ensuring_Validity_of_NCLEX_With_DIF_Analysis.pdf

II. INTEGRATING TCN CONCEPTS IN FOUNDATION COURSES

CHAPTER

Introductory Nursing Courses

6

Priscilla Limbo Sagar and Ann D. Corcoran

Priscilla Limbo Sagar and Ann D. Corcoran

KEY TERMS

Acculturation
Bafa Bafa
Barnga
Cultural competence
Culture
Ethnicity
Ethnocentrism

General informants
Journaling
Key informants
Linguistic competence
Reflection
Shadowing
Transcultural nursing

LEARNING OBJECTIVES

At the completion of this chapter, the learner will be able to

1. Describe the concepts of culture and cultural diversity encountered within nursing and health care professions that needs to be integrated in an introductory nonclinical course.
2. Implement creative teaching methods to spark interest in cultural diversity and promotion of cultural competence.
3. Identify basic current government and accrediting bodies regarding diversity and cultural competence.
4. Analyze important teaching and learning strategies for beginning nursing students.
5. Identify culturally congruent interventions for clients in health care settings.

OVERVIEW

The progression through a nursing program includes many levels of knowledge acquisition and understanding. Students who enter college with an interest in nursing may not have a complete comprehension of what the concept of nursing is; in many cases, their initial impetus to pursue this career includes a desire to help people or care for the sick. It is not until they have become immersed in the didactics of nursing education and clinical practice that beginning nursing students truly become acquainted with the image of a registered professional nurse.

Prior to the basic foundation blocks of nursing practice such as bedside care and assessment, students need to be introduced to the concept of nursing and its relationship to "opportunities of a lifetime" (Dentzer, 2003, p. 61). Dentzer emphasized three key points in these opportunities: nursing profession as service to fellow human beings and to oneself, nursing research and its capacity to make a difference in major health care challenges facing society, and nursing body of knowledge from research to make real difference in health care. There is strength in the sheer number of nurses—3,163, 063 (United States Department of Health and Human Services [USDHHS], Health Resources Services Administration [HRSA], 2010), a strength not fully capitalized on by this largest group of health care professionals. Sagar (2012) called upon the three million plus nurses to integrate **cultural competence** in all settings of nursing practice, education, administration, and research.

Cultural diversity and cultural competence need to be integrated in nursing curricula at all levels. This integration needs to be done in the first nursing course, whether or not the curriculum requires a separate **transcultural nursing** (TCN) course or courses. Nursing students care for a widely diverse cultural population in the clinical setting. In addition, nursing programs also include a variety of culturally diverse students. According to the 2012 statistics of the American Association of Colleges of Nursing (AACN), of the students enrolled in a generic entry level baccalaureate degree program, minorities account for 28% of the population (AACN, 2012). Nurse educators are responsible for stimulating an awareness of the concept of cultural sensitivity to clients, to students, and to our colleagues. In addition, nurse educators must encourage critical thinking skills in these beginning nursing students.

Difficulties exist when incorporating cultural competency and its many facets and considerations into nursing curricula. Issues include lack of consensus on what should be taught, lack of standards, as well as a need for and support from faculty prepared in TCN (Campesino, 2008; Campinha-Bacote, 2006; Lipson & DeSantis, 2007; Mixer, 2008). In addition, Campinha-Bacote (2008) noted that when evaluating cultural competency in nursing students, faculty may not have the experience in utilizing evaluation tools (Campinha-Bacote, 2006). It is, therefore, a mammoth task for nursing faculty to introduce cultural competence and carry the concept across the curriculum. The ethnonursing research by Mixer (2008) in EBP 6.1 not only showed how faculty provide generic and professional care to students in order to promote healthy ways of life but also attested to the lack of conceptual framework in integrating culturally competent concepts in nursing curricula.

EBP 6.1

Mixer (2008) conducted an ethnonursing research study to explore the nursing faculty expressions, patterns, and practices related to teaching culture care in an urban baccalaureate nursing program located in a public university at a southeastern U.S. city. As the theoretical framework of this pilot study, the researcher chose Leininger's (2006) Culture Care Theory (CCT) along with the sunrise enabler.

(continued)

Key informants are individuals with the most knowledge regarding the domain of inquiry; **general informants** provide general knowledge, reflections, and cultural insights (Leininger, 2006, p. 28). Three key informants (all full-time tenured nursing faculty) and three general informants (full-time and nontenure track adjunct faculty) participated in this study. The participants' ages ranged from 27 to 55 years and their teaching experiences were between 1.5 to 27 years. Four of the participants were African Americans and two were Anglo Americans.

Three major themes emerged from the study: 1) "faculty provided generic and professional care to nursing students to maintain and promote healthy and beneficial ways of life; 2) faculty taught students culture care...in classroom, online, and clinical...but without an organizing framework; [and] 3) care is essential for faculty health and well-being and to enable faculty to teach culture care to...students" (Mixer, 2008, p. 33).

According to Mixer (2008), discoveries from this study included application of the three modes of action: preservation/maintenance, accommodation/ negotiation, and repatterning/ restructuring (Leininger, 2006). Although all the informants value teaching culture care, the school had no formal TCN course, had limited cultural concepts taught, and had no integration of culture care content across the curriculum. Mixer further suggested that faculty maintain their initiative to provide each student with opportunities to care for ethnically diverse clients; negotiate to integrate culture care into existing nursing courses; develop required and elective courses to teach culture care; and use repatterning to utilize the CCT as an organizing framework for classroom, online, and clinical teaching.

The CCT, the sunrise enabler, and the ethnonursing method served as a solid framework and method for this pilot study. Mixer (2008) predicted that the conduct of a larger study will further support the CCT and contribute to the body of nursing knowledge, especially in nursing education and to the promotion of culturally congruent care.

Applications to Practice

■ Investigate your nursing program's recruitment, retention, and graduation plan for all students. Is there a difference in the attrition rates between majority and minority students? Do you have minority students?

■ Are faculty part of the recruitment efforts at the middle and high schools?

■ Do you involve graduates of your program in the recruitment, retention, and success of minority students?

■ If you were to replicate this study, how would you conduct it? What would you change in terms of conceptual framework, method, sampling, and analysis of findings?

Source: Leininger (2006); and Mixer (2008).

Integration of TCN Concepts

The introduction of cultural competency in a 1- to 3-credit foundation nursing course may aim to meet some of the *Standards of Practice for Culturally Competent Nursing Care* (Douglas et al., 2011; Transcultural Nursing Society, 2012). At this level, fundamental terms and concepts centering on one's own critical reflection (Standard #2), knowledge of cultures (Standard #3), and cross-cultural communication (Standard #9) can be included. The practice of **reflection**, the examination of an individual's own cultural values which could potentially conflict with others' values and hence hinder "therapeutic relationships and effective patient outcomes" (Douglas et al., 2011, p. 319), could be initiated with the novice student as he or she learns critical thinking.

Schuessler, Wilder, and Byrd (2012) identified that reflection nurtures thinking that changes practice. In addition, when the practice of reflection is combined with **journaling**, students can develop self-analysis, leading to an enhanced awareness of their environment (Schuessler et al., 2012). Students in the foundational level of their nursing education may not have insight into the concept of cultural competence. A broad spectrum of information introduced at this level can be very overwhelming. As identified in the *Standards of Practice for Culturally Competent Nursing Care*, suggestions to implement this standard of critical reflection includes hosting programs to enhance understanding of different cultures and customs, as well as the use of role modeling (Douglas et al., 2011; Transcultural Nursing Society, 2012).

Adopting consistent definitions of culture, cultural and linguistic competence, and other related terms that the school will use in all its nursing programs can be introduced in this course. For example, the school may choose the definition of **culture** as the "integrated patterns of human behavior that include the language, thoughts, communications, actions, customs, beliefs, values, and institutions of racial, ethnic, religious, or social groups" (USDHHS, Office of Minority Health [OMH], 2000, p. vi.). In addition the USDHHS, OMH (2000) definition of cultural and linguistic competence is "a set of congruent behaviors, attitudes, and policies that come together in a system, agency, or among professionals that enables effective work in cross-cultural situations" (p. vi). Using basic case studies and applying the enhanced standards of the culturally and linguistically appropriate services ([CLAS]; USDHHS, OMH, 2013) standards would be appropriate in this course, especially the delineation of Standards 5, 6, 7, and 8 for agencies receiving federal funding. Emphasis on the history of CLAS standards may be included, since legislation requiring cultural competence training has been already signed into law in the states of Washington, California, Connecticut, New Jersey, and New Mexico and is strongly recommended in Maryland (USDHHS, OMH, 2013). In other states, the proposition was referred to committee, is currently under consideration, has died in committee, or was vetoed. Module 3.1, Culturally and Linguistically Appropriate Services (CLAS) Standards, may be assigned as group work with student presentations in class for every standard. An alternative and inclusive definition of **linguistic competence** may be adopted from the National Center for Cultural Competence (2009):

> The capacity of an organization and its personnel to communicate effectively, and convey information in a manner that is easily understood by diverse audiences including persons of limited English proficiency, those who have low literacy skills or are not literate, individuals with disabilities, and those who are deaf or hard of hearing. (2009, para 1)

As students are introduced to the building blocks of cultural competency, topics such as acculturation, ethnicity, and ethnocentrism can be presented. The concept of **acculturation** can have a wide variety of interpretations. The *Faculty Toolkit for Integrating Cultural Competence in Baccalaureate Nursing Education* defined acculturation as "incorporating some cultural attributes of the larger society by diverse individuals, peoples, or groups" (AACN, 2008, p. 14). Spector's (2013) description of **ethnicity,** identification with or affiliation in a distinct racial, national, or cultural group including the observance of that group's customs, beliefs, and language (p. 23), may be used. The concept of **ethnocentrism** can be simply defined as the "universal tendency of human beings to think that their ways of thinking and believing are the only right way..." (Purnell, 2013, p. 6). There may exist diversity in culture, ethnicity, gender, or gender orientation among nursing students; this may be an avenue where open dialogue and discussion is worthwhile. Students can be encouraged to share their own culture from personal, family, and community perspectives at the onset of this lecture component; this helps the faculty in identifying students' existing knowledge base on the subject.

At the freshman level of a baccalaureate degree nursing program, students may not yet be exposed to the clinical component of the curriculum. It is at this vantage point that an introduction to the concept of cultural competence can be presented. The opportunity to identify key terms and concepts at this level can prepare the novice nursing student for the culturally centered situations that may arise when providing patient care. The question exists, however: How do we introduce this concept in a motivating and stimulating manner?

Teaching and Learning Strategies

As nursing educators, we need to present course content in a manner that stimulates thinking, maintains interest, and fuels discussion. Students enrolled in a foundation or fundamental nursing course are novice to the many concepts and theories that help mould and develop future professional registered nurses (RNs). It is imperative that nurse educators demonstrate confidence, knowledge, and creativity when fostering cultural diversity and promoting cultural competence. Teaching students concepts of culture and cultural diversity lends itself to a variety of ways to present this material in a stimulating manner.

LECTURE

Lecture, a commonly used presentation of content to learners, is usually enhanced by handouts, study guides, or visual aids. To increase student involvement, Rowles (2005) proposed group discussions; for example, using two 10-minute discussions in between two 20-minute lectures.

Methods traditionally in existence include the classroom lecture. Introducing culture in a lecture session may aid students in identifying definitions and key concepts. The disadvantage with the lecture method for this topic—as in any other lecture topics—may be the issue of waning student attention; the material may become boring, especially if poorly delivered or lacking an impetus for creative thinking on the part of the instructor (Caputi, 2005).

DISCUSSION

A foundation level nursing course can initiate communication among students and faculty regarding their interests in nursing, as well as questions regarding the academic nursing program and the professional role of the nurse. The opportunity also exists for open discussion among students and faculty in an informal or formal manner. The topic of culture can open a colorful discussion among students at this level. Students may be quite willing to share personal reflections on their own culture and how this affects their lives. With a potential classroom of culturally diverse students, many may already identify ways in which culture affects health, spirituality, birth and death rituals, diet, and communication.

The danger that exists with an open discussion forum is the potential for one person or a few people to monopolize the session. In this case, the faculty skills of facilitation and drawing the quiet students into the discussion may control the situation. In addition, the faculty should plan ahead and employ clear objectives for this discussion forum. Techniques recommended for a discussion period include: (1) maintaining the role of facilitator, (2) encouraging group participation, (3) preventing monopolization of time, and (4) keeping discussions on track (DeYoung, 2009).

MULTIMEDIA

The current generation exists in a world of Internet communication and entertainment. Can nursing education incorporate this media component into an effective teaching method? A fundamental concern prior to the use of any web-based information is the evaluation of its appropriateness and relevance to the topic. Educators must be able to discriminate between commercialized, inaccurate media and well-developed information (Baumlein, 2005).

Websites such as YouTube provide a variety of media clips regarding cultural diversity. Students may be given an exercise in which to navigate through these sites to find one of interest and relevance to culture and health care. This can be an in-class group assignment, or one in which they can investigate independently and present their feedback to the class. The instructor must keep in mind that, along with the Internet-based information, this teaching–learning format should aim to meet the objectives and outcomes of the course.

GAMES

The use of games as a teaching–learning strategy may be effective for a freshman introductory course. Games are an effective learning method, sustaining the learner's attention and providing him or her active learning strategies to enhance the learning process (Caputi, 2005). Games have been used in education for many years, and in many disciplines not limited to nursing. Games have been found to enhance motivation and learning (Blakely, Skirton, Cooper, Allum, & Nelmes, 2008; Fawcett & Dodd, 2009; Henderson, 2005), foster teamwork and collaboration (McLafferty, Dingwall, & Halkett, 2010), and promote learning in a nonthreatening and stress-reduced environment (Henderson, 2005; Glendon & Ulrich, 2005), among others. Games can be presented in a variety of methods; however, there are also disadvantages to gaming in the classroom setting such as increased competition, time-consuming preparation, and potential for stress and embarrassment among players (Graham & Richardson, 2008; Henderson, 2005). In addition, game construction and use must have a valid purpose in teaching the required course content (DeYoung, 2009).

The use of games has been implemented to enhance cultural awareness. Haupt (2006) presented her creation of a *Diversity Bingo* game among nursing students. The author acknowledged that nurse educators need to be aware of student needs and the changing demographics of nursing students. This game allowed for learning in the affective domain, as students were able to reflect on their own personal experiences during class. This game can be utilized for a student population that has many English language learners (ELL) as well as those entering nursing as a second career. Established games such as *Barnga* and *Bafa Bafa* create interactive learning on cultural awareness, the ability to debrief and discuss findings, and have been used not only in nursing education, but also in the industrial and business settings (Graham & Richardson, 2008).

Barnga (Thiagarajan, 1990) is an established card game that is used in a variety of settings to present cultural awareness. During this game, participants are not allowed to talk to one another; instead, they rely only on gestures and drawing to communicate. At the completion of the game, the outcome is to demonstrate that moving from one culture to another can cause a conflict of emotions (Graham & Richardson, 2008; Koskinen, Abdelhamid, & Likitalo, 2008). A participant may feel that he or she is aware of the rules when moving from one group to another; however, each group is given different rules. The lack of a common verbal language among groups may lead to confusion in communication. Barnga is an effective card game in that several numbers of students can participate, from a minimum of nine people to as many as a full classroom setting. In addition, there is time upon completion of the game for debriefing and discussion (Koskinen et al., 2008).

Bafa Bafa (Shirts, 1969) is another game used to present cultural awareness. Bafa Bafa, unlike Barnga, is more of a simulation game. Students are divided into one of two groups representing cultures: the alphas and betas. Students are given instructions on the rules of each culture. One culture is based on trading, competition, and code language, while the other is more male-dominated and values close physical contact (Graham & Richardson, 2008). As with Barnga, this game entails orientation, game playing, and debriefing (Koskinen et al., 2008).

SHADOWING AND OBSERVATION

Observing or **shadowing** professional RNs in various practice settings may provide essential learning experiences that connect theory to practice, foster aim for a particular niche or nursing specialty, or stimulate passion for the profession. Although shadowing is more commonly used in elementary, middle, and high-school programs, beginning nursing students may get clarification about the roles and responsibilities of the professional RN (Briggs, Merk, & Mitchell, 2003). Reflection on agency or institution compliance with CLAS standards may be integrated in the shadowing experience.

In a research study by Fougner and Horntvedt (2011), students were exposed to real-life experiences in hospitals or home-based rehabilitation settings. The participants consisted of physiotherapy, occupational therapy, and nursing students. The authors noted that upon completion of the shadowing experience, students were provided with examples of good role models and had the opportunity to observe the real world in practice (Fougner & Horntvedt, 2011). It is important to keep in mind that a shadowing/observational experience needs to be developed with specific directions and outcomes. The student as well as the professional should be prepared as to their roles and expectations. The opportunity for a student to shadow a professional nurse can help to formulate ways of thinking, secure new insights and skills, and gain confidence in learning in the clinical setting (Price & Price, 2009).

The Sample Role Play Scenario 6.1 illustrates the vital role of communication, both verbal and nonverbal, in all human interactions. Approximately 90% of all problems in nurse–client interactions developed from miscommunications (Andrews, 2012). About 12% to 19% of the U.S. population are non-English speakers; that equates to 52 million people ages 5 and older (Andrews, 2008; Berry-Caban & Crespo, 2008). This is a huge concern; language is vital in the navigation of any health care system. After the role play, the basic elements of the CLAS standards can be reviewed here.

SAMPLE ROLE PLAY SCENARIO 6.1

American Tourists: Student A (female) and Student B (male) are dressed as American tourists. As the Americans travel and explore various locations, they become tired and hungry, so they decide to return to their hotel. Unfortunately, they have walked far, lost their way, and will need public transportation to take them back to the hotel. They decide to ask two native citizens for help. The Americans need to figure out a proper way to ask questions from the natives. If they fail to understand how things are done in these lands, the natives will not provide assistance. Neither tourist speaks Hsilgne.

Native Citizens: Two students, C and D, will represent each of the locations (students can pick a unique name for their locations). In these imaginary locations, there are certain ways of doing things. In location 2, natives use a different language.

◾ Location #1. Natives here shake hands with their left; the right hand is only used for ablutions.
◾ Location #2. Natives here speak a different language called Hsilgne, a combination of German, Latin, and French.

Student E is the certified transcultural nurse. She will moderate the discussion following the role playing and use the following questions as a guide:

1. Examine nonverbal communication issues in these scenarios.
2. Have you ever experienced being in a location where you do not speak the language? Describe your experience.
3. Discuss the possible applications of this role play in client situations.

Instructor/Educator: Debriefing

1. Reflect on each of the different location scenarios. How did you feel?
2. Discuss what you learned. What other learning needs do you have? Explain.
3. Reflect on the changes needed in your own knowledge.
4. In client situations, why do you think interpreters or translators are necessary?

Source: Adapted from Kodotchigova (2002).

CRITICAL THINKING EXERCISES 6.1

Undergraduate Student

1. You have an assignment about beginning reflection in your Intro to Nursing course. Discuss what you have prepared so far in terms of your own cultural values that may interfere with your therapeutic relationships with clients. Has this helped you in preparing to interact with clients? If yes, why? If no, why not?
2. Do you think there is enough content of cultural diversity and promotion of cultural competence integrated in your beginning nursing course? Does this course include observational experience or shadowing-of-a-nurse experience in the hospital or in the community?
3. If you were to add an observational or shadowing-of-a-nurse experience, what would you add? Why?
4. Would you be in favor of including a 3-credit TCN course in your current curriculum? If yes, which course would you be in favor of deleting from your BS in Nursing curriculum? Why?

Faculty in Academia

1. How many credits do you have in your Introduction to Nursing course?
2. Do you have a separate TCN course in the undergraduate program? How many credits is that TCN course? Are there TCN courses in the graduate program?
3. If you were to add a 3-credit TCN course in the undergraduate program, which current course would you delete? Why?

Staff Development Educator

1. Do you have beginning student observational rotation or "shadowing" RNs in your institution? How many hours does the rotation entail?
2. If you have the above rotation, who serves as preceptors? If the preceptors are not paid, what kind of motivational incentives do you or the school of nursing offer preceptors?
3. What continuing competence workshops do you offer preceptors? Are these workshops over and above those required for staff nurses who do not serve as preceptors?

SUMMARY

The progression through nursing education begins with the introduction of many concepts to a student: pathophysiology, pharmacology, assessment, and nursing skills at the bedside, to name a few. The provision of nursing care to an individual, family, and community also requires an awareness of culture with the considerations and respect each culture deserves. It is imperative that this concept of culturally and linguistically appropriate care be presented to the nursing student at each level of his or her education. The foundation nursing courses provide the opportunity to address basic concepts and definitions and their application to client care. This chapter identifies the primary terms and concepts that can be developed in a foundation nursing course. Teaching and learning strategies across a variety of formats are discussed. Evidence-based practice (EBP) examples and critical thinking exercises are provided to guide the educator in presenting this important topic to nursing students.

REFERENCES

American Association of Colleges of Nursing. (2008). *Cultural competency in baccalaureate nursing education.* Washington, DC: Author.

American Association of Colleges of Nursing. (2012). *Race/ethnicity of students enrolled in generic (entry level) baccalaureate, master's, and doctoral (research–focused) programs in nursing, 2002–2011.* Retrieved May 24, 2013, from www.aacn.nche.edu/research-data/EthnicityTbl.pdf

Andrews, M. M. (2008). Cultural diversity in the health care workforce. In M. M. Andrews & J. S. Boyle (Eds.), *Transcultural concepts in nursing care* (5th ed., pp. 297–326). Philadelphia, PA: Wolters Kluwer/Lippincott Williams & Wilkins.

Andrews, M. M. (2012). Culturally competent nursing care. In M. M. Andrews & J. S. Boyle (Eds.), *Transcultural concepts in nursing care* (6th ed., pp. 17–37). Philadelphia, PA: Wolters Kluwer Health /Lippincott Williams & Wilkins.

Baumlein, G. K. (2005). Creative technology in the classroom. In L. Caputi & L. Engelmann (Eds.), *Teaching nursing: The art and science* (pp. 59–83). Glen Ellyn, IL: College of DuPage Press.

Berry-Caban, C. S., & Crespo, H. (2008). Cultural competency as a skill for health care providers. *Hispanic Health International, 6*(3), 115–121.

Blakely, G., Skirton, H., Cooper, S., Allum, P., & Nelmes, P. (2008). Educational gaming in the health sciences: Systematic review. *Journal of Advanced Nursing, 65*(2), 259–269. doi:10.1111/j.1365-2648.2008.04843.x

Briggs, L., Merk, S. E., & Mitchell, B. (2003). *Collaboration for the promotion of nursing: Building partnerships for the future.* Indianapolis, IN: Sigma Theta Tau International Honor Society of Nursing.

Campesino, M. (2008). Beyond transculturalism: Critiques of cultural education in nursing. *Journal of Nursing Education, 47*(7), 298–304.

Campinha-Bacote, J. (2006). Cultural competence in nursing curricula: How are we doing 20 years later? *Journal of Nursing Education, 45*(7), 243–244.

Caputi, L. (2005). Teaching in the classroom. In L. Caputi & L. Engelmann (Eds.), *Teaching nursing: The art and science* (pp. 38–58). Glen Ellyn, IL: College of DuPage Press.

Dentzer, S. (2003). Nursing and the opportunities of a lifetime. *Journal of Professional Nursing, 19*(2), 61–65.

DeYoung, S. (2009). *Teaching strategies for nurse educators* (2nd ed.). Upper Saddle River, NJ: Prentice-Hall.

Douglas, M. K., Pierce, J. U., Rosenkoetter, M., Pacquiao, D F., Callister, L. C., Hattar-Pollara,...& Purnell, L. D. (2011). Standards of practice for culturally competent nursing: 2011 update. *Journal of Transcultural Nursing, 22*(4), 317–333. doi:10.1177/1043659611412965

Fawcett, D. L., & Dodd, C. (2009). Periopardy: The 21st century. *AORN Journal, 89*(3), 565–571.

Fougner, M., & Horntvedt, T. (2011). Students' perceptions on shadowing interprofessional teamwork: A Norwegian case study. *Journal of Interprofessional Care, 25,* 33–38. doi:10.3109/1356182 0.2010.490504

Glendon, K., & Ulrich, D. (2005). Using games as a teaching strategy. *Journal of Nursing Education, 44*(7), 338–339.

Graham, I., & Richardson, E. (2008). Experiential gaming to facilitate cultural awareness: Its implication for developing emotional caring in nursing. *Learning in Health and Social Care, 7*(1), 37–45.

Haupt, B. (2006). Diversity bingo: A strategy to increase awareness of diversity in the classroom. *Nurse Educator, 31*(6), 242–243.

Henderson, D. (2005). Games: Making learning fun. *Annual Review of Nursing Education, 3,* 165–183.

Kodotchigova, M. (2002). Role play in teaching culture: Six quick steps for classroom implementation. *The Internet TESL Journal, VIII*(7). Retrieved July 18, 2013, from http://iteslj.org/Techniques/Kodotchigova-RolePlay.html

Koskinen, L., Abdelhamid, P., & Likitalo, H. (2008). The simulation method for learning cultural awareness in nursing. *Diversity in Health and Social Care, 5,* 55–63.

Leininger, M. M. (2006). Culture care diversity and universality theory and evolution of the ethnonursing method. In M. Leininger & M. McFarland (Eds.), *Culture care diversity and universality: A worldwide nursing theory* (2nd ed., pp. 1–41). Boston, MA: Jones & Bartlett.

Lipson, J. G., & DeSantis, L. A. (2007). Current approaches to integrating elements of cultural competence in nursing education. *Journal of Transcultural Nursing, 18*(1), 10S–20S. doi:10.1177/1043659606295498

McLafferty, E., Dingwall, L., & Halkett, A. (2010). Using gaming workshops to prepare nursing students for caring for older people in clinical practice. *International Journal of Older People Nursing, 5*(1), 51–60. doi:10.1111/jl740–3743.2009.00176x

Mixer, S. J. (2008). Use of the culture care theory and ethnonursing method to discover how nursing faculty teach culture care. *Contemporary Nurse, 28*, 23–36.

National Center for Cultural Competence. (2009). *Linguistic competence.* Retrieved June 29, 2013, from http://nccc.georgetown.edu/documents/Definition%20of%20Linguistic%20Competence.pdf

Price, A., & Price, B. (2009). Role modelling practice with students on clinical placements. *Nursing Standard, 24*(11), 51–56.

Purnell, L. D. (2013). Transcultural diversity and health care. In L. D. Purnell (Ed.), *Transcultural health care: A culturally competent approach* (4th ed., pp. 3–14). Philadelphia, PA: F. A. Davis.

Rowles, C. J. (2005). Strategies to promote critical thinking and active learning. In D. M. Billings & J. A. Halstead (Ed.), *Teaching in nursing: A guide for faculty* (2nd ed., pp. 283–324). St. Louis, MO: Elsevier Saunders.

Sagar, P. L. (2012). *Transcultural nursing theory and models: Application in nursing education, practice, and administration.* New York, NY: Springer Publishing.

Schuessler, J. B., Wilder, B., & Byrd, L. W. (2012). Reflective journaling and development of cultural humility in students. *Nursing Education Perspectives, 33*(2), 96–99. doi:10.5480/1536–5026-33.2.96

Shirts, R. G. (1969). *History of BaFa' BaFa:' A cross cultural/diversity/inclusion simulation.* San Diego, CA: Simulation Training Systems. Retrieved September 1, 2013, from www.stsintl.com/business/articles/History-of-BaFa-2.pdf

Spector, R. E. (2013). *Cultural diversity in health and illness* (8th ed.). Upper Saddle River, NJ: Pearson Education.

Thiagarajan, S. (1990). *Barnga.* Yarmouth, ME: Intercultural Press.

Transcultural Nursing Society. (2012). *Standards of practice for culturally competent care: Executive summary.* Retrieved March 23, 2013, from www.tcns.org/files/Standards_of_Practice_for_Cult_Comp_Nsg_care-2011_Update_FINAL_printed_copy_2_.pdf

U.S. Department of Health and Human Services, Health Resources Services Administration. (2010). *The registered nurse population: Initial findings from the 2008 National Sample Survey of registered nurses.* Retrieved January 18, 2013, from bhpr.hrsa.gov/healthworkforce/rnsurveys/rnsurveyinitial2008.pdf

U.S. Department of Health and Human Services, Office of Minority Health. (2000). *Culturally and linguistically appropriate services.* Retrieved January 6, 2011, from http://minorityhealth.hhs.gov/templates/browse.aspx?lvl=2&lvlID=15

U.S. Department of Health and Human Services, Office of Minority Health. (2013). *The national standards for culturally and linguistically appropriate services in health and health care* (the *National CLAS Standards*). Retrieved July 16, 2013, from https://www.thinkculturalhealth.hhs.gov/pdfs/EnhancedNationalCLASStandards.pdf

Nursing Skills

Priscilla Limbo Sagar and Teresa V. Hurley

KEY TERMS

Debriefing
Demonstration
Interprofessional learning
Learning resource center
Purnell Model for Cultural Competence

Return demonstration
Role playing
Simulation
Skills laboratory
Unfolding case scenario

LEARNING OBJECTIVES

At the completion of this chapter, the learner will be able to

1. Integrate diversity and culturally congruent care when performing basic nursing skills.
2. Analyze biological variations in specific ethnocultural groups and safety in the administration of medications.
3. Utilize creative strategies in teaching and learning activities when integrating diversity and cultural competence content in a nursing skills course.
4. Apply collaboration with the interprofessional team in providing safe care to patients.

OVERVIEW

The integration of transcultural nursing (TCN) concepts into a nursing skills course begins with laying a foundation for students to build upon. Learning about various cultures and the provision of culturally sensitive care is contingent on the nurse educator's passion, inquisitiveness, enthusiasm, and creativity. These qualities enable the educator to construct an interactive learning environment that captures and holds the students' attention, inspires them to learn more about cultural diversity, and implements culturally congruent care in their classroom and clinical learning.

Integration of TCN Concepts

Culturally competent care is mandated by academic as well as organizational accreditation. Early on, students studying nursing skills need to know the imperatives for including cultural diversity in the course; for complying with the enhanced culturally and linguistically appropriate services (CLAS) standards (U.S. Department of Health and Human Services [USDHHS], Office of Minority Health [OMH], 2013); and for eliminating disparities in health and health care access and quality (USDHHS, OMH, 2010).

Cultural influences affect people's view of health, illness, and health care (Taylor, Lillis, LeMone, & Lynn, 2011; Wilkinson & Treas, 2011). The glaring disparities in health and health care quality (Edberg, 2013; Rose, 2011) and the lack of minorities among health care professionals (Sullivan Commission, 2004) continue to be of concern to all stakeholders. Although skills textbooks such as those written by Taylor et al. (2008) and Wilkinson and Treas (2011) have incorporated cultural aspects of care, there is a very important decision to adopt a theoretical framework upon which to base the teaching of diversity and promotion of cultural competence. Culture care, furthermore, calls for vertical and horizontal threading in the nursing curricula in both classroom and clinical learning.

Analysis of the health care setting where the students will be having their clinical experience provides insight into the planning aspect of the course. Students who will be practicing in rural areas will have far different experiences than students practicing in an urban setting. Opportunities for the students to care for culturally diverse clients may be limited by the available clinical sites. But planning for diverse and unusual experiences should not be hampered by limitations when nurse educators use their imagination, their desire, and their commitment to diversity and promotion of cultural competence.

There are endless possibilities of teaching foundational skills and transcultural concepts by using effective teaching–learning strategies in the classroom, clinical, and **learning resource center** (LRC) or **skills laboratory**. In these arenas, the educator's creativity can be at play to plan participatory interactions to assist the students in gaining insight into cultures other than their own. In the classroom, strategies such as discussions, case studies, and role playing can be employed. While in clinical, discussions during pre- and postconferences, role plays, and case studies can be used.

The LRC is the site of most initial skills learning, from basic skills such as hygiene to the more complicated procedures of administration of medications and intravenous fluids; this is a fertile ground from which to integrate TCN concepts. The faculty could **demonstrate** skills and then ask for a **return demonstration** of the skills. Whether using a specific theory or model or employing an eclectic approach, faculty teaching in a foundational skills course is in a strategic position to develop awareness, skills, and competencies in providing culturally congruent care for all clients.

TEACHING AND LEARNING STRATEGIES

There are various teaching and learning strategies nurse educators may use to integrate cultural awareness and competence into a nursing skills course. These include, but are not limited to, unfolding case scenarios, **interprofessional learning**, role playing, and **simulation**. These strategies are based on active learning principles to facilitate the students' acquisition of knowledge.

A culture-based scenario is an example of an interactive strategy. This will enable the nurse educator to use creativity to facilitate the students' learning of content and foster their critical thinking within a clinical context. A singular culture or multiple cultures may be used to promote the students' understanding using a variety of strategies such as classroom discussions, clinical assessments, group presentations, poster presentations, role playing, simulation, and interprofessional projects.

Unfolding Case Scenarios

When employing **unfolding case scenarios**, the nurse educator may use the same situations throughout the semester by including additional information. These situations allow the students to grow in their ability to critically think and develop clinical judgment. Succeeding scenarios may use any of these questions: What if the biopsy was positive? Who would make the decision regarding mastectomy? Who should be assigned to care for her in the hospital? What if the only specialist is a male surgeon? What are her spiritual needs? How could you accommodate her religious practices? Are there dietary restrictions? What does the nurse need to know about medications?

Health care providers perceive the care of Muslim women as a challenge; in addition, these women see health care providers as not comprehending their spirituality or culture (Hasnain, Connell, Menon, & Tranmer, 2011). The major areas of concern are communication (Hasnain et al., 2011; Sheets & El-Azhary, 2000), hygiene, food and medication restrictions (Sheets & El-Azhary, 2000), fasting (Aadil, Houti, & Moussamih, 2004; Pathy, Mills, Gazzeley, Ridgley, & Kiran, 2011), modesty, and family involvement in health care (Aadil et al., 2004; Pathy et al., 2011). These areas have been identified as reasons why these women will not seek health care (Hasnain et al., 2011; Pathy et al., 2011).

Bringing cultural awareness to the above areas are foundational topics addressed in a nursing skills course. The initial case scenario should incorporate areas identified in the literature as problematic, especially those related to communication and modesty in the case of the female Muslim Arab client. Thus, when making initial contact, the nurse needs to realize that eye contact between the female client and a male provider is prohibited and will be avoided. The nurse should extend his/her right hand and, if not reciprocated, understand that it is based on belief system and not as a sign of rudeness. The nurse should also seek permission to enter a room and wait for the client to cover her head. The unfolding case scenario is in Box 7.1.

These questions provide a framework for the students to seek additional knowledge in order to make clinical decisions. For example, the students need to consider how an Arab Muslim woman might view surgical removal of her breast. Her cultural beliefs and values affect her decision making regarding mastectomy, chemotherapy, pain management, nutritional management, and palliative care. Extending the scenario in this way opens the door to learning activities that place emphasis on the meaning of suffering as atonement for sins, alleviation of pain as a virtue, and preparation of the client for her afterlife. It also provides a jumping point to address ethical principles.

The inclusion of ethical principles provides the nursing students with an opportunity to reflect and discuss how they would react in situations. One of the most challenging issues concerning the Arab Muslim clients is the delay in seeking treatment and/or their refusal

---

BOX 7.1   UNFOLDING CASE SCENARIO: CARING FOR A TRADITIONAL ARAB MUSLIM FEMALE CLIENT

A 44-year-old Muslim woman visits your health care facility accompanied by her sister, aunt, husband, father, and father-in-law. She is a homemaker with four children ranging in age from 4 to 12 years. Her appointment was scheduled for 11:00 a.m., but she does not show up until 1:00 p.m. She is wearing a head scarf, partial veil, and loose fitting clothing that cover her legs, arms, and body.

1. How would you address the fact that the woman showed up 2 hours late for her appointment?

2. How would you introduce yourself to the client and her family?

3. Would you ask the family members to leave the room during your initial assessment?

4. What major factors would you need to include in your assessment?

5. How would you safeguard the client's modesty in preparation for the biopsy, during, and after the procedure? What if the biopsy was being performed by a male provider?

6. What would you need to include in discharge teaching? Who would you include in the process?

7. What factors may limit the women's ability to seek follow-up care? How would you assist the client in overcoming those limitations you have identified?

---

to accept treatment based on a male provider's decision. Although the teachings within Islam permit clients to make choices concerning their care, the decision-making power usually has a hierarchal order with most authority relegated to the male parent, spouse, and elder children (Sheets & El-Azhary, 2000). The nursing student needs to understand these family dynamics in order to advocate on behalf of the client in a Western health care system where the value is an individual autonomy.

Wiggins (1998) contends that authentic understanding needs to be assessed using a variety of strategies in order to uncover the multifaceted nature of the concept. The use of real-life patient care scenarios is one way students' understanding may be assessed. Higher order thinking is revealed by their demonstration of ability to interpret, apply, and analyze data needed to provide safe and humanistic care to clients with diverse cultural backgrounds.

Ultimately, the goal of nursing education is to prepare the next generation of professionals to critically think as they care for people in need of health care in diverse practice areas.

Interactive assessments and reiterative assessments of performance will help students to reflect upon their performance and make changes in their behavior (Wiggins, 1998). The culture-based scenario enables students to demonstrate their clinical reasoning ability, which can be seen as a "coherence of cluster knowledge" (Kiel et al., 2008). The students' performance provides feedback and an understanding that it is not enough for them to know the procedural steps of a skill, but to know how to interpret, apply, and analyze the client care situation.

Wiggins (1998) contends that authentic understanding needs to be assessed using a variety of strategies in order to uncover the multifaceted nature of the concept. The use of real-life client care scenarios is one way students' understanding may be assessed. Higher order thinking is revealed by their ability to interpret, apply, and analyze data needed to provide safe and humanistic care to clients with diverse backgrounds.

Interprofessional Learning

The American Association of the Colleges of Nursing (AACN, 1995) position statement on *Interdisciplinary Education* stressed the importance of providing collaborative experiences, especially early on in the curricula. The Institute of Medicine (2010) had emphasized this in its report titled *Future of Nursing: Leading Change, Advancing Health*. Heller, Oros, and Durney-Cowley (2011) concurred and emphasized the role of nursing practice, education, and research in embracing the changing demographics and in focusing on holistic care.

With the explosion of technological advancements in health care and the field of informatics, an interprofessional strategy provides an arena for students from different disciplines to learn from each other and appreciate each other's contributions. As they work together, students may learn critical management concepts such as decision making, team work, delegation, and conflict management. As an example, nursing skills students could create a scenario. They then could invite premedicine, dental, physical therapy, human services, and information technology students to participate in the scenario that, which is filmed by communication majors. The students have the opportunity to learn the value of collaboration to meet the cultural and spiritual needs of diverse groups in addition to acquiring skills they will need as they face the challenges of 21st century health care. This also provides an opportunity to celebrate the students' own cultures by having a festival of sharing that includes dress, music, dancing, and food.

The use of technology supports thinking processes such as problem solving and understanding complex concepts; induces student motivation and fosters sense of self-esteem; promotes equity among the social classes; prepares students for the future; and changes school structures (U.S. Department of Education, 2010). The National Research Council (2000) emphasized the use of technology as a means for an educator to address real world problems, to use scaffolding to promote understanding, to give feedback and assist in promoting reflection, and to develop learning communities for students.

Role Playing

Role playing, a strategy whereby individuals enter into the role of others while observers analyze and interpret (Rowles & Brigham, 2005), is another approach that allows students the opportunity to use their creativity in applying TCN concepts (Shearer & Davidhizar, 2003). Briefly, the faculty role centers on developing objectives, providing guidelines for the roles and time frame, monitoring the process, and facilitating analysis and debriefing (Rowles & Brigham, 2005; Shearer & Davidhizar, 2003). There is more discussion on role play in Chapter 2. The foundational scenario can be used throughout the semester and developed to include more complex health care issues. The students need to use previously learned knowledge and skills. As they actively engage in playing the role of the Arab Muslim woman, as well as her husband, family, provider, nurse, and ancillary personnel, they will have an experiential learning that promotes understanding and higher order thinking.

The scenario need not be long to be effective as the clinical application of the content unfolds. As an example, students can be assigned into groups to present a 5-minute scenario. The students should be given the latitude to create culturally sensitive or insensitive exchanges. The latter calls upon them to create nuances that may not be known such as eye contact, space orientation, decision-making processes, written informed consents, intravenous placement, and dietary restrictions. The planned feedback at the end of the role play or simulation is referred to as **debriefing;** this provides an opportunity for participants to analyze their actions, address emotional reactions to the role play, and receive constructive comments (Decker, Gore, & Feken, 2011). Inclusive of the debriefing are learning outcomes, application to practice, further learning needed, and changes necessary to improve client care (Gaberson & Oermann, 1999).

Simulation

Simulation is being used in nursing education programs as both a teaching strategy and an assessment method (Rauen, 2001). It is a student-centered experiential teaching method that can be adapted to the multiple learning needs of students (Li, 2007; Rauen, 2001). The simulated experience places students in a real-life clinical experience where they will have to critically think (Billings & Halstead, 2005; Rauen, 2001). Their involvement in the scenario group may also provide a means to fulfill the social and collaborative needs of an adult learner as they engage in finding solutions to client problems. Chapter 19 contains a thorough discussion of simulated learning.

As with role playing, a simulated experience may be developed for the LRC to include the performance of procedural skills that reflect the provision of culturally sensitive care. Using the case of the Arab Muslim women as an example, a variety of skills may be integrated into the simulation, such as the foundational knowledge about communication and family/nurse interactions. The procedural skills may include assessments of vital signs, hydration status, glucose testing, insertion of an indwelling urethral catheter, wound care, tube feedings, oxygen administration, and medication administration.

APPLICATION: PURNELL MODEL FOR CULTURAL COMPETENCE

The **Purnell Model for Cultural Competence (MCC**, 2013) is one of the most widely used models in nursing and allied health. The MCC is highly applicable in foundation courses. The 12 domains of the MCC can be used in their entirety or selectively. For example, in a basic skills course the MCC domains of biocultural ecology, communication, family roles and organizations, health care practices, nutrition, and spirituality may be integrated in all skill modules and work in harmony with literature on caring for a traditional Arab Muslim client (Box 7.1). Course outcomes need to reflect the students' ability to gain awareness, knowledge, and skills about different cultures and the provision of culturally congruent care. Table 7.1 highlights five domains of the MCC: beliefs and values, health care practices, communication, family roles and relationships, and nutrition.

There is increasing evidence and various tools to measure cultural competence among students, faculty, and staff. The study by Hughes and Hood (2007) illustrates a college of nursing's (CON) systematic approach to integrating TCN concepts in its curriculum and measuring cultural sensitivity among its baccalaureate students (EBP 7.1).

TABLE 7.1 Suggestions for Client Care of an Arab Muslim Female Client Using Domains of the Purnell Model for Cultural Competence

Cultural Domains	Suggestions for Client Care
Spirituality **(Beliefs and Values: Islamic Tenets** (Ahmed, 1981) ▪ Recitation of the *Profession of Faith.* ▪ Praying five times a day facing Mecca in Saudi Arabia. ▪ Fasting during Ramadan from dawn to dusk. Exempt are children under 13 years of age, the elderly (Sheets & El-Azhary, 2000), diabetics, pregnant women, those with mental illness (Pathy et al., 2011). Clients may still fast due to the belief that doing so will gain greater eternal rewards (Pathy et al., 2011; Sheets & El-Azhary, 2000). If exempt during an illness, one must fast the number of days missed (Sheets & El- Azhary, 2000). Family will fast on behalf of the mentally ill. ▪ Giving alms to the poor. ▪ Making a pilgrimage to Mecca during one's lifetime.	Facilitate ability to practice faith by doing the following: Arrange care around prayer times. Arrange bed or furniture facing East; assist client in assuming bodily positions and in placing prayer rugs on the floor; provide water for ablutions prior to prayer and after urinary and bowel eliminations (Lawrence & Razmus, 2001). Assess whether client has fasted, is currently fasting, or intends to fast (Pathy et al., 2011; Sheets & El-Azhary, 2000); include medications. Assess if client has history of diabetes, cardiac disease, or asthma including use of medications (Aadil et al., 2004; Pathy et al., 2011; Sheets & El-Azhary, 2000). Diabetic, cardiac (Pathy et al., 2011), and asthmatic clients are at high risk for complications (Sheets & El-Azhary, 2000).
Health care Practices ▪ Relationships valued over tasks. ▪ Courtesy and hospitality. ▪ Extended family over the individual social obligation to be part of the care of an ill member. ▪ Female modesty including partial or complete facial veil (Lawrence & Razmus, 2001; Pathy et al., 2011; Sheets & El-Azhary, 2000).	Provide enough time to develop and maintain trust. Do not rush interactions. Expect frequent visits and requests from immediate and extended family and neighbors as a demonstration of their support for the ill member (Sheets & El-Azhary, 2000). Provide privacy and maintain modesty by covering body parts. Assign female staff (Sheets) and have a female nurse in attendance during exams and procedures by male health care providers (Hasnain et al., 2011; Lawrence & Razmus, 2001).

(continued)

TABLE 7.1 Suggestions for Client Care of an Arab Muslim Female Client Using Domains of the Purnell Model for Cultural Competence   (continued)

Cultural Domains	Suggestions for Client Care
Communication ■ Arabic speaking. ■ Distance between communicants should be 2 feet apart with direct eye contact to observe pupil response (Sheets & El-Azhary, 2000). ■ Female modesty. ■ Left hand used for washing after elimination and considered dirty. Right hand is considered clean. ■ Verbal consent highly valued over the written word, which is distrusted. ■ Present time orientation.	Provide interpreter of same-gender. Assess ability to read and write Arabic and/or English and use open-ended questions to avoid closing down communication (Hasnain et al., 2011). Close distance and touch by the same-sex providers helps in reducing stress (Sheets & El-Azhary, 2000). Assign females to provide care and, if possible, one of the same ethnicity or religion (Hasnain et al., 2011). Do not use the left hand when taking or receiving objects. Insert intravenous access devices on the left side. Shake hands by extending the right hand and administer medications using the right hand Written consent involves legalities. Avoid conflict by offering a compromise; ask a female client to sign the consent and male provider to cosign. Late and missed appointments may be addressed by notifying the clients by telephone. Arrange care around the male's ability to transport the female client
Family Roles and Relationships Males are protectors and providers and females are caregivers who attend to children and the home (Sheets & El-Azhary, 2000). Extended family and friends provide spiritual care and support (Lawrence & Razmus, 2001).	Include males in health care decisions. Seek out the cooperation and assistance of the patriarchal leader (Lawrence & Razmus, 2001). Acknowledge the client's need to have family and friends present for healing prayers and arrange for them to participate in client's care (Lawrence & Razmus, 2001).
Nutrition Consuming pork, pork byproducts, alcohol, and blood are not permitted. Follow a ritual slaughtering of animals; client may refuse to eat foods prepared at health care facility (Lawrence & Razmus, 2001; Sheets & El-Azhary, 2000).	Consult with dietician. Vegetarian or Kosher foods maybe consumed (Lawrence & Razmus, 2001). Arrange to have family bring in foods prepared at home. Determine if client is permitted to take medications that have alcohol- or pork-based products such as gelatin and heparin, insulin (Sheets & El-Azhary, 2000).

Source: Cultural domains adapted from Purnell (2013).

As schools continue to systematically include cultural concepts in their curricula, they will need to utilize tools to measure outcomes of students' cultural competence. Among 212 baccalaureate students from four diverse programs in the United States surveyed with Campinha-Bacote's (2007) *Inventory for Assessing the Process of Cultural Competency Among Healthcare Professionals (IAPCC-R)* prior to graduation, the scores consisted mainly in the awareness level (Kardong-Edgreen & Campinha-Bacote, 2008). In 2008, Campinha-Bacote developed the student version of the IAPCC-SV to measure the cultural desire of students. Campinha-Bacote also recommended qualitative measures such as journals and field notes alongside the IAPCC-SV.

EBP 7.1

Hughes and Hood (2007) described the development, implementation, and evaluation of a multicultural curriculum at St. Luke's College of Nursing (SLCON) in Missouri and its journey to educate future nurses, develop their skills, and deliver culturally congruent care. Students at SLCON are mostly middle class, European American women. Dominant ethnic groups in the community consist of African Americans, Latinos, Native Americans, and Asians. The adoption of a transcultural nursing (TCN) content in the curriculum was part of the SLCON evolution from an associate degree to a baccalaureate program. To guide its curriculum, SLCON adopted the eclectic conceptual frameworks of Betty Neumann, Jean Watson, Leininger, and Giger and Davidhizar.

The Giger and Davidhizar (2008) Transcultural Assessment Model (TAM) was used for its practicality and evidence-based, culture-focused care (Hughes & Hood) in six areas of communication, biological variations, environmental control, space, social organizations, and time (Giger & Davidhizar, 2008). Hughes and Hood indicated that biological variations among cultural groups was incorporated in the physical assessment course; the cultural groups included represented those in the local community as well as nationally.

The SLCON used the *Cross Cultural Evaluation Tool* by Freeman (1993, as cited in Hughes & Hood, 2007). The *CCET* provides a cross-cultural interaction score (CIS), which measures the change in behavior and attitude among students from the courses' TCN content. The researchers administered the *CCET* in the beginning and at the end of the five classes with TCN content.

The student pre- and posttest scores and paired *t*-test results indicated a consistent increase in cultural sensitivity after the implementation of teaching strategies. Some student interventions—such as not considering it unusual if an Asian patient requested warm instead of cold water, obtaining a generator for an Amish patient on mechanical ventilation, and assisting a Moslem patient to face Mecca for prayers—also reflected some depth of cultural sensitivity.

(continued)

EBP 7.1 (continued)

Applications to Practice

Analyze the course you are taking/teaching. How are cultural concepts integrated throughout the baccalaureate curriculum?

■ If you were to replicate this study, how would you conduct it? What would you change in terms of conceptual framework, method, sampling, and analysis of findings?

■ What other tools could you think of that could measure cultural competence among students and faculty? Would you have used it in this study instead of the CCT? Why?

———————

Source: Hughes & Hood (2007).

CRITICAL THINKING EXERCISES 7.1

Undergraduate Student
1. You often hear faculty at your school say that you need to develop cultural awareness as you begin to care for culturally diverse clients in your clinical rotations and when you graduate. How comfortable are you when working with clients from cultures other than your own?
2. Do you think there is enough content of cultural diversity and promotion of cultural competence integrated in your skills modules, in LRC learning, and in clinical?
3. Have you had opportunities to care for culturally diverse clients during your clinical rotation? Describe.

Faculty in Academia
1. How many credits do you have in this skills course? Do you think you have enough hours in this course to weave in TCN content?
2. Is it possible to add a credit or credits in the current skills course? If yes, how? If not, why?
3. How do you critically appraise diversity and promotion of cultural competence in your current skills course?

Staff Development Educator
1. Do you have students in skills courses on clinical rotation at your facility? In what units are they placed?
2. What clinical activities do these students engage in?
3. Do these students have opportunities to care for culturally diverse clients? Are there additional learning activities such as interprofessional planning of care where cultural care is integrated?
4. Are you planning to provide a workshop/conference on cultural diversity? Who will be attending this workshop?

SUMMARY

In this chapter, the authors explored both integration of TCN concepts and teaching strategies for nursing and some interprofessional collaboration with students from allied health. It is imperative that cultural diversity and promotion of cultural competence be woven and threaded into nursing skills and foundational courses. These lay the groundwork for beginning students in their journey to becoming registered nurses who are ready to meet the challenges of health care in the 21st century.

REFERENCES

Aadil, N., Houti, I. E., & Moussamih, S. (2004). Drug intake during Ramadan. *British Medical Journal, 129,* 778–782.

American Association of Colleges of Nursing. (1995). *Interdisciplinary education and practice.* Retrieved May 30, 2012, from http//www.accn.nche.edu/publication/position/interdisciplinary

Billings, D. M., & Halstead, J. A. (2005). *Teaching in nursing: A guide for faculty* (2nd ed.). St. Louis, MO: Elsevier Saunders.

Campinha-Bacote, J. (2007). *The process of cultural competence in the delivery of healthcare services: The journey continues.* Cincinnati, OH: Transcultural C.A.R.E. Resources.

Decker, S., Gore, T., & Feken, C. (2011). Simulation. In T. J. Bristol & J. Zerwekh (Eds.), *Essentials for e-learning for nurse educators* (pp. 277–294). Philadelphia, PA: FA Davis.

Edberg, M. (2013). *Essentials of health, culture, and diversity: Understanding people, reducing disparities.* Burlington, VT: Jones & Bartlett Learning.

Gaberson, K. B., & Oermann, M. H. (1999). *Clinical teaching strategies in nursing.* New York, NY: Springer Publishing.

Giger, J. N., & Davidhizar, R. E. (2008). *Transcultural nursing: Assessment and intervention* (5th ed.). St. Louis, MO: Mosby Elsevier.

Hasnain, M., Connel, K. J., Menon, L., & Tranmer, P. A. (2011). Patient-centered care for Muslim women: Provider and patient perspectives. *Journal of Women's Health, 20*(1), 73–83.

Heller, B. R., Oros, M. T., & Durney-Cowley, J. (2011). *The future of nursing education: Ten trends to watch.* Retrieved May 30, 2012, from www.nln.org/nlnjournal/infotrends.htm#2

Hughes, K. H., & Hood, L. J. (2007). Teaching methods and an outcome tool for measuring cultural sensitivity in undergraduate nursing students. *Journal of Transcultural Nursing, 18*(1), 57–62. doi:10.1177/1043659606294196

Institute of Medicine. (2010, October 5). *The future of nursing: Leading change, advancing health.* Washington, DC: National Academies Press.

Kardong-Edgreen, S., & Campinha-Bacote, J. (2008). Cultural competency of graduating US Bachelor of Science nursing students. *Contemporary Nurse, 28,* 37–44.

Kiel, C., Stein, C., Webb, L., Billings, V., & Rozenblitt, L. (2008). Discerning the division of cognitive labor: An emerging understanding of how knowledge is clustered in other minds. *Cognitive Science, 32,* 259–300. doi:10.1080/03640210701863339

Lawrence, P., & Razmus, C. (2001). Culturally sensitive care of the Muslim patient. *Journal of Transcultural Nursing, 12,* 228–233.

Li, S. (2007, April). *The role of simulation in nursing education: A regulatory perspective.* Powerpoint presentation at the AACN Hot Issues Conference, Denver, CO. Retrieved June 15, 2013, from www.google.com/search?hl=en&rls=commicrosoft%3Aenus&q=simulation+and+nursing+education&btnG=Search&aq=f&aqi=g1&aql=&oq=&gs_rfai=

National Research Council. (2000). *How people learn: Brain, mind, experience, and school.* Washington, DC: National Academies Press.

Pathy, R., Mills, K. E., Gazzeley, S., Ridgley, A., & Kiran, T. (2011). Health is a spiritual thing: Perspectives of health care professionals and female Somali and Bangladeshi women on the health impacts of fasting during Ramadan. *Ethnicity & Health, 16*(1), 47–56.

Purnell, L. D. (2013). *Transcultural health care: A culturally competent approach*. Philadelphia, PA: F. A. Davis.

Rauen, C. (2001). Using simulation to teach critical thinking skills: You can't just throw the book at them. *Critical Care Nurse Clinics North America, 13*, 93–103.

Rose, P. R. (2011). *Cultural competency for health administration and public health*. Boston, MA: Jones & Bartlett.

Rowles, C. J., & Brigham, C. (2005). Strategies to promote critical thinking and active learning. In D. Billings & J. Halstead (Eds.), *Teaching nursing: A guide for faculty* (2nd ed., pp. 283–315). St. Louis, MO: Elsevier/Saunders.

Shearer, R. G., & Davidhizar, R. (2003). Using role play to develop cultural competence. *Journal of Nursing Education, 42*(6), 273–276.

Sheets, D. L., & El-Azhary, R. A. (2000). The Arab Muslim client: Implications for anesthesia. *Journal of the American Association of Nurse Anesthetists, 66*(7), 304–312.

Sullivan Commission. (2004). *Missing persons: Minorities in the health professions: A report of the Sullivan Commission on diversity in the health care workforce*. Retrieved July 26, 2013, from http://health-equity.pitt.edu/40/1/Sullivan_Final_Report_000.pdf

Taylor, C., Lillis, C., LeMone, P., & Lynn, P. (2011). *Fundamentals of nursing: The art and science of nursing care* (7th ed.). Philadelphia, PA: Lippincott Williams & Wilkins.

U.S. Department of Education Office of Education and Improvement. (2010). *Technology and educational reform*. Retrieved May 20, 2012, from www2.ed.gov/pubs/EdReform Studies/EdTech/index.html.

U.S. Department of Health and Human Services, & Office of Minority Health. (2010). *National partnership for action to end health disparities*. Retrieved February 2, 2013, from www.healthypeople.gov/2020/about/DisparitiesAbout.aspx

U.S. Department of Health and Human Services, & Office of Minority Health. (2013). *The national standards for culturally and linguistically appropriate services in health and health care* (the *national CLAS standards*). Retrieved May 25, 2013, from https://www.thinkculturalhealth.hhs.gov/pdfs/EnhancedNationalCLASStandards.pdf

Wiggins, G. (1998). *Educative assessment: Designing assessments to inform and improve student performance*. San Francisco, CA: Jossey-Bass.

Wilkinson, J. M., & Treas, L. S. (2011). *Fundamentals of nursing: Volume 1. Theory, concepts, and applications*. Philadelphia, PA: F. A. Davis.

Health Assessment and Physical Examination

Drew Y. Sagar and Priscilla Limbo Sagar

CHAPTER

8

KEY TERMS

Apocrine
Biocultural variations
Bisexual
Blood pressure (BP)
Chloasma
Cultural assessment
Culture-bound syndromes
Culturologic nursing assessment
Cyanosis
Ecchymosis
Erythema
Ethnicity
Ethnohistory
Folk diseases
Folk healing
Folk illnesses
Gay

Icteric
Jaundice
Keloid
Lesbian
Lesbian, gay, bisexual, and transgender
Leukoedema
Limited English proficiency
Melisma
Mongolian spots
Objective data
Pallor
Petechiae
Pseudofolliculitis
Race
Subjective data
Transgender
Vitiligo

LEARNING OBJECTIVES

At the completion of this chapter, the learner will be able to

1. Discuss the process of obtaining a cultural history and performing a comprehensive health assessment for an individual, family, or group from a diverse cultural background.
2. Identify biocultural differences affecting the appearance of individuals or groups of diverse ethnicities.
3. Analyze cultural factors influencing the perception of health and illness among individuals of divergent ethnic groups.

4. Propose strategies used when caring for gender and sexual minorities.
5. Discuss methods of patient/client care delivery congruent to culturally competent care.
6. Describe the concept of culture and cultural diversity.
7. Distinguish between culture and ethnicity.

OVERVIEW

Cultural assessment or *culturologic nursing assessment* is performed to determine the client's health care needs and to provide culturally congruent care (Leininger, 2002; Leininger & McFarland, 2006). Cultural assessment needs to be integrated in all health assessment and physical assessment courses. It is paramount that this cultural assessment be linguistically appropriate.

The population of the United States is progressively becoming more culturally and ethnically diverse. Currently at 37%, the U.S. minority populations are projected to be the majority by the year 2060 at 57% (U.S. Census Bureau, 2012). About 12% to 19% of the U.S. population is non-English speakers; this translates to 52 million people from age 5 years and older (Andrews & Boyle, 2008; Berry-Caban & Crespo, 2008). The Sullivan Commission (2004) stated that 2 out of 10 Americans speak a language other than English at home. These are alarming statistics and an enormous concern—considering that language is fundamental in navigating the health care system (Stanhope & Lancaster, 2010) and is cited most frequently as the primary barrier to health care (Berry-Caban & Crespo, 2008).

The culturally and linguistically appropriate services (CLAS) standards mandates that every agency or institution that receives federal funding use interpreters (for spoken language) or a translator (for written language) for people who are unable to speak English or for those with **limited English proficiency (LEP)** (U.S. Department of Health and Human Services, Office of Minority Health, 2013). For more information about CLAS standards, see Chapter 3. In concordance with CLAS standards, The Joint Commission (TJC, 2010a, 2010b) released new and revised standards in 2010 for client-focused communication as part of a program to advocate for effective communication, enhance cultural competence, and uphold client and family-centered interventions. TJC devised client-focused communication to expand client safety and quality of care as well as to motivate hospitals to foster practices promoting improved communication and client engagement.

Integration of TCN Concepts

When planning revisions to existing health assessment and physical examination courses, concepts of race, ethnicity, and relationship between ethnicity and incidence of illness need to be integrated. The variations in physical examination and laboratory results must also be included. The discussion in this chapter is not meant to replace coverage of an inclusive, thorough health and physical assessment; this covers suggestions as to transcultural nursing (TCN) areas of inclusion for culturally and linguistically appropriate care.

Race is a division of a species which differs from other divisions by the frequency with which certain hereditary traits occur among its members (Brues, 1977, as cited by Overfield, 1985). Leininger (1995, 2006) describes **ethnicity** as a term that refers to an individual's or group's social identity or past origins as related to language, religion, and national origins, and considers the word to be a vague and ill-defined term in its present usage. She prefers instead to use the term *culture* in its place, because it has well-defined characteristics and is more inclusive, as it refers to both people's ways of life and their biologic racial characteristics.

Biocultural Variations in Diseases

Research evidence reveals a relationship between ethnicity and the incidence of illness across the life span. Having the knowledge of normal **biocultural variations** as well as variations during illness will assist health care professionals to organize a more accurate, systematic, and comprehensive health assessment and physical examination (Andrews, 2012a). Table 8.1 shows common illnesses among selected ethnic groups.

TABLE 8.1 Commonly Occurring Genetic Disorders Among Selected Ethnic Groups

Ethnic Groups	Commonly Occurring Genetic Disorder
Amish	Ocular albinism Limb Girdle muscular dystrophy Ellis Van-Creveld syndrome (dwarfism) Pyruvate kinase deficiency Cartilage hair hyperplasia Phenylketonuria Glutamic aciduria
Blacks	Sickle-cell disease Hemoglobin C disorder G-6-PD deficiency, African type Adult lactase deficiency Systemic lupus erythematosus Beta thalassemia
Chinese	Alpha thalassemia G-6-PD deficiency, Chinese type Adult lactase deficiency
English	Cystic fibrosis Hereditary amyloidosis
Jews, Ashkenazi Jews, Sephardi	Tay Sach's disease (infantile) Niemann-Pick disease (infantile) Gaucher disease (adult) Factor XI deficiency Familial Mediterranean fever Ataxia-telangiectasia
Scots	Phenylketonuria Cystic fibrosis

Sources: Andrews (2012a); Giger & Davidhizar (2008); and Wenger & Wenger (2013).

Cultural Health Assessment

According to Andrews (2012a), there are two components to cultural assessment: the *process* component and the *content* component. The process component consists of the nurse's method of data gathering, attention to both verbal and nonverbal communication, and the system and order of data gathering. The content component consists of data groupings under which information about the client is collected. The two major sections of cultural assessment comprise both the health history and the physical examination (Andrews, 2012a).

The health history is aimed at gathering **subjective data,** which is what people say or convey about themselves. **Objective data** are obtained by observation through inspection, percussion, and auscultation, and by using laboratory results along with the physical examination (Andrews, 2012a; Jarvis, 2012).

Sources of information. When obtaining the health history, it is important to note the source of information. Mention the specific language or dialect spoken by the client as well as the use of an interpreter. Document the client's cultural affiliation and **ethnohistory**. The ethnohistory is not only helpful in assessment of risk factors for hereditary and acquired diseases but also in determining cultural heritage (Andrews, 2012a).

Reasons for seeking care. Since the time of birth, people develop perspectives about health and illness within their culture, including the sick role. In the client's own statement, document the client's reason for seeking the health care provider. The client's description of symptoms will vary according to the client's perception of his or her illness based on his or her own sociocultural and ethnohistorical concept (Andrews, 2012a, 2012b). Health care providers must partner with socioculturally and economically diverse clients in the context of gender identity, religious and spiritual beliefs, and the role of being sick (Anderson, Andrews, et al., 2010).

Current and past illnesses. Some diseases have increased prevalence among specific cultural groups. An evolving knowledge of biocultural aspects of illnesses will be vital in the assessment, planning, implementation, and evaluation of care that is linguistically and culturally appropriate.

Religious and spiritual beliefs. Religious and spiritual beliefs, interwoven with culture, profoundly affect the health and illness experience and outcome (Anderson, Andrews, et al., 2010). Recognizing, accepting, and respecting this will be instrumental in the accurate health assessment and physical examination, thus gathering a database for planning, implementation, and evaluation of care that culturally and linguistically fit the client's needs.

Culture-Bound Syndromes

Culture-bound syndromes (CBS), sometimes referred to as **folk illnesses** or **folk diseases,** denote disorders limited to a specific culture or group of cultures (Andrews, 2012a). Although some of the syndromes do not significantly affect health, some could actually be serious, in which case they are often fatal (Basuray, 2013). Aimed at assisting practitioners with culturally congruent care, the *Diagnostic and Statistical Manual of Mental Disorders (DSM-IV)* of the American Psychiatric Association (APA, 2000) developed a glossary of CBS. Table 8.2 shows a selected listing of CBS. The complete listing and discussion of CBS can be found on pp. 897–903 (APA, 2000). Furthermore, the *DSM-5* (APA, 2013) expanded its *Cultural Formulation* (CF) in the assessment and management of mental health problems. The *DSM-5* (APA, 2013) includes the *Cultural Formulation Interview (CFI),* an approach to assessment that has been field tested for usefulness and client acceptability.

TABLE 8.2   A Selection of Cultural Bound Syndromes

	Characteristics	Locality
Amok	Prevalent among males; brooding; outbursts of violent, aggressive, or homicidal behavior aimed at people and objects	Malaysia, Laos, Philippines, Polynesia (cafard or cathard), Papua New Guinea, Puerto Rico, and among Navajo (iich'aa)
Anorexia nervosa, bulimia	Excessive preoccupation with thinness; self-imposed starvation Gross overeating, then vomiting and fasting	Whites
Ataque de nervios	Usually occurs after a stressful family event; uncontrollable shouting, crying, heat in the chest rising to the head; verbal or physical aggression; being out of control; amnesia; return to usual level of functioning	Caribbean Latinos; Latin Americans; Latin Mediterranean
Boufe'e delirante	Sudden outburst of agitated and aggressive behavior, marked confusion, psychomotor excitement; sometimes with visual and auditory hallucinations or paranoid ideation	West Africa, Haiti
Hwa-byung (also wool-hwa-byung)	Anger syndrome; may be due to suppression of anger; insomnia, fatigue, panic, fear of impending death, anorexia, dyspnea, among others; feeling of mass in the epigastrium	Korea
Koro	Sudden and intense anxiety that the penis (vulva and nipples in females) will recede into the body and may cause death; may be in localized epidemic form	Southeast Asia (China, shuk yang, shook yong, suo yang; Thailand, rok-joo)
Mal de ojo (evil eye)	Children are especially at risk; fitful sleep; crying without cause, diarrhea, vomiting, fever. Sometimes occurs in adult females	Mediterranean
Pibloktoq	Abrupt dissociative episode with severe excitement; usually followed by convulsions and coma for 12 hours; complete amnesia of the attack; tearing of own clothes, breaking of furniture, eating feces	Arctic and subarctic Eskimo communities
Spell	Trance state; may "communicate with dead relatives or spirits"; short periods of personality change	Blacks and EuroAmericans from the southern United States
Susto (fright or soul loss, pasmo)	Attributed to a terrifying event that causes the soul to leave the body, resulting in unhappiness and illness. Somatic: muscle aches and pains, headache, diarrhea. Ritual healing: calling the soul back to the body and cleansing the individual to reestablish bodily and spiritual balance. Differing experience may be connected to major depressive or post-traumatic stress disorders.	Latinos in the United States; Mexico, Central America, South America

Source: Adapted from American Psychiatric Association (2000).

VARIATIONS IN GENDER IDENTITY: LESBIAN, GAY, BISEXUAL, TRANSGENDER HEALTH

It is imperative that care of **lesbian, gay, bisexual, or transgender (LGBT)** individuals be integrated in the content of nursing and allied health curricula. In addition, LGBT training for staff needs to be planned, implemented, and evaluated to ensure that this important content is part of the continuing competence of all health care professionals. There is a marked need for curricular content in the health care needs of the LGBT population in medicine (Rutherford, McIntyre, Daley, & Ross, 2012).

According to the USDHHS (2010), in 2002, about 4% of the U.S. population between the ages of 18 to 44 years acknowledged themselves as LGBT. Individuals who identify in the gender and sexual minorities undergo continuing stigma, discrimination, and threats to safety even early in life. In a survey of 8,584 students ages 13 through 20 years from all 50 states and the District of Columbia, the Gay, Lesbian, and Straight Education Network (GLSEN, 2011) revealed overwhelming hostility of the school environment. LGBT students experience painful homophobic remarks (up to 84.9%), discrimination, harassment (81%), and assault at school (38.3%; GLSEN, 2011). For more information about this landmark study, see EBP 8.1.

EBP 8.1

The National School Climate Survey (2011), conducted by the Gay Lesbian Straight Education Network (GLSEN), included 8,584 students of lesbian, gay, bisexual, or transgender (LGBT) identity. The respondents to the survey comprised a sample that represented students between the ages of 13 and 20 years old from grades 6 through 12 and were from the 50 states as well as the District of Columbia. More than two-thirds of students identified themselves as White (67.9%), slightly less than one-half were female (49.6%), and more than half identified themselves as gay or lesbian (GLSEN, 2011). In order to gain a representative sample of the nation's youth, participants were recruited for the survey using both advertisements through the popular social networking Internet website Facebook as well as implementing outreach through groups providing support services to LGBT youth on local, regional, and national levels (GLSEN, 2011).

The study examines multiple aspects of personal experience that are negatively affected by bias and discrimination related to LGBT identity. It also explores interventions that have been effective in promoting positive change in the social environment encountered by students and, by extension, their sense of well-being and self-image. Some of the areas of negative impact in which LGBT students experience bias include (1) hearing hostile or homophobic remarks; (2) fearing for personal safety associated with assault and harassment; and (3) resorting to truancy from classes and school days because of feeling threatened or unsafe, resulting from their LGBT identity and or racial/ethnic heritage.

Other areas addressed in the study were the impact of the bias experience on students' academic performance and aspirations for pursuit of college or technical

(continued)

school education, reporting of incidents of harassment/bullying by students to school officials and/or other adults, as well as their respective responses to reported incidents (GLSEN, 2011).

Additionally, the study explores accessibility of various supports available to LGBT students such as Gay Straight Alliance Groups (GSAs) and access to materials related to LGBT issues within the school library or school computers. Additional measures include the frequency with which the addition of LGBT issues such as the Stonewall riots of 1969 in Greenwich Village, New York, and prominent gay/lesbian persons in history are included in school curriculum (GLSEN, 2011).

The GLSEN study proposes multiple solutions to address the issue of LGBT bias and harassment and its sequelae. Among the solutions proposed are the formation of GSAs for students in the schools, providing an inclusive curriculum, strict antibias bullying and harassment policies, and supportive educators.

The survey reported that students who attend schools with an active GSA were less likely to hear derogatory remarks such as "faggot" or "dyke" or the word "gay" used in a negative manner. LGBT students were also less likely to feel unsafe based on their sexuality, and staff members and faculty were more likely to intervene when incidents of harassment or bullying related to issues of sexual identity were witnessed in a school with an active GSA and effective policies against bullying (GLSEN, 2011).

The presence of an inclusive curriculum in the school encourages a supportive environment and a sense of belonging for LGBT students; this results in less absenteeism and harassment of students. Students supported by faculty demonstrate better grades and improved prospects for tertiary education.

Applications to Practice

■ Investigate your nursing program mission and philosophy in terms of diversity and cultural competence. Are these actually threaded in the curriculum? Do you see LGBT content in various nursing courses?
■ Analyze the course you are taking/teaching. How is diversity in theory and in clinical?
■ If you were to replicate this study, how would you conduct it? What would you change in terms of conceptual framework, sampling, and analysis of findings?

Source: Gay, Lesbian, & Straight Education Network (2011).

Physical Examination

It is important to note biocultural variations when performing cultural assessment as well as when conducting the head to toe physical examination. In some cultures, **folk healing** practices such as coining and cupping may leave skin marks similar to bruising. The health care providers' awareness of these practices will be helpful when distinguishing markings from folk practices and from possible abuse. See Chapter 14 for discussions of generic folk healing practices.

Variations in Skin Color

Skin color is the most obvious characteristic among groups of people and is determined by the presence of melanin within the epidermal layer of the skin. Melanocytes originate in the neural crest near the embryonic central nervous system, then migrate to the epidermis during fetal development (Wasserman, 1974, as cited by Overfield, 1985). Melanocytes produce melanosomes, which inject melanin particles into the skin. It is generally accepted that darker skin tones have a greater degree of protection from the harmful effects of sun exposure. The melanosomes of Black people are longer and broader than those of Whites, Asians, and Native Americans, presenting a more even distribution under the skin that provides better protection (Overfield, 1985).

The darker the client's skin, the more challenging it is to assess for changes in color (Giger & Davidhizar, 2008). Establishing a baseline skin color is vital. The best light source is daylight (Anderson, Boyle, et al., 2010; Giger & Davidhizar, 2008).

Mongolian spots. Mongolian spots are areas of dark pigmentation presenting with a bluish hue; they are caused by melanocytes that remain in deeper layers of tissue, particularly in the lumbosacral area. These spots can most often be seen on the buttocks of the lower back but are sometimes found on the arms, thighs, and abdomen (Jarvis, 2012). Because of their color, appearance, and location, Mongolian spots can be mistaken for bruises and consequently raise suspicions of child abuse among health care professionals unfamiliar with their appearance (Anderson, Boyle, et al., 2010). Mongolian spots occur most frequently in dark-skinned people with a frequency of approximately 90% among Blacks, 80% among Asians and the indigenous people of North America, and 9% among Caucasians (Walton, 1976, as cited by Overfield, 1985; Giger & Davidhizar, 2008; Overfield, 1995, as cited by Andrews, 2012a).

Vitiligo. Vitiligo, or nonpigmented areas on the skin surface, is a condition whereby the melanocytes become nonfunctional and present with the appearance of colorless areas of the skin. Appearing on the face, neck, hands, feet, and body orifices, the presence of vitiligo has the greatest effect on dark-skinned people and may cause disturbances in body image (Jarvis, 2012). This condition is also statistically linked with an increased incidence of hyperthyroidism, diabetes mellitus, and pernicious anemia (Overfield, 1995, as cited by Andrews, 2012a; Overfield, 1985).

Leukoedema. Leukoedema appears as grayish-white lesions that may be present on the buccal mucosa. Leukoedema may be found among Blacks (68–90%) and Whites (43%); this may be mistaken for pathologic conditions such as thrush (Overfield, 1995, as cited by Andrews, 2012; Overfield, 1985). Oral hyperpigmentation is a condition thought to be related to an accumulation of postinflammatory changes that increases in frequency with age. This condition affects up to 10% of White and 90% of Black peoples. Leukoedema is also common among East Indians (Jarvis, 2012).

Cyanosis. Cyanosis is defined as the abnormal blue color of skin, which may be difficult to assess in people with dark skin pigmentation (Andrews, 2012a; Spector, 2013). The bluish mottling indicates decreased perfusion; this could occur in shock, heart failure, bronchitis, and congenital heart disease (Jarvis, 2012). Other signs are ashen gray lips and tongue (Spector, 2013). In darkly pigmented people, it is best to examine the palms of the hands, soles of the feet, lips, tongue, and conjunctiva, and may be assessed by pressing on the palms; a slow blood return indicates cyanosis (Spector, 2013). Accompanying signs such as tachypnea, the use of accessory respiratory muscles, and complaints of dyspnea should be included in the observation (Overfield, 1995, as cited by Andrews, 2012).

Jaundice. Jaundice, abnormal yellow color of the skin and eyes, is best assessed in the sclera of both light- and dark-skinned people. One thing that needs to be considered, however, is that the sclera of many dark-skinned people may have fat deposits containing high levels of carotene, causing a yellow discoloration to the sclera (Overfield, 1995, as cited by Andrews, 2012; Spector, 2013). The palate may be assessed in darkly pigmented people. If the surface of the palate is free from heavy melanin deposits, the presence of jaundice may be determined there. The absence of jaundice to the palate when the sclera appears yellow is indicative of carotene pigmentation rather than jaundice (Overfield, 1995, as cited by Andrews, 2012).

The tongue and the mucosa may have oral hyperpigmentation; this alters the value of the oral mucosa as a site for assessment (Anderson, Boyle, et al., 2010). Compared to Whites at 10% to 50%, 50% to 90% of Blacks may have oral hyperpigmentation (Giger & Davidhizar, 2008).

Pallor. Pallor, or colorless appearance, presents as an absence of underlying red pink skin tones from the oxygenated hemoglobin in the blood, taking on the color of connective tissue which is mostly white (Jarvis, 2012). Brown-skinned people show a yellowish-brown appearance; black-skinned people present with an ashen gray appearance (Spector, 2013). The lips, oral mucosa, and nail beds should also be assessed (Anderson, Boyle, et al., 2010; Overfield, 1995, as cited by Andrews, 2012a; Spector, 2013).

Erythema. Erythema, or redness due to excess blood in dilated superficial capillaries, may be difficult to assess in dark-complexioned people. It may be associated with inflammation, localized swelling, and increased skin temperatures. The hands may be used to assess for warmth, for firmness in underlying tissue, and for tightness of stretched skin surfaces associated with swelling (Jarvis, 2012). The dorsal aspects of the hands are more sensitive than the palmar surface and may be used to assess skin temperature that may be increased with inflammation (Overfield, 1995, as cited by Andrews, 2012a; Spector, 2013).

Petechiae. Petechiae are small hemorrhagic spots in the skin. These are difficult to assess in dark-complexioned people and it is best assessed in less-pigmented areas such as the abdomen and buttocks. In Black or very dark-skinned people it may not be identifiable on skin surfaces and is seen on the surfaces of mucous membranes in the oral cavity or on the conjunctival surface (Anderson, Boyle, et al., 2010; Overfield, 1995, as cited by Andrews, 2012a).

Ecchymosis. Ecchymosis, hemorrhagic areas in the skin larger than petechiae, is assessed similarly to petechiae in the same locations. In order to differentiate between erythema, petechiae, and ecchymosis, the application of light pressure to tissue surfaces will blanche erythema but not ecchymosis or petechiae (Overfield, 1995, as cited by Andrews, 2012a). Ecchymosis denotes a history of trauma to a specific area and can be detected from swelling of that area (Spector, 2013).

Melasma or Chloasma. Melasma or chloasma, mask of pregnancy, is a patchy tan or dark brown discoloration of the face that is more common in dark-skinned women (Spector, 2013) and is possibly due to hyperestrogenemia (Jarvis, 2012). This may present as hyperpigmentation, particularly on the forehead, cheek bones, and upper lip in women who are pregnant or in women using birth control pills. The cause is unknown, but if it occurs as a result of pregnancy it generally fades within 6 months postpartum; if it is related to the use of oral contraceptive use it may never fade (Overfield, 1985). In contrast, Jarvis (2012) asserted that this condition could fade after stopping the pills.

Keloid. A keloid is a scar formation that develops at the site of surface wounds or incisions. The scar tissue formation is unusually large, extending beyond the dimensions of the wound in area and elevation, and may continue to enlarge after healing occurs (Spector, 2013). The hypertrophic scar appears smooth, akin to rubber, and claw-like; this has a higher incidence among Blacks but may also occur among Whites (Jarvis, 2012). In some instances, the scars from trauma, surgical incision, ear piercing, or intravenous infusion may be ropelike and represent the wound healing process (Giger & Davidhizar, 2008).

Pseudofolliculitis. Pseudofolliculitis is ingrown hairs and razor bumps that are common to Blacks (Jarvis, 2012; Spector, 2013). As the name implies, these occur in areas where shaving is performed either with an electric or blade razor. This occurs as the result of an immune response triggered when hair is shaved too closely, causing the end to enter the skin; this triggers a range of responses including inflammation, papules, pustules, and even keloid formation (Spector, 2013).

Variations in Secretions

There are approximately 2–3 million eccrine glands that open through pores onto the surface of the skin. These glands play a key role in both thermoregulations through the process of sweating, and fluid and electrolyte balance through chlorides that are contained in sweat (Overfield, 1995, as cited by Andrews, 2012a; Overfield, 1985).

The **apocrine** sweat glands are largely responsible for body odor and are located in the axillary, perineal, anal, and areola areas, becoming active during puberty. The number of both types of sweat glands is variable by race. In Eskimo peoples, the majority of eccrine glands are located on their faces with relatively few located on other surfaces. This appears to be an adaptive response to a cold environment, allowing more sweat production from the face in order to keep clothing dry, thus reducing the risk of associated hypothermia (Andrews, 2012a). Native American and Asian peoples have relatively few apocrine glands in comparison to Whites and Blacks and consequently have relatively or no body odor by contrast (Overfield, 1985).

Musculoskeletal Variations in Trunk and Extremities

Black and White men are similar in height; however, the sitting or standing height of White men is greater than Blacks because of greater trunk length. The legs of both Black men and women are longer than in Whites. Because of greater trunk length, Whites tend to have greater body fat than Blacks (Overfield, 1985). Additionally, Black men have the longest and narrowest bones of any other group. Asian and Native American peoples have the least bone density of the groups that have been studied (Overfield, 1995, as cited by Andrews, 2012a).

White men have bone density similar to that of Black women, and White women have a bone density that is below that of either group (Overfield, 1985). The greater bone density of Black men appears to correspond to comparatively low rates of osteoporosis in this group (Jarvis, 2012; Overfield, 1995, as cited by Andrews, 2012a). Interestingly, despite lower bone mass densities Asian women demonstrate lower incidence of bone fractures than Whites. The reasons for this are not fully understood, but it may be related to micro bone structure development and cultural and environmental factors associated with muscle strength and fall risk (Cooper & Ballard, 2011).

There is a wide variance of the curvature of the long bones of people from diverse cultures. Comparatively, it is interesting to look at these femoral characteristics: Native Americans and first Nation People of Canada (anteriorly convex), Blacks (straight), and Whites (intermediate; Andrews, 2012a; Jarvis, 2012). The heavier density of bones among Blacks may possibly help protect them from increased curvature related to obesity (Andrews, 2012a; Jarvis, 2012).

Variations in Measurements

In the performance of health assessment of multicultural and multiethnic people, variation in vital signs needs to be considered. It is well documented that in the United States Black Americans experience a greater morbidity and mortality from chronic diseases such as hypertension and related cardiovascular diseases. Thirty-five to 40% of Blacks have hypertension; this accounts for 20% of Black deaths (Giger & Davidhizar, 2008).

In order to reduce risks of cardiovascular events, patient education about **blood pressure (BP)** needs to be integrated in health assessment and physical examination courses. The blood pressure categories of the American Heart Association (AHA; American Heart Association, 2012) indicate these guidelines: normal BP (120 systolic, less than 80 diastolic); prehypertension (systolic 120–139 and diastolic 80–89); and high BP (140–159 systolic and diastolic 90–99). However, there are recommendations to maintain blood pressure controls with systolic blood pressure less than 130 and diastolic less than 80 with inherent risk factors for coronary artery disease or diabetes mellitus present (Bertoia, Waring, Gupta, Roberts, & Eaton, 2011). This is the standard for care regardless of ethnic or racial heritage.

It is likely that ethnic variations in cardiovascular status are apparent quite early in life. The pulse rate among Black neonates averages 6–9 beats per minute more than among White American neonates with and without socioeconomic control, respectively. The tendency for higher pulse rates in neonates is possibly linked to later trends in blood pressure elevation (Schacter, Lachin, & Wimberly, 1976, as cited by Overfield, 1985).

Comparison of BP reading indicates that as adults Black Americans have higher blood pressure than White or European American people (Giger & Davidhizar, 2008; Reed, 1981; Rowland & Roberts, 1982; as cited by Overfield, 1985). While it has been accepted that Black males in late adolescence and early adulthood possess a tendency for lower blood pressure than their White male counterparts until their mid-30s, at which time this trend reverses and the average blood pressure for Black males is approximately 5 mmHg higher. This tendency remains constant until the age of 65 when it approximately equalizes for both groups (Overfield, 1995, as cited by Andrews, 2012a). Interestingly, however, there is evidence to suggest that this trend may begin significantly earlier. A recent 15-year longitudinal study by Wang et al. (2006) of ambulatory blood pressure monitoring demonstrated that Black Americans experience higher systolic and diastolic blood pressure at a much younger age than previously thought. Additionally, nocturnal blood pressure recordings were significantly higher with systolic blood pressure readings of 1.5 and 4 mm day and night, respectively. Diastolic blood pressure recordings were similarly higher at 1 and 3 mm day and night, respectively, than among White American counterparts (Wang et al., 2006).

CRITICAL THINKING EXERCISES 8.1

Undergraduate Student

1. How comfortable are you with taking a health history and performing a physical examination?
2. Do you think there is enough content of cultural diversity and promotion of cultural competence integrated in your physical assessment classes (theory) and in clinical?
3. Would you be in favor of taking SLMs in health history and performance of physical assessment? Why?

Graduate Student

1. How many advanced physical assessment course(s) do you have in your graduate program? Are concepts in diversity integrated in those courses, both in the didactic and practicum portions?
2. Do you have opportunities to manage care for culturally diverse clients and their families?
3. How comfortable are you in implementing culturally and linguistically appropriate services? Is this type of care a focus at your institution?
4. How often do you come across LGBT families? Are you comfortable managing their care? Describe.

Faculty in Academia

1. Have you woven diversity and cultural competence in your health history and physical assessment courses, both in didactic and in practice portions? Describe.
2. Is the care of LGBT families threaded in your curriculum? Analyze.
3. How do you critically appraise culturally and linguistically appropriate concepts in your courses?

Staff Development Educator

1. How do you measure continuing competence in history and performance of physical assessment among nurses in your institution?
2. Do you have a simulation laboratory for staff practice of skills?
3. Do the staff development specialists supervise some of these practice sessions? Are staff members reimbursed for their time to complete required CE in client assessment and physical examination? How many hours are eligible for reimbursement?

SUMMARY

The United States is progressively becoming culturally and ethnically diverse. People who do not speak English as well as those with LEP are increasing. A comprehensive, culturally and linguistically appropriate health assessment and physical examination is key to achieving positive client outcomes. Students need a sound background in these skills, and practicing nurses require intrinsic and extrinsic motivation to pursue this as continuing competence. There are wide biological variations in between and among racial and ethnic groups; knowing these variations will assist students and health care professionals to hone their skills of health assessment and physical examination.

REFERENCES

American Heart Association. (2012). *About high blood pressure*. Retrieved July 7, 2013, from www. heart.org/HEARTORG/Conditions/HighBloodPressure/AboutHighBloodPressure/Understanding-Blood-Pressure-Readings_UCM_301764_Article.jsp

American Psychiatric Association. (2000). *Diagnostic and statistical manual of mental disorders* (4th ed., text rev.; Arlington, VA: American Psychiatric Publishing.

American Psychiatric Association. (2013). *Diagnostic and statistical manual of mental disorders* (5th ed., text rev.; *DSM-V-TR*). Arlington, VA: American Psychiatric Publishing.

Anderson, N. L. R., Boyle, J. S., Davidhizar, R. E., Giger, J. N., McFarland, M. R., Papadopoulos, R.,...Wehbe-Alamah, H. (2010). Cultural health assessment. In M. K. Douglas & D. F. Pacquiao (Eds.), *Core curriculum for transcultural nursing and health care*. Thousand Oaks, CA: Dual printing as supplement to *Journal of Transcultural Nursing, 21*(1), 307S–336S.

Anderson, N. L. R., Andrews, M. M., Bent, K. N., Douglas, M. K., Elhamoummi, C., Keenan, C.,...Mattson, S. (2010). Culturally based health and illness beliefs and practices across the lifespan. In M. K. Douglas & D. F. Pacquiao (Eds.), *Core curriculum for transcultural nursing and health care*. Thousand Oaks, CA: Sage. Dual printing as supplement to *Journal of Transcultural Nursing, 21*(1), 152S–235S.

Andrews, M. M. (2012a). Cultural competence in the health history and physical examination. In M. M. Andrews & J. S. Boyle (Eds.), *Transcultural concepts in nursing care* (6th ed., pp. 38–72). Philadelphia PA: Wolters Kluwer Health/Lippincott Williams & Wilkins.

Andrews, M. M. (2012b). The influence of cultural and health belief systems on health care practices. In M. M. Andrews & J. S. Boyle (Eds.), *Transcultural concepts in nursing care* (6th ed., pp. 73–88). Philadelphia, PA: Wolters Kluwer/Lippincott Williams & Wilkins.

Andrews, M. M., & Boyle, J. S. (2008). *Transcultural concepts in nursing care* (5th ed.). Philadelphia, PA: Wolters Kluwer/Lippincott Williams & Wilkins.

Basuray, J. M. (2013). Health beliefs across cultures: Understanding transcultural care. In J. M. Basuray (Eds.), *Culture & health: Concept and practice* (Rev. ed., pp. 58–84). Ronkonkoma, NY: Linus.

Bertoia, M.,Waring, M., Gupta, P., Roberts, M., & Eaton, C. (2011). Implications of new hypertension guidelines in the United States. *Hypertension, 58,* 361–366. Retrieved June 6, 2013, from http://hyper.ahajournals.org/content/58/3/361.long

Berry-Caban, C. S., & Crespo, H. (2008). Cultural competency as a skill for health care providers. *Hispanic Health International, 6*(3), 115–121.

Cooper, C. M., & Ballard, J. E. (2011). Bone mineral density in Hispanic women: A review of literature with implications for promoting culturally relevant osteoporosis education. *Journal of Healthcare for the Poor and Underserved, 22*(2), 450–468.

Gay Lesbian Straight Education Network. (2011). *The 2011 national school climate survey: Key findings on the experiences of lesbian, gay, bisexual, and transgender youth in our nation's school*. Retrieved May 15, 2013, from www.glsen.org/binary-data/GLSEN_ATTACHMENTS/file/000/002/2106–1.pdf

Giger, J. N., & Davidhizar, R. E. (2008). *Transcultural nursing: Assessment and intervention* (5th ed.). St. Louis, MO: Mosby Elsevier.

Jarvis, C. (2012). *Physical examination and health assessment* (6th ed.). St. Louis, MO: Elsevier Saunders.

Leininger, M. M. (2002). Culture care assessments for congruent competency practice. In M. Leininger & M. R. McFarland (Eds.), *Transcultural nursing: Concepts, theories, research, and practice* (3rd ed., pp. 117–143). New York, NY: McGraw-Hill.

Leininger, M. M. (2006). Culture care diversity and universality theory and evolution of the ethnonursing method. In M. M. Leininger & M. R. McFarland (Eds.), *Culture care diversity and universality: A worldwide nursing theory* (2nd ed., pp. 1–41). Sudbury, MA: Jones & Bartlett.

Leininger, M. M., & McFarland, M. R. (2006). *Culture care diversity and universality: A worldwide nursing theory* (2nd ed.). Sudbury, MA: Jones & Bartlett.

Overfield, T. (1985). *Biologic variation in health and illness: Race, age, and sex differences*. Menlo Park, CA: Addison-Wesley.

Rutherford, K., McIntyre, J., Daley, A., & Ross, L. (2012). Development of expertise in mental health service provision for lesbian, gay, bisexual, and transgender communities. *Medical Education, 46,* 903–913. doi:10.1111/j.1365–2923.2012.04272.x

Spector, R. E. (2013). *Cultural diversity in health and illness* (8th ed.). Upper Saddle River, NJ: Pearson Education.

Stanhope, M., & Lancaster, J. (2010). *Foundations of nursing in the community: Community-oriented practice* (3rd ed.). St. Louis, MO: Mosby/Elsevier.

Sullivan Commission. (2004). *Missing persons: Minorities in the health professions: A report of the Sullivan Commission on diversity in the health care workforce.* Retrieved July 9, 2013, from http://depts.washington.edu/ccph/pdf_files/Sullivan_Report_ES.pdf

The Joint Commission. (2010a). *Advancing effective communication, cultural competence, and patient- and family-centered care: A roadmap for hospitals.* Oakbrook Terrace, IL: Author.

The Joint Commission. (2010b). *Cultural and linguistic care in area hospitals.* Oakbrook Terrace, IL: Author.

U.S. Census Bureau. (2012). *U.S. Census Bureau projections show a slower growing, older, more diverse nation a half century from now.* Retrieved August 3, 2013, from www.census.gov/newsroom/releases/archives/population/cb12–243.html

U.S. Department of Health and Human Services, Office of Minority Health. (2010). *National partnership for action to end health disparities.* Retrieved February 2, 2013, from www.healthypeople.gov/2020/about/DisparitiesAbout.aspx

U.S. Department of Health and Human Services, Office of Minority Health. (2013). *The national standards for culturally and linguistically appropriate services in health and health care* (the *national CLAS standards*). Retrieved May 25, 2013, from https://www.thinkculturalhealth.hhs.gov/pdfs/EnhancedNationalCLASStandards.pdf

Wang, X., Poole, J., Treiber, F., Harshfield, G., Hanevold, C., & Schneider, H. (2006). Ethnic and gender differences in ambulatory blood pressure trajectories: Results from a 15-year longitudinal study in youth and young adults. *Circulation, 114*(25), 2780–2787.

Wenger, A. F., & Wenger, M. R. (2013). The Amish. In L. D. Purnell (Ed.), *Transcultural healthcare: A culturally competent approach* (pp. 115–136). Philadelphia, PA: F. A. Davis.

III. INTEGRATING TCN CONCEPTS ACROSS THE LIFE SPAN

TCN Concepts in Childbearing Courses

Priscilla Limbo Sagar and Debra A. Hrelic

KEY TERMS

Binder
Childbearing
Childbearing women
Decision making
Female circumcision (FC)
Female genital mutilation (FGM)
Hot and cold theory
Lesbian, gay, bisexual, transgender

Naming the baby
Perinatal period
Pica
Placenta
Prescriptive behavior
Restrictive behavior
Taboo
Time orientation (past, present, future)

LEARNING OBJECTIVES

At the completion of this chapter, the learner will be able to

1. Discuss the importance of integrating transcultural concepts in childbearing courses.
2. Analyze important transcultural concepts to include in childbearing courses.
3. Organize three activities to promote cultural sensitivity among students when caring for childbearing clients.
4. Compare and contrast childbearing practices among diverse cultures.
5. Identify at least three issues requiring transcultural awareness in perinatal nursing.

OVERVIEW

Improving maternal health is one of the eight millennium goals of the United Nations (UN) to be achieved by the year 2015 (United Nations, 2000). Nurse educators are in a unique position to affect the next generation of nurses and to bring about awareness, knowledge, and skills in fostering culturally congruent care for **childbearing women**. It is estimated that by the year 2050, more than 50% of the population in the United States will be made up of minorities (Martin et al., 2006; U.S. Census Bureau, 2012). This shift in population composition will increase expectations and demands on health care providers to provide culturally and linguistically appropriate services (CLAS; United States Department of Health and Human Services [USDHHS], Office of Minority Health [OMH], 2013). Muñoz & Luckmann, 2005) to childbearing women and families in the United States.

Surrounding a woman's pregnancy and childbirth are times heavily laden with ritual and health-related traditions; each cultural group has specific practices and approaches (Basuray & Macias, 2013). Health care providers need to be aware that each culture has its own prescriptions, restrictions, and taboos related to pregnancy and childbirth; when followed, these are believed to result in healthy outcomes for both mother and baby (Purnell, 2013b). Culturally **prescriptive behavior** is that which is expected of, advised, about or imposed upon the woman during her pregnancy or **childbearing** period. In contrast, **restrictive behavior** refers to a behavior that is limited or curbed during the **perinatal period**. A behavior that is **taboo** is culturally forbidden or not permitted, and is believed to have grave supernatural implications to both mother and baby.

Childbearing is a period of intense challenges not only for the pregnant woman but also for her family and her support system. There are culturally approved and culturally disapproved practices regarding fertility, pregnancy, birthing, and postpartum; some of these practices may be "prescriptive, restrictive, and taboo" (Purnell, 2013a, p. 34). Every culture has unique beliefs about the phases of childbearing. These beliefs may be similar or different from those of other cultures. Despite the many differences, health care workers erroneously assume that this hugely important phase in a family life have similar impact to all people.

Questions such as the following may clarify the childbearing family's cultural preferences and are helpful tools for nurses and other health care workers: "How could I be of help to you in maintaining your traditional customs, beliefs, and practices while hospitalized? Are there things I need to know so my care is consistent with your needs?"

Integration of TCN Concepts

The question exists as to what transcultural areas to integrate when planning the course syllabus. Nursing faculty need to be creative in their approach to transcultural nursing (TCN) education strategies in childbearing courses. Concepts such as **decision making**, time, nutrition, hot and cold theory, placenta, female circumcision and female genital mutilation, naming the baby, communication, period of recuperation of the mother, pica, breastfeeding, and weaning are just a few of the culturally impacted issues that nursing students need to learn. Students must consider the perceptions and expression of pain during childbirth, as experienced in different cultures. In addition, they need to be sensitive to the issue of cultural impact on postpartum maternal hygiene as well as newborn care and bonding in the immediate postpartum period.

DISPARITIES IN HEALTH CARE, ACCESS, AND QUALITY

It is imperative that disparities in infant and maternal mortality be included in the course content of childbearing courses. The United States—despite spending more than any other country on health care—has a maternal mortality rate of 13.3 deaths per 1,000 live births, a rate that is behind 40 other countries (Lauderdale, 2012). In addition, the World

Health Organization (WHO) reported that 15 million babies, more than 1 in 10 births, are born prematurely (WHO, 2012). Over a million premature births die shortly after birth; those who survive may have chronic disabilities at huge cost to the families and to society (WHO, 2012). In the United States, 12%, or more than one in nine births, are premature, ranking 6th among 10 nations with premature births (WHO, 2012). There are some glaring disparities and marked differences in infant mortality by race and ethnicity. African American women have four times the risk of dying from pregnancy-related complications than White women (Lauderdale, 2012). Particularly in 2006, the overall U.S. infant mortality rate was 6.68 infant deaths per 1,000 live births (Mathews & MacDorman, 2011). The highest infant mortality rate was 13.35 for non-Hispanic Black women with a rate 2.4 times that for non-Hispanic White women (5.58); 8.28 or higher for American Indian/Alaska Native (AI/AN) women; and 8.01 higher for Puerto Rican women (Mathews & MacDorman, 2011).

Decision Making

Among some cultures such as Mexican Americans, decision making resides in the male authority; nurses need to be respectful of this (Lauderdale, 2012). Among Hispanics, the "family" is the primary support, particularly during the childbearing period (Galanti, 2003; Moore, Moos, & Callister, 2010). It is not uncommon for a woman in labor to arrive in the hospital with a group of supporters, who are often introduced as her "family" but may include nonblood relatives and friends (Moore et al., 2010). Gender roles are traditional in the Hispanic family; the eldest male is seen as the authority figure and head of household (Galanti, 2003, 2004). The role of running the household and child-rearing is primarily the woman's role (Galanti, 2003, 2004). Extended family also plays an important role. Elders are shown respect at home and in the community, and often take on the role of caregivers for the grandchildren (Chapman & Durham, 2010; Galanti, 2003). Decisions regarding important matters are generally made by the family as a whole. This can often be a source of difficulty in labor since Hispanic fathers frequently choose not to participate in the labor process due to modesty issues; women are hesitant to make decisions without their input (Andrews, 2006; Carteret, 2011; Galanti, 2003, 2004; Oria de Quinzanos, 2003). The nature of labor and delivery frequently requires that decisions be made rapidly.

Among Hmong families, decisions about a family member of either gender usually reside with the husband's family elders (Purnell, 2013b). Hmong girls generally marry in their teens. Since these are ceremonial marriages, they do not violate state laws (Purnell, 2013b). Purnell (2013b) further added that during pregnancies in their teens, Hmong women tend to be healthy. Extended families are common among the Hmong; young families live with the in-laws. In terms of decisions, other references suggested that the pregnant woman might wish to consult with her grandparents regarding labor induction or cesarean section (Giger & Davidhizar, 2013; Moore et al., 2010; Ritter & Hoffman, 2010).

The nursing implications are vital and vary in complexity. Often times parents wish to look further than family members present for decision-making guidance. Spiritual leaders, additional family members, friends, or others may be called upon before the family is willing or able to commit to a decision. It is a nursing responsibility to identify if there is a person or persons who the client regularly consults with for informal or formal decisions. Upon admission to the labor and delivery unit, each client should be asked these questions as part of her admission assessment: "Is there someone you rely upon to assist you with health-related decisions? Could he or she be easily reached? Do you have a contact number for him or her? What is the best way to reach him or her?"

Time

Another cultural consideration is **time orientation**: (**past, present, and future**). The dominant western culture in the United States is future-oriented. The focus of health care is in prevention and future planning, and the concept of punctuality is valued (Chapman & Durham, 2010; Moore et al., 2010). In perinatal nursing, women frequently seek out preconception care and most always obtain prenatal care from early in their pregnancy. A **future-oriented** belief is based on the societal view that leaves very little to fate and powers outside of individual control (Chapman & Durham, 2010; Moore et al., 2010). Basically, one might believe that eating well, exercising, and taking care of oneself will result in good health. Other groups, such as Mexican Americans, frequently do not seek prenatal care because pregnancy is seen as a natural event and a part of life (Moore et al., 2010). Arab women also tend to not participate in prenatal care, with traditional medicine and remedies dominating throughout the Arabic pregnancy (Chapman & Durham, 2010). Generally, Chinese Americans are **past-oriented**—viewing the past with great importance and revering their ancestors. They may frequently be late for appointments (Callister, 2005; Callister et al., 2011). By and large, African Americans are **present-oriented**, caring more for what is happening in the here and now (Moore et al., 2010; Ritter & Hoffman, 2010).

Many cultural groups are much more relaxed about the concept of time, as evidenced by the timeliness of keeping perinatal clinic appointments. The message needs to be clear that medical appointments do not afford the same flexibility as perhaps one's personal schedule; missing and arriving very late for appointments may mean that appointments have to be rescheduled to allow for care of other patients. Health care providers may build in some flexibility in scheduling to better accommodate clients. This may include longer time slots for appointments or perhaps a numbering system where clients receive a number when they arrive and are then seen in the order of arrival.

Nutrition: Food Cravings and Pica

It is a belief in many cultures that the pregnant woman should be given food that she craves; otherwise, it will adversely affect the baby. In some Filipinos, there is a belief that eating certain foods may later be physically manifested in the baby; for example, eating purple eggplant may result in a dark birthmark or darker skin tone on the baby. **Pica** is the craving for and ingestion of nonfood matter. Three main pica substances consumed are soil, ice, and laundry or corn starch (Basuray, 2013; Lauderdale, 2012). Other substances such as sand, burnt matches, plastic, and coffee grounds may also be ingested (Campinha-Bacote, 2013). Pica is most common among African American women in the south (Campinha-Bacote, 2013), in women from lower socioeconomic status, and in some Hispanic women who prefer solid milk of magnesia from Mexico (Lauderdale, 2012). Some women who ingest nonfood elements claim that this practice reduces nausea and fosters easy birth (Campinha-Bacote, 2013).

Hot and Cold Theory

Hot and cold theory—or the belief in harmony and balance—is based on the Greek concept of the four body humors, namely yellow bile, black bile, phlegm, and blood (Andrews, 2012). To restore equilibrium, these two opposing forces need to be adjusted

(Mattson, 2013). Medications, herbs, foods, and beverages are deemed hot or cold not because of their physical temperature but for their effects. Illnesses are also classified as hot or cold, and hence should be treated with the subtraction or addition of a remedy that is opposite in effect (Spector, 2013). Therefore, if childbirth is classified as a hot illness, then the postpartum woman may avoid cold beverages, air, raw fruits and vegetables, and showers—since most of the heat has been lost during the birthing process (Lauderdale, 2012; Mattson, 2013). Please review Module 3.2 in Chapter 3 to learn more about the theory of hot and cold.

Placenta

In some cultural groups, the **placenta** is considered important as an organ that connected the mother and baby prior to birth (Basuray & Macias, 2013). Other cultures believe that the placenta is part of the newborn, or is related to and a friend of the baby; these cultures, such as Native Hawaiians and the Igbo tribe of Nigeria, may celebrate to honor that relationship (Basuray & Macias, 2013). Generally, in the western culture, the placenta is disposed of or incinerated. In some indigenous cultures in the Philippines, however, the placenta has a special place for burial or is buried with other objects such as books in order to foster intelligence (Basuray & Macias, 2013) or pencils or other office supplies to encourage a liking for academia in the child (S. Veluz, Personal Communication, June 12, 2012).

Female Circumcision and Female Genital Mutilation

Female circumcision (FC), also interchangeably referred to as **female genital mutilation** (FGM), involves the partial or total removal of the external female genitalia (Basuray & Macias, 2013). This practice is believed to have originated in Africa and is done on newborn girls or on young women before marriage. FC is usually performed by illiterate and untrained individuals; complications abound such as hemorrhage, infection, urinary retention, sepsis, shock, and death (Basuray & Macias, 2013). FC is believed to increase fertility and ease childbirth (Anuforo, Oyedele, & Pacquiao, 2004). In Nigeria, stillbirth is associated with uncircumcised women, specifying that death occurs when the baby's head touches the mother's clitoris. Anuforo et al. (2004) suggested massive public education regarding FC complications, education about the myths concerning FC, and promoting awareness of acceptable alternatives to FC such as clitoral flattening or cutting of pubic hair.

Naming the Baby

Throughout recorded history, man has used a series of sounds or words to identify each another. These "names" are but one of the characteristics of how we distinguish one another from the crowd. Names can provide a sense of individuality and identity, set the tone for a child's destiny by providing strength or direction, and reveal a family history or a legacy. Names can be meant to honor a beloved friend, a music idol, or a superhero. Nothing is more personal than one's name.

Parents-to-be in every culture ponder the question of **naming the baby** for many months, sometimes planning names years before the child is even conceived. Yet, what is in a name? This question can be answered differently by any number of families, and is influenced by any number of factors. Many cultures have specific preferences that impact the baby-naming process after childbirth. The Western European cultures primarily follow the same cultural patterns in the naming of infants (Horlacher, 2000; Moore & Moos, 2003; Rockler-Gladen, 2007). Names may be chosen for any variety of reasons, such as family factors, religious aims, or even the sound of the name. Infants are given a primary and middle name, which is followed by the surname of the father if the mother is married or chooses to give the infant the father's surname. If she is unmarried, the infant may have her last name (Horlacher, 2000; Moore & Moos, 2003, Rockler-Gladen, 2007).

Chinese and some Southeast Asian cultures reverse their names. The surname precedes the given name (Callister, 2005; Callister et al., 2011; Kim-Godwin, 2003). For obvious reasons, this can prove confounding and even dangerous when referring to medical records. The admitting nurse and record keeper needs to make careful notation on the patient's chart of first and last name, as well as how the patient wishes to be referred to. Errors in the recording may also occur on the birth certificate information, so nurses should be aware of this potential complication. In the Chinese culture, there is recognition that the given name of an infant is a guide to a life of spirituality and meaning (Callister, 2005; Callister et al., 2011; Kim-Godwin, 2003). To honor that, they may partake in some variation of an ancient traditional baby-naming ceremony called the *Red Egg and Ginger Ceremony*, where the infant is given his/her name and is introduced to the world of family and friends (Popovic, 2009–2012). This ceremony happens when the infant is 30 days of age, and is often celebrated in a modified form today. Traditionally, infant girls are given names that represent beauty and nature; male infants are more often awarded names denoting strength and good health (Popovic, 2009–2012).

Traditions differ somewhat in different parts of Africa. There is a naming festival approximately a week or so after the infant's birth. The infant's name is generally given by an elder, who first whispers it to the baby before announcing it to others. The thought behind this tradition is that one should know his/her name before anyone else does (Horlacher, 2000). When performing a family history, nurses need to take careful note of each person and his or her name; when applicable, write each name a person has been known by to avoid unnecessary confusion and potential errors.

Lesbian, Gay, Bisexual, and Transgender Families

Although usually associated with a stigma, homosexuality occurs in many societies, including those that deny its presence (Purnell, 2013a). The care for lesbian, gay, bisexual, and transgender (**LGBT**) families is an important concept to include in existing or developing courses in childbearing families.

The USDHHS (2010) estimated that in 2002, about 4% of the U.S. population between the ages of 18 to 44 years have acknowledged themselves as LGBT. Commonly, individuals belonging to gender and sexual minorities experience continuing stigma, discrimination, and threats to safety even early in life (Gay, Lesbian, and Straight Education Network [GLSEN], 2011). There is an obvious need for content integration of the health care needs of the LGBT population in nursing and allied health care curricula. Chapter 8 provides more discussion regarding LGBT families.

Other Important Concepts

There is a wide range of cultural prescriptions regarding when a woman can return to full activity after childbirth; this time frame varies from culture to culture and can last from as short as 2 weeks to as long as a few months (Lauderdale, 2012). Diagnosis-related groupings in the United States will make activity time frame determination difficult. Other cultures may restrict fathers from involvement in the delivery room (Noble, Rom, Newsome-Wicks, Englehardt, & Woloski-Wruble, 2009) or immediately after birth. In some cultures, wearing a **binder** on the infant's abdomen is believed to prevent the umbilicus from protrusion and herniation (Purnell, 2013a). It will be helpful to emphasize these variations on the syllabus, hence promoting culturally congruent care.

When planning a syllabus for a childbearing course, TCN concepts that need to be integrated may be presented as a table (Table 9.1). This handout will be helpful when planning culturally congruent interventions in both classroom discussions and clinical experiences in the perinatal clinic, in home visits, at the delivery room, and in neonatal rotations.

The use of evidence-based practice (EBP) will improve the health care of childbearing women and their families. The study by Anuforo et al. (2004) in EBP 9.1 can be included as an assignment for reflection for nursing students. In staff development settings, this or other research articles may be discussed during staff meetings or used when revising policies and procedure guides.

TABLE 9.1 Prescriptive, Restrictive, and Taboo Practices Among Selected Cultures

Clients	Prescriptive Practices	Restrictive Practices	Taboo Practices
African Americans	To initiate labor: ride on bumpy road, ingest castor oil, sniff pepper Avoid cold during the postpartum period; place bellyband and coin on umbilicus to prevent protrusion	Do not drink too much liquid (this will drown the baby)	Taking pictures (may cause stillbirth) and not having their picture taken (captures the soul); not reaching above their head to prevent the umbilical cord from wrapping around the baby's neck; craving for and ingestion of nonfood items such as clay; purchasing clothing for the infant
Jewish	Place bed from north to south; pregnant woman carries a preserving stone; men pray on holy days that woman does not miscarry	Husband stands at woman's head to avoid viewing wife's genitals; some husbands do not attend delivery	Not touching wife during labor after water breaks and with bleeding; not saying the baby's name prior to the naming ceremony or harm may befall baby; naming on the 7th day (8th day for a male child). Avoidance of baby shower (Orthodox Jews)

(continued)

TABLE 9.1   Prescriptive, Restrictive, and Taboo Practices Among Selected Cultures *(continued)*

Clients	Prescriptive Practices	Restrictive Practices	Taboo Practices
Vietnamese Americans	Avoid weddings and funerals; may bring bad fortune to the baby	Avoid cold air, food, and beverages after birth and increase consumption of hot foods; in some Asian cultures, steam from hot stones are administered; reduce raw fruits and vegetables after birth	The head is considered sacred. Touching the mother or infant's head is taboo.
Navajo Indians Other Native Americans	Happiness will bring joy and good fortune	Avoid knots or braids; may cause difficult labor	Avoid participation in traditional ceremonies or dances; spirits will harm the baby. Placenta is buried outside the home to keep away evil spirits and to symbolize connection between the child and the earth.

Sources: Developed from Campinha-Bacote (2013); Basuray & Macias (2013); Lauderdale (2012); Mattson (2013); Noble, Rom, Newsome-Wicks, Engelhardt, & Woloski-Wruble (2009); and Purnell (2013).

EBP 9.1

Anuforo, Oyedele, and Pacquaio (2004) conducted an ethnographic study to explore meanings, beliefs, and practices of female circumcision (FC) among the three main Nigerian tribes, namely the Igbos, Yorubas, and Hausas in the United States and Nigeria. This study addressed three issues: (1) meanings, beliefs, and practices related to FC; (2) similarities and differences existing among the three tribes between those residing in the United States and those in Nigeria; and (3) factors influencing the participants' attitudes toward FC.

The researchers used Leininger's CCT as a conceptual framework and ethnography as the method of choice since FC, being imbedded into the Nigerian culture, required the act to be studied in its naturalistic setting (Anuforo et al., 2004). Institutional approval from Kean University was obtained prior to data collection. Two of the researchers travelled to Nigeria to conduct the interviews. One researcher was from the Ibo and the other from the Yoruba tribe.

The 50 participants in this study, obtained by snowball sampling, consisted of 30 from the Hausa, Igbo, and Yoruba tribes in Nigeria and 20 from the United States from the Igbo and Yoruba tribes (members of Hausa tribes usually do not emigrate from Nigeria). A total of three sites each in Nigeria and in the United States were

(continued)

EBP 9.1 *(continued)*

used for participant observations. The three sites in Essex County, New Jersey, were used because the participants had families in the Nigerian sites.

The researchers interviewed participants between 2 to 3 times over a 1-month period; each interview lasted 45 minutes to an hour. The researchers translated the interview questions to the Ibo and Yoruba languages. In addition, a translator was hired to translate the interview questions into Hausa. The three versions of the questions were then translated back to English.

Five themes emerged from the study: (1) The FC practice stems from social, cultural, and religious factors; (2) FC practices reveal tribal similarities and differences; (3) personal and occupational experiences affect perceptions of complications of FC; (4) educational and generational factors affect concepts of sexual role and relationships; and (5) groups vary in their response regarding continuation of FC. All informants viewed FC as a "rite to womanhood" (p. 108) and an act that increases the woman's value for marriage. Furthermore, uncircumcised females in the small villages and rural areas face stronger social sanctions compared to those in urban areas.

Applications to Practice

■ Have you had female clients who had undergone FC, FGM, or both? How were you able to come across this information? Describe.
■ How will you characterize the experiences of these women in terms of FC, FGM, or both?
■ If you were to replicate this study, how would you conduct it? What would you change in terms of conceptual framework, sampling, and analysis of findings?

Source: Anuforo, Oyedele, & Pacquaio (2004).

APPLICATION

Aimed at providing culturally competent care, Dr. Josepha-Campinha-Bacote (2003, 2007, 2011) developed the ASKED model, wherein "A" stands for awareness, "S' for skill, "K" for knowledge, "E" for encounters, and "D" for desire. Dr. Campinha-Bacote's (2005) *Biblically Based Model for Cultural Competence (BASKED)* included "B" for the Bible—symbolic of being asked as a health care worker for one's readiness to provide appropriate care for clients. Table 9.2 illustrates a sample workshop assignment in a 4-credit childbearing course assignment that utilizes Campinha-Bacote's *Process of Cultural Competence in the Delivery of Healthcare Services Model.*

This application shows how well Campinha-Bacote's model lends itself in planning care and encouraging reflection on one's journey to cultural competence in the care of individuals from a given, distinct cultural group. The assignment in Critical Thinking Exercise 9.1 could be adapted for doctoral, master's, baccalaureate, or associate and diploma programs.

TABLE 9.2 A Sample Workshop Assignment in a 4-Credit NUR 3000-Caring for the Childbearing Family Course at Mount Eden College, Anytown, USA, That Applies Campinha-Bacote's Biblically Based Model of Cultural Competence as Well as Current Research About Childbearing Practices Among Jewish Clients

Assignment 1-My Journey to Cultural Competence: Caring for Childbearing Jewish Families
Cultural Awareness. Am I aware of my personal biases against Jewish clients?   Is there research showing racist practices against this group? Discuss day to day events showing prejudice, discrimination, and violence against the Jews.
Cultural Knowledge   **Read:**   Basuray, J. M., & Macias, K. (2013). Recognizing, respecting, and addressing valued traditions and celebration. In J. M. Basuray (Ed.), *Culture & health: Concept and practice* (Rev. ed., pp. 151–166). Ronkonkoma, NY: Linus, Inc.   Lauderdale, J. (2012). Transcultural perspectives in childbearing. In M. M. Andrews & J. S. Boyle (Eds.), *Transcultural concepts in nursing care* (pp. 91–122). Philadelphia, PA: Wolters Kluwer/Lippincott Williams & Wilkins.   Noble, A., Rom, M., Newsome-Wicks, M., Engelhardt, K., & Woloski-Wruble, A. (2009). Jewish laws, customs, and practice in labor, delivery, and postpartum care. *Journal of Transcultural Nursing, 20*(3), 323–333. doi:10.1177/1043659609334930   Other relevant research articles
Cultural Encounter   Patient care assignment of Jewish clients or   interview: First generation Jewish American woman of childbearing age.   According to this book, Jewish Americans place high emphasis on_____ during the perinatal period. Is this correct according to your experiences and knowledge? If yes, please explain. If no, please add more information.   According to this article, Jewish Americans prefer to_____. Is this correct? If yes, please explain. If no, kindly add more information.   According to the research studies and book(s) I reviewed, Jewish Americans are hesitant to sign organ donation cards. Is this true? If yes, please explain. If no, kindly add more information.
Assignment 1-My Journey to Cultural Competence: Caring for Childbearing Jewish Families
Be creative in using variations of these questions.   If you had asked some creative questions during the interviews, please include them.   You may include the whole interview as an appendix at the end of the paper after the Reference List. However, include enough on the *Brief Interview* portion of the paper to be understood.
Cultural Skill   Discuss a minimum of two (2) research studies involving practices performed by maternal and childbearing Jewish clients. Compare and contrast the research studies. Discuss their strengths and limitations. Despite the weaknesses and limitations, are these research studies helpful in your case study and in your development of a culturally competent care plan for a pregnant Jewish woman?   Discuss culturally competent nursing interventions utilizing Campinha-Bacote's Biblical Model of Cultural Competence and findings from research studies.
Cultural Desire. Do I want to be competent in caring for Jewish clients? What is the next step in my journey? How do I sustain my cultural desire here and for other cultural groups?

CRITICAL THINKING EXERCISES 9.1

Undergraduate Student

1. You often hear faculty at your school say that you need to be prepared to care for culturally diverse childbearing clients for your clinical rotations and beyond. As you progress in the program, do you feel more confident when caring for childbearing clients?
2. Do you think you are ready to provide culturally congruent care of the childbearing family during your clinical rotations and upon graduation?
3. To add to your educational preparation, what concepts would you add in your present care of childbearing family course? What concepts would you be in favor of deleting from your current course? Why?

Graduate Student

1. Are TCN concepts in the care of the childbearing family integrated in your master's curriculum?
2. If you are in a family nurse practitioner (FNP) tract, how many courses do you have in the childbearing family?
3. Do the above courses contain culturally congruent care of diverse families? Describe.

Faculty in Academia

1. Describe the strategies for integration of TCN concepts into the childbearing course that you teach. Have you examined the effectiveness of those strategies?
2. How would you characterize student feedback to the above strategies? Have you incorporated student feedback into the course? If yes, how? If not, why?
3. Have you attended any workshop or conference on cultural competence? Was it helpful in your integration of diversity and cultural competence in your childbearing courses?

Staff Development Educator

1. Do you require a yearly module in cultural diversity and promotion of cultural competence among your nurses in labor and delivery, in the newborn unit, and in units with clients experiencing reproductive and women's issues?
2. If you have no modules, are the nurses above required to earn continuing education credits (CEs) for available face-to-face or online classes?
3. How long has it been since you attended a workshop/conference on cultural diversity and promotion of cultural competence among women with reproductive and health issues? When are you planning to attend a workshop/conference on this topic?

SUMMARY

This chapter discussed important concepts for inclusion into existing childbearing courses, for developing new childbearing courses, or for planning integration of TCN concepts in the curricula with or without specific use of TCN models. The nurse needs to examine his or her own journey to cultural competence in the care of the perinatal client and her family. This reflection will assist in developing genuine empathy, concern, and respect for clients, families, and the community. This will also be a tool for planning, implementing, and evaluating culturally and linguistically congruent care for diverse families.

REFERENCES

Andrews, C. (2006, July). Modesty and healthcare for women: Understanding cultural sensitivities. *Community Oncology, 3*(7), 443–445.

Andrews, M. (2012). The influence of cultural and health belief systems on health care practices. In M. M. Andrews & J. S. Boyle (Eds.), *Transcultural concepts in nursing care* (6th ed., pp. 73–88). Philadelphia, PA: Wolters Kluwer/Lippincott Williams & Wilkins.

Anuforo, P. O., Oyedele, L., & Pacquiao, D. F. (2004). Comparative study of meanings, beliefs, and practices of female circumcision among three Nigerian tribes in the United States and Nigeria. *Journal of Transcultural Nursing, 15*(2), 103–113.

Basuray, J. M. (2013). Health beliefs across cultures: Understanding transcultural care. In J. M. Basuray (Ed.), *Culture & health: Concept and practice* (Rev. ed., pp. 58–84). Ronkonkoma, NY: Linus.

Basuray, J. M., & Macias, K. (2013). Recognizing, respecting, and addressing valued traditions and celebration. In J. M. Basuray (Ed.), *Culture & health: Concept and practice* (Rev. ed., pp. 151–166). Ronkonkoma, NY: Linus, Inc.

Blencowe, H., Cousens, S., Oestergaard, M., Chou, D., Moller, A. B., Narwal, R. L., & Lawn, J. E. (2012). National, regional and worldwide estimates of preterm birth: Estimates from 2010. *The Lancet, 379*(9832), 2162–2172.

Callister, L. C. (2005, November/December). What has the literature taught us about culturally competent care of women and children. *MCN: Maternal Child Nursing, 30*(6), 380–388.

Callister, L. C., Ead, M., & Yeung Diehl, J. (2011, Nov-Dec). Perceptions of giving birth and adherence to cultural practices in Chinese women. *MCN: The American Journal of Maternal/Child Nursing, 36*(6), 387–394.

Campinha-Bacote, J. (2003). *The process cultural competence in the delivery of healthcare services: A culturally competent model of care.* Cincinnati, OH: Transcultural C.A.R.E. Associates.

Campinha-Bacote, J. (2005). *A Biblically based model of cultural competence in the delivery of healthcare services.* Cincinnati, OH: Transcultural C.A.R.E. Associates.

Campinha-Bacote, J. (2011). *The process of cultural competence in the delivery of healthcare services.* Retrieved March 10, 2011, from http://transculturalcare.net/

Campinha-Bacote, J. (2013). People of African American heritage. In L. D. Purnell, *Transcultural health care: A culturally competent approach* (4th ed., pp. 91–114). Philadelphia, PA: FA Davis.

Carteret, M. (2011, March). *Modesty in health care: A cross-cultural perspective. Dimensions of culture: Cross cultural communications for healthcare professionals.* Retrieved June 15, 2012, from www.dimensionsofculture.com/2010/11/modesty-in-health-care-a-cross-cultural-perspective

Chapman, L., & Durham, R. (2010). *Maternal-newborn nursing: The critical components of nursing care.* Philadelphia: FA Davis.

Galanti, G. (2003, July). The Hispanic family and male-female relationships: An overview. *Journal of Transcultural Nursing, 14*(3), 180–185.

Galanti, G. (2004). *Caring for patients from different cultures* (3rd ed.). Philadelphia, PA: University of Pennsylvania Press.

Gay, Lesbian, & Straight Education Network. (2011). *The 2011 national school climate survey: Key findings on the experiences of lesbian, gay, bisexual, and transgender youth in our nation's school.* Retrieved May 15, 2013, from www.glsen.org/binary-data/GLSEN_ATTACHMENTS/file/000/002/2106–1.pdf

Giger, J. N., & Davidhizar, R. E. (2013). *Transcultural nursing: Assessment and intervention* (6th ed.). St. Louis, MO: Elsevier Mosby.

Horlacher, G. T. (2000, Sep). *Various country and ethnic naming customs.* Retrieved June 18, 2012, from www.progenealogists.com/namingpatterns.htm

Kim-Godwin, Y. S. (2003, March/April). Postpartum beliefs & practices among non-western cultures. *MCN: American Journal of Maternal Child Nursing, 28*(2), 74–80.

Lauderdale, J. (2012). Transcultural perspectives in childbearing. In M. M. Andrews & J. S. Boyle (Eds.), *Transcultural concepts in nursing care* (6th ed., pp. 91–122). Philadelphia, PA: Wolters Kluwer/Lippincott Williams & Wilkins.

Martin, J. A., Hamilton, B. E., Sutton, P. D., Ventura, S., Menacker, F., & Kimeyer, S. (2006). Births: Final data for 2004. *National Vital Statistics Reports, 55*(1). Hyattsville, MD: National Center for Health Statistics, Center for Disease Control. Retrieved July 26, 2013, from www.cdc.gov/nchs/data/nvsr/nvsr55/nvsr55_01.pdf

Mathews, T. J., & MacDorman, M. F. (2011). *Infant deaths: United States, 2000–2007*. Hyattsville, MD: Center for Disease Control. Division of Vital Statistics, National Center for Health Statistics, Center for Disease Control, *60*(1), 49–51. Retrieved January 26, 2013, from www.cdc.gov/mmwr/preview/mmwrhtml/su6001a9.htm

Mattson, S. (2013). People of Vietnamese heritage. In L. D. Purnell (Ed.), *Transcultural health care: A culturally competent approach* (4th ed., pp. 479–480). Philadelphia, PA: FA Davis.

Moore, M. L., & Moos, M. K. (2003). *Cultural competence in the care of childbearing families*. White Plains, NY: March of Dimes Foundation.

Moore, M. L., Moos, M. K., & Callister, L. C. (2010). March of Dimes continuing nursing education. In M. O. Dimes (Ed.), *Cultural competence: An essential journey for perinatal nurses* (pp. 1–95). White Plains, NY: Education & Health Promotion.

Muñoz, C., & Luckmann, J. (2005). *Transcultural communication in nursing,* 2nd ed. Clifton Park, NY: Thomson Delmar Learning.

Noble, A., Rom, M., Newsome-Wicks, M., Engelhardt, K., & Woloski-Wruble, A. (2009). Jewish laws, customs, and practice in labor, delivery, and post partum care. *Journal of Transcultural Nursing, 20*(3), 323–333. doi:10.1177/1043659609334930

Oria de Quinzanos, G. (2003). A Mexican perspective. In M. L. Moore & M. K. Moos (Eds.), *Cultural competence in the care of childbearing families* (p. 128). White Plains, NY: March of Dimes Foundation.

Popovic, M. (2009–2012). *Traditions and customs from all over the world*. Retrieved July 20, 2013, from http://traditionscustoms.com/coming-of-age/red-egg-and-ginger-party

Purnell, L. D. (2013a). The Purnell Model for Cultural Competence. In L. D. Purnell, *Transcultural health care: A culturally competent approach* (4th ed., pp. 15–44). Philadelphia, PA: F. A. Davis.

Purnell, L. D. (2013b). People of Hmong heritage. In L. D. Purnell, *Transcultural health care: A culturally competent approach* (4th ed., pp. 310–318). Philadelphia, PA: F. A. Davis.

Ritter, L. A., & Hoffman, N. A. (2010). *Multicultural health*. Sudbury, MA: Jones & Bartlett.

Rockler-Gladen, N. (2007, February 20). *Pregnancy & childbirth@Suite101: Jewish baby naming traditions: A brief lesson in Hebrew and Yiddish names and how they are chosen*. Retrieved June 18, 2012, from http://suite101.com/article/jewish-baby-girl-names-a14298#B

Spector, R. E. (2013). *Cultural diversity in health and illness* (8th ed.). Boston, MA: Pearson.

United Nations. (2000). *Millenium development goals: Improve maternal health*. Retrieved January 23, 2013, from www.un.org/millenniumgoals/maternal.shtml

U.S. Census Bureau. (2010). *Overview of race and hispanic origin: 2010*. Retrieved July 20, 2013, from www.census.gov/prod/cen2010/briefs/c2010br-02.pdf

U.S. Census Bureau. (2012). *Annual estimates of the resident population: April 2010 to July 1, 2012: 2012 Population estimates*. Retrieved May 14, 2013, from http://factfinder2.census.gov/faces/tableservices/jsf/pages/productview.xhtml?pid=PEP_2012_PEPANNRES&prodType=table

U.S. Department of Health and Human Services, Office of Minority Health. (2010). *National partnership for action to end health disparities*. Retrieved February 2, 2013, from www.healthypeople.gov/2020/about/DisparitiesAbout.aspx

U.S. Department of Health and Human Services, Office of Minority Health. (2013). *Enhanced national CLAS standards*. Retrieved August 16, 2013, from https://www.thinkculturalhealth.hhs.gov/Content/clas.asp

World Health Organization. (2012). *15 million babies born too soon*. Retrieved January 26, 2013, from www.who.int/mediacentre/news/releases/2012/preterm_20120502/en

TCN Concepts in Child-Rearing Courses, From Infancy to Adolescence

Priscilla Limbo Sagar

KEY TERMS

Acculturation
Cultural marginality
Curandero, curandera
Extended family

Lesbian/gay/bisexual/transgender family
Nuclear family
Parenting
Sobadores

LEARNING OBJECTIVES

At the completion of this chapter, the learner will be able to

1. Discuss the importance of integrating transcultural concepts in child-rearing courses.
2. Analyze three activities to promote cultural sensitivity among students when caring for children.
3. Compare and contrast child-rearing practices of diverse cultures.
4. Identify at least three issues that impact the care of children.
5. Devise culturally congruent care for children and their families.

OVERVIEW

The U.S. Census Bureau (2012) projected that the United States will be more diverse in 2060, with the minority population increasing from the current 37% to 57%. The U.S. Census Bureau also estimated that in 2012, 52.7% of non-Hispanic White people were below 18 years old; that number will decrease to 32.9% in 2060. There also will be a reduction of the overall population below 18 years old from the current 23.5% to 21.2% in 2060, secondary to recent trends in fertility and reduced migration (U.S. Census Bureau, 2012).

Woodring and Andrews (2012) emphasized the central role children play in cultural survival through transmission of customs and values from one generation to the next.

Today's children are tomorrow's future. According to the U.S. Census Bureau American Community Survey in 2011, there is a 21.6% poverty rate among children; this translates to one out of five children in poverty and is the highest rate since the survey was started in 2001. People who earn slightly above the poverty level have difficulty with living expenses yet are unable to qualify for assistance.

Integration of TCN Concepts

There are vital areas that need to be integrated in nursing care of children such as acculturation, family, poverty and health disparity, generic folk practices, and growth and development. These concepts need to be integrated in existing courses, in course revisions, and in planning new courses in the culturally and linguistically appropriate care of children.

The Process of Acculturation

Acculturation refers to modifications of attitudes and behaviors from an original culture because of contact with another culture. Acculturation is a two-way, concurrent process of acquisition, retention, and relinquishment of characteristics of both the old and new cultures (Anderson et al., 1993; de la Cruz, Padilla, & Agustin, 2000; Purnell, 2013). In the *multidimensional* aspect of acculturation, there is uneven acculturation across areas of social life (Choi, 2001, 2008, 2013). For example, a Filipino adolescent may speak mainly English and involve socially with peers at school while concurrently maintaining familial cultural traditions and rituals at home. In the *orthogonal* aspect of acculturation, the person can simultaneously keep two cultural identities without choosing one or the other (Choi, 2001). *Marginalized* individuals are neither at ease with their old or new culture (Choi, 2013; Purnell, 2013). During acculturation, the individual undergoes two types of stress: process-oriented stress and discrimination from being "different" (Choi, 2001, p. 197). Choi (2001, 2013) viewed **cultural marginality** as a transition where an individual feels as though he or she is in between two cultures yet belongs to neither one.

The Evolving Concept of Family

The **extended family** is characteristic of many African, Asian, and Latin American families whereby parents share the household with grandparents, aunts, uncles, and other relatives. Many hospitals have adopted flexible visiting hours to accommodate extended family members. **Nuclear families** are now rare; there are implications in health care since the majority of programs are tailored for nuclear families (Woodring & Andrews, 2012).

Lesbian, gay, bisexual, and transgender families (LGBT) are increasing. An LGBT family is composed of two adults of the same sex living together as domestic partners; the couple may be childless or raising a child or children (Ball, Bindler, & Cowen, 2010). An individual with LGBT identity may also be a single parent. These types of families require the same respect and acceptance, not discrimination, from health care workers. It is of prime importance that health care providers recognize the nurturing capacity of LGBT families (Ball et al., 2010). For more discussion about LGBT individuals, refer to Chapter 8, including EBP 8.1.

Parenting refers to the leadership role in the family through guidance of children in learning appropriate behavior, beliefs, morals, and system of rites and in developing social responsibility and becoming productive members of society (Ball et al., 2010). Parenting styles vary from family to family and from culture to culture.

Poverty and Health Disparities

In the United States, one in five children ages 0 to 17 years lives in poverty (U.S. Census Bureau, 2011). Compared to Whites (17%) and Asians (13%), Black (38.2%) and Hispanic (32.3%) children have much higher poverty rates (U.S. Census Bureau, 2011). Poverty has a cumulative impact on children and perpetuates the cycle of poverty. Children living in poverty, particularly young children, have increased incidence of cognitive and behavioral problems, reduced likelihood to stay in school, and, as they grow up, more possibility of years being unemployed (U.S. Census Bureau, 2011). One of the goals of *Healthy People 2020* (U.S. Department of Health and Human Services [USDHHS], Office of Minority Health [OMH], 2010) is elimination of health disparities. This is a content that needs to be integrated in all nursing courses. Immigrant children in first generation families face poverty along with other stresses of migration.

In a study that utilized the third National Health and Nutrition Examination Survey (NHANES), Burgos, Schetzina, Dixon, and Mendoza (2005) used 4,372 (Mexican Americans [MAs] in three generational groups), 4,138 (non-Hispanic Black), and 4,594 (non-Hispanic White) children ages 2 months to 16 years. The Burgos et al. (2005) study showed that first generation MA families had a substantial burden in regards to poverty level, educational attainment, and language. Hispanics make up the largest group of minority children in the United States; MAs are the largest subgroup among Hispanics (Burgos et al., 2005). Hispanic parents cited (1) language difficulties, (2) extended wait at the physician's office, (3) inadequate health insurance, (4) problems paying bills, and (5) struggle finding transportation as the foremost barriers to seeking health care (Burgos et al., 2005).

Generic Folk-Healing Practices

Many cultural groups and families practice generic folk healing exclusively or alongside western medicine. For example, among Southeast Asians, there are practices such as coining and pinching that leave marks on the skin (Woodring & Andrews, 2012); these marks may appear as bruises and may be mistaken for physical abuse.

The family may use folk healers in the community; these may vary according to the cultural groups. Mexican Americans and other Hispanics may go to a **curandera** (female) or **curandero** (male) for simple or more complicated ailments (Spector, 2013). They may also seek the **sobadores**, healers that use massage and manipulation (Purnell, 2013). Puerto Ricans may use an *espiritista*, a healer who communicates with spirits, for mental illness (Ball et al., 2010).

Growth and Development

As the child matures, they undergo expected physical growth, cognitive abilities, and psychosocial development (Ball et al., 2010). There are cultural and individual variations regarding size. Many growth development parameters have been normed on European American children and may not be applicable for minority children. Generally, Asian children are shorter than African American and White children (Woodring & Andrews, 2012). Nurses and other health care professionals must keep these variations in mind when performing a health history, measurements, and physical assessment of children.

TEACHING AND LEARNING STRATEGIES

Some learning strategies that may be helpful in teaching child-rearing courses include: self-learning modules (SLMs), clinical conferences, and written assignments. Other teaching and learning strategies are discussed in Chapter 2; some of those specific teaching and learning strategies may be applicable to enhance learning in child-rearing courses.

Self-Learning Modules

SLMs allow great flexibility for independent learning; these may be in hard copies, on compact discs (CDs), on the intranet or Internet, at the school of nursing (SON), or available at the affiliating agencies. With the current trend of partnerships between SONs and affiliating institutions, sharing of resources will be beneficial to both students and staff.

SLMs can be assigned prior to the clinical rotation or during the rotation. They may also be assigned to students as a makeup assignment for clinical absences. Chapter 3 has two and Chapter 13 has one full-length SLM. This chapter has an SLM in the care of a child with asthma, Self-Learning Module 10.1.

Clinical Conferences

During pre- and postclinical conferences, the faculty can integrate concepts about diversity and promotion of cultural competence to complement didactic learning in the classroom. Some strategies might include a 10-minute presentation of care for a child from a diverse culture, sexual orientation, or religion, among others.

During the course of the rotation, each student can be assigned to do a presentation and to answer questions from classmates. Assigning a certain number of points that can be added to the lowest exam grade may increase each student's motivation to learn and prepare for the presentation; for example, assigning up to 5 points, depending on the quality of the presentation as specified on the grading rubrics. A specific grading rubric would help the students prepare for the assignment and assist the faculty in objectively grading each presentation.

Written Assignments

An example of a written assignment in this course is a cultural assessment of a family that is different from one's own. Some questions that may be asked in the interview include: Please describe the healing practices in your culture; in other words, what do you do to keep well? Do you use a healing practitioner in the community prior to seeing a western practitioner? What are the conditions wherein you go to the folk healer?

In terms of assignments or multicultural activity, the faculty may review the admission assessment tool in the agency with the students. To stimulate creativity, students may be asked to analyze additional areas that could be added to the admission tool to gain more knowledge about the child and her family's cultural values, beliefs, and practices. These cultural values, beliefs, and practices influence health and health-seeking behaviors. Written assignments need specific guidelines to help students maximize their grades on the assignment (Chapter 2 contains a discussion about grading rubrics).

Having guest speakers for class or during clinical conferences is another way of integrating diversity and cultural competence. Some possibilities for a guest speaker are a certified transcultural nurse, religious leader, community leader, or a public health nurse.

EBP 10.1

Choi, Meininger, and Roberts (2006) conducted a cross-sectional study of 316 adolescents grades 6–8 in three middle schools in the southwest United States. This study aimed to measure somatic symptoms as well as general symptoms of depression in adolescents.

After IRB approval, consent forms in both English and Spanish were sent to parents of adolescents in participating schools, along with the principal's letter of endorsement. The researchers calculated that the response rates were 27% for European Americans and 10% for ethnic minorities. The low return rate for minorities is consistent with other studies (Choi et al., 2006).

The 316 participants—consisting of 66 African Americans (AAs), 144 European Americans (EAs), 77 Hispanic Americans (HAs), 20 Asian Americans (AAs), and 6 other adolescents—responded to the Diagnostic Statistical Manual Scale for Depression (DSD); Somatic Symptom Scale; the modified Social, Attitudinal, Familial, and Environmental Scale for Children (SAFE-C); Family Environment Scale (FES); and a 6-item Coping Scale. The Somatic Symptom Scale has 11 items that relate to the most common signs and symptoms of adolescents with depression including headache, chest pain, stomach ache, and dizziness.

Findings indicate that Asian Americans and HAs showed markedly higher scores on social stress and mental distress and lower scores on resources than EAs (Choi et al., 2006). In comparison to EAs, AAs and HAs were more apt to experience social stress ($2.2 < OR < 4.3$) and HAs were more prone to have suicidal ideation ($OR = 2.04$; 95% CI = 1.04–3.98). Compared to EAs, AAs, HAs, and Asian American adolescents showed a lack of resources to protect them from mental distress. Ethnic minority adolescents also reported problems with family relationships. Asian Americans reported the utmost somatic scores. Adolescents manifesting a high level of somatic symptoms have a tendency to have a high level of depression (Rhee, 2003, as cited in Choi et al., 2006).

Choi et al. (2006) acknowledged the following limitations: (1) inability to pin point a causal relationship among variables since this was a cross-sectional study and (2) small sample size and possible bias in selecting participants due to parental consent. For future studies, the researchers suggested more active and culturally sensitive recruitment procedures.

(continued)

EBP 10.1 *(continued)*

Applications to Practice

■ Investigate the availability of resources for adolescents and their families in your community.

■ Is there additional support for immigrant adolescents and their families?

■ If you were to replicate this study, how would you conduct it? What would you change in terms of conceptual framework, sampling, and analysis of findings?

Source: Choi, Meininger, & Roberts (2003).

SELF-LEARNING MODULE 10.1 AN ORTHODOX JEWISH CHILD WITH ASTHMA

Barbara J. Joslyn, EdD, RN
Former Assistant Professor, Mount Saint Mary College, Newburgh, NY

Take Pretest (Appendix 11)

OVERVIEW

This module calls for culturally and linguistically appropriate care for an 18-month-old girl with exacerbation of asthma. Asthma is one of the most common chronic respiratory conditions affecting children in the United States. In 2005, 12.7% (9 million) of all children in the United States had been diagnosed with asthma; 70% of these children had an asthmatic episode within the last 12 months (Ball, Bindler, & Cowen, 2010). Nurses and other health care providers need to partner with families regarding health maintenance; child and family education; and prevention of exacerbation (Ball et al., 2010).

The child's parents are Orthodox Jews who live in the community 18 miles away from the hospital. Orthodox Jews observe the Sabbath, which begins before sunset on Friday and ends after sunset on Saturday (Selekman, 2013). On the Sabbath, observant Jews do not perform work and there are prohibitions including those that pertain to operating equipment requiring electricity; this may impact adherence to recommended medical treatment. Referral to the rabbi may be necessary to explore exemptions from prohibitions for the sick child (Schwartz, 2008). Furthermore, the module requires critical thinking and clinical judgment for the nurse in providing patient education to the mother and in communicating with this young child who does not understand English.

This activity can be adapted to small groups in a classroom, a large classroom discussion, or a discussion question in an online format. In the classroom, this activity can include role playing to illustrate nonverbal behavior in establishing rapport with a non-English-speaking toddler.

(continued)

SELF-LEARNING MODULE 10.1   AN ORTHODOX JEWISH CHILD WITH ASTHMA   *(continued)*

OBJECTIVES

At the completion of this module, the learner will:

1. Discuss the prohibitions on the Sabbath considering administration of medication using a device that requires electricity to operate.
2. Explore solutions to a problem with a parent about adapting or seeking exemption from the Sabbath prohibitions concerning electrical medical equipment.
3. State the language restrictions that impact communication with young Orthodox Jewish children.
4. Model or state the nonverbal behaviors you can use to demonstrate acceptance of a toddler who does not understand English.

CONTENT

1. Assigned pediatric text: Look up sections discussing asthma discharge teaching, normal toddler behavior in a hospital setting, and communication with toddlers.

Learning Resources

SUGGESTED READINGS

1. Ball, J. W., Bindler, R. C., & Cowen, K. J. (2010). *Child health nursing: Partnering with children and families.* [Chapter 25. Alterations in respiratory function]. New York, NY: Pearson.
2. Coleman-Bruckheimer, K., &. Dein, S. (2011). Health care behaviors and beliefs in Hasidic Jewish populations: A systematic review of the literature. *Journal of Religion and Health, 50,* 422–436.
3. Schwartz, E. A. (2008). Jewish Americans. In J. N. Giger & R. E. Davidhizar (Eds.), *Transcultural nursing: Assessment and intervention* (5th ed., pp. 592–618). St. Louis, MO: Mosby Elsevier.
4. Selekman, J. (2013). People of Jewish heritage. In L. D. Purnell (Ed.), *Transcultural healthcare: A culturally competent approach* (4th ed., pp. 339–356). Philadelphia: F. A. Davis.
5. Woodring, B. C., & Andrews, M. M. (2012). Transcultural perspectives in the nursing care of children. In M. M. Andrews & J. S. Boyle (Eds.), *Transcultural concepts in nursing care* (6th ed., pp. 123–156). Philadelphia, PA: Wolters Kluwer/ Lippincott Williams & Wilkins.

You are a staff nurse on a busy pediatric unit on a Friday morning. You just received the report from the night nurse. One of your patients is an 18-month-old girl with exacerbation of asthma; she is from a practicing Orthodox Jewish family. The patient's mother is 19 years old and is 6 months pregnant with her second child. This is the child's fifth hospital admission in the last 4 months. She has been improving and her albuterol treatments were advanced to every 4 hours last night. Overnight, she had minimal wheezing. Her oxygen saturations are 94% on room air. The child breastfed overnight, but refused solid food yesterday. Read

(continued)

this module and review the questions at the end as you plan for culturally congruent interventions for the young mother and her daughter.

Your assessment. When you enter the room of the 18-month-old girl for your initial nursing assessment, the child is awake and watches you but does not respond to your smiling face or your friendly comment: "Hi, how are you this morning? You look very pretty in your pink pajamas." Seeing that her mother is already up and dressed, you introduce yourself. The mother tells you that she needs to go home early today because she needs to prepare for the Sabbath. She says her child is getting better and should be discharged this morning. She further states her absolute deadline for discharge today is 2:30 p.m. because the last shuttle bus to the Jewish community leaves at 3:00 p.m. You explain that the physicians will make rounds this morning and make the decision about discharge. She asks you if the physicians can first see her daughter prior to the other patients.

Later that morning after rounds, the physician in charge of this child's care tells you the child can be discharged home today. You check the discharge orders, including the order that the child receive around the clock (ATC) albuterol treatments by nebulizer throughout the weekend. The order also specifies that the child should be seen by her pediatrician on Monday.

Discharge

As you review the discharge orders with the mother, she interrupts you to say she is not allowed to touch anything mechanical that requires electricity on the Sabbath. The mother adds that she cannot give the albuterol inhalation treatments, but she will be taking the child home with her. She asks you how she can give this medication.

As you problem solve with this mother, you should consider the following questions:

■ Why is it necessary for albuterol to continue to be given every 4 hours at home for the next 2 days?
■ Is there an alternative delivery system not requiring electricity?
■ What might happen if the child does not receive the albuterol in the next 24 hours?
■ What are the religious prohibitions affecting this mother's concerns?
■ What steps can the mother make at this time to resolve this situation to satisfy the religious prohibitions? What are her options?
■ Would consulting with the rabbi help the mother? Why?

Self-Assessment

1. List the usual discharge teaching recommended in your inpatient setting for children hospitalized with asthma.
2. State the pharmaceutical action of albuterol as used in asthma. Why is albuterol used in posthospital treatment? Explain.

(continued)

SELF-LEARNING MODULE 10.1   AN ORTHODOX JEWISH CHILD WITH ASTHMA *(continued)*

3. What are the child's personal asthma triggers? Have you included these in your teaching plan to her mother?
4. Enumerate areas of Orthodox Jewish prohibitions that directly impact using medical equipment requiring electricity.
5. Discuss the probable reason this toddler did not react to you when you spoke to her?
6. Demonstrate acceptance and interest in a toddler who does not understand English.

Take Posttest (Appendix 12; the key to pretest and posttest is available in Appendix 13.)

LESSON EVALUATION

1. Complete Module Evaluation (Appendix 3).
2. Pre- and posttest questions can used to evaluate the knowledge the student has obtained.
3. Any of the questions in this module can be used as online discussion questions (DQ). The evaluation is dependent on your institutional policy.
4. Short (2–3 pages) papers can be assigned. It is suggested that instructors develop their own grading rubrics.
5. Students in small groups can present this information to the larger class. It is suggested that instructors develop their own grading rubrics.

CRITICAL THINKING EXERCISES 10.1

Undergraduate Student
1. How comfortable are you when caring for a culturally diverse child?
2. Using what you have learned, how would you develop a culturally congruent care plan for the asthmatic child in Module 10.1?
3. Do you think there is enough content of cultural diversity and promotion of cultural competence in caring for children integrated in your classes (theory) and in clinical?

Graduate Student
1. If you are in the family nurse practitioner track, how many credits do you have in the care of children and families?
2. Do you use a conceptual model in caring for children and families? Elaborate.
3. Do you feel that your education, including your practice, will prepare you to manage care for diverse children and their families?

Faculty in Academia
1. Do you use a specific theory or model in teaching nursing care of children and families? Explain.
2. How many hours do you spend in teaching about lesbian/gay/bisexual/transgender families in your child-rearing course? Discuss?
3. How do you critically appraise diversity in your child-rearing course? Have you recently revised your course to keep abreast with culturally and linguistically appropriate care standards and guidelines?

(continued)

CRITICAL THINKING EXERCISES 10.1 *(continued)*

Staff Development Educator

1. What continuing education credits (CEs) are offered in the institution to develop culturally competent care of children?
2. Are there CEs offered online to develop culturally competent care of children?
3. Do you require a yearly module in cultural diversity and promotion of cultural competence in the care of children?
4. How long has it been since you attended a workshop/conference on cultural diversity and promotion of cultural competence among children? When are you planning to attend a workshop/conference on this topic?

SUMMARY

This chapter explores child-rearing and areas suggested for inclusion in courses dealing with nursing care of children. The United States is increasingly becoming more culturally and ethnically diverse, and by 2060 the current minority population is projected to make up 57% of the general population (U.S. Census Bureau, 2012). At a poverty rate of 21.6%, one in every five children lives in poverty. The poverty rate is much higher among Black and Hispanic children. The *Healthy People 2020* initiative aims to eliminate disparities in health care. All these important concepts must be included in child-rearing courses. The end goal is culturally congruent care for children and their families.

REFERENCES

Anderson, J., Moeschberger, M., Chen, M. S., Kunn, P., Wewers, M. E., & Guthrie, R. (1993). An acculturation scale for Southeast Asians. *Social Psychiatry and Psychiatric Epidemiology, 28*(3), 134–141.

Ball, J. W., Bindler, R. C., & Cowen, K. J. (2010). *Child health nursing: Partnering with children and families.* New York, NY: Pearson.

Burgos, A. E, Schetzina, K. E., Dixon, B., & Mendoza, F. S. (March, 2005). Importance of generational status in examining access to and utilization of health care services by Mexican American children. *Pediatrics, 115*(3), 322–330.

Choi, H. (2001). Cultural marginality: A concept analysis with implications for immigrant adolescents. *Issues in Comprehensive Pediatric Nursing, 24,* 193–206.

Choi, H. (2008). Theory of cultural marginality. In M. J. Smith & P. R. Liehr (Eds.), *Middle range theory for nursing* (pp. 243–259). New York, NY: Springer Publishing.

Choi, H. (2013). Theory of cultural marginality. In M. J. Smith & P. R. Liehr (Eds.), *Middle range theory for nursing* (pp. 289–307). New York, NY: Springer Publishing.

Choi, H., Meininger, J. C., & Roberts, R. E. (2006). Ethnic differences in adolescents' mental distress, social stress, and resources. *Adolescence, 41*(162), 263–283.

Coleman-Brueckheimer, K., &. Dein, S. (2011). Health care behaviors and beliefs in Hasidic Jewish populations: A systemic review of the literature. *Journal of Religion and Health, 50,* 422–436.

de la Cruz, F. A., Padilla, G. V., & Agustin, E. O. (2000). Adapting a measure of acculturation for cross cultural research. *Journal of Transcultural Nursing, 11*(3), 191–198.

Purnell, L. D. (2013). *Transcultural health care: A culturally competent approach.* Philadelphia, PA: F. A. Davis.

Selekman, J. (2013). People of Jewish heritage. In L. D. Purnell (Ed.), *Transcultural healthcare: A culturally competent approach* (4th ed., pp. 339–356). Philadelphia: F. A. Davis.

Spector, R. E. (2013). *Cultural diversity in health and illness* (8th ed.). Boston, MA: Pearson Education.

U.S. Census Bureau. (2011). *Child poverty in the United States 2009 and 2010: Selected race groups and Hispanic origin*. Retrieved July 4, 2013, from www.census.gov/prod/2011pubs/acsbr10–05.pdf

U.S. Census Bureau. (2012). *U.S. Census Bureau projections show a slower growing, older, more diverse nation a half century from now*. Retrieved August 3, 2013, from www.census.gov/newsroom/releases/archives/population/cb12–243.html

U.S. Department of Health and Human Services, Office of Minority Health. (2010). *National partnership for action to end health disparities*. Retrieved February 2, 2013, from www.healthypeople.gov/2020/about/DisparitiesAbout.aspx

Woodring, B. C., & Andrews, M. M. (2012). Transcultural perspectives in the nursing care of children. In M. M. Andrews & J. S. Boyle (Eds.), *Transcultural concepts in nursing care* (6th ed., pp. 123–156). Philadelphia, PA: Wolters Kluwer/Lippincott Williams & Wilkins.

TCN Concepts in Adult Health Courses

Priscilla Limbo Sagar and Drew Y. Sagar

KEY TERMS

Acculturation
Autonomy
Biological variations
Caregiving
Communications
Environmental control
Future orientation
Giger and Davidhizar Transcultural
  Assessment Model
Past orientation

Present orientation
Privacy
Respite
Safety
Sandwich generation
Self-identity
Social organization
Space
Territoriality
Time orientation

LEARNING OBJECTIVES

At the completion of this chapter, the learner will be able to

1. Analyze cultural influences in adult development.
2. Compare and contrast the influences of culture in caregiving between and among cultural groups.
3. Analyze biological variations between and among cultural groups and how these variations are integrated in providing culturally congruent care for adults.
4. Collaborate with an interprofessional team in the safe administration of medications.
5. Apply the Giger and Davidhizar Transcultural Assessment Model in planning integration of transcultural concepts in adult health courses.

OVERVIEW

Adulthood, though initially characterized as a long plateau separating childhood and old age, is now viewed as a dynamic stage with challenges and transformations (Boyle, 2012). There is a tremendous influence of culture in this dynamic, most productive stage of life.

When planning a course in adult health nursing, transcultural perspectives need to be woven into the course. There is a heavy weight allotted in adult health courses in undergraduate programs; these offer fertile grounds of transcultural (TCN) content to alleviate disparities in health care. Ideally, a separate course in TCN is recommended. In baccalaureate programs with no separate TCN course, faculty need to be creative in integrating TCN concepts. The **Giger and Davidhizar Transcultural Assessment Model** ([*TAM*], 2008, 2013) is applied in the care of the adult client.

Integration of TCN Concepts

Building on the work of Freud, Erik Erikson's stages of development (1963, 1968, as cited in Schwecke, 2003) cover the life cycle from birth to death. The adult life stage and developmental task is "generative lifestyle versus stagnation," which entails personal and professional growth (Schwecke, 2003, p. 28).

Peoples' cultural values and beliefs affect the way they practice health promotion, illness prevention, and treatment acceptance for diseases. The Giger and Davidhizar TAM has six cultural phenomena, namely *biological variation, communication, environmental control, space, social orientation,* and *time* (Giger & Davidhizar, 2008, 2013). These six cultural phenomena (see Chapter 1 for a review of the TAM) are highly applicable in the care of adults and can be woven in adult health nursing courses. Thoughtful integration of TCN concepts are imperative in preparing practitioners ready to care for multicultural adult clients.

There are many variations within and outside of specific cultures when dealing with the concepts of biological variations, communication, environmental control, space, social orientation, and **time orientation** (Giger & Davidhizar, 2008, 2013). These six areas of Giger and Davidhizar's (2008, 2013) TAM can be integrated—in part or in its totality—in all modules of adult health courses. The TAM is practical, simple, straightforward, and lends itself well in academic applications in nursing (Davidhizar & Giger, 2001; Sagar, 2012) and allied health (Dowd, Giger, & Davidhizar, 1998; Ryan, Carlton, & Ali, 2000). Spector (2013) continues to include the six areas of the TAM in her *Health Traditions Model*.

Biological Variations

There has been increasing evidence that a connection exists between ethnicity and the incidence of illness. Health care professionals who are knowledgeable about biocultural variations during illness are able to organize a thorough, systematic, and accurate assessment and physical examination (Andrews, 2012); this is crucial in planning, implementation, and evaluation of culturally congruent care. A more thorough discussion about **biological variations** is in Chapter 8.

For adult clients, it is an eye opener to look at two of the most prevalent illnesses, diabetes and hypertension, as well as the glaring disparities in health care access and quality among vulnerable populations. Giger and Davidhizar (2008) pointed out not only the

50% to 100% mortality from diabetes among Blacks, Hispanics, and American Indians but also the profound evidence of undermanagement of this disease among such vulnerable groups.

The research by Tsugawa, Mukamal, Davis, Taylor, and Wee (2012) showed that diabetic retinopathy is more prevalent among Blacks at Hb A1c levels between 5% and 7% (see EBP 11.1). This has significant implications to the assessment, planning, implementation, and evaluation of care of adults with diabetes. It is imperative that health care professionals include this in the patient education that is so vital in preventing complications of retinopathy.

EBP 11.1

Diabetes mellitus is a major health concern affecting the population in the United States. Hemoglobin A1c (HbA1c) is used extensively as an indicator of average serum glucose levels to assess the degree of risk for development of complications for diabetes as well as the degree of control in management of diabetes (Herman, 2009).

Tsugawa, Mukamal, Davis, Taylor, and Wee (2012) conducted a cross-sectional study among 2,804 White persons and 1,008 Black persons 40 years of age or older in the United States from 2005 through 2008. The study was performed in order to examine the relationship between HbA1c level and the incidence of retinopathy in participants.

There have been numerous studies to indicate that HbA1c levels are higher in Blacks, Asians, and Hispanics than in Whites in spite of factors including fasting serum glucose levels, duration of medication use, or compliance amount of adiposity (Herman, 2009). Because of the increasing evidence demonstrating HbA1c levels are higher among Black Americans than among Whites, recent proposals have been made to raise baseline cutoffs for HbA1c in determining the presence of diabetes and associated risks in Black Americans.

Tsugawa et al. (2012) performed the study to address proposals for raising the HbA1c baseline, analyzing data from a nationally representative sample from the National Health and Nutrition Examination Survey (NHANES), National Health Statistics, Center for Disease Control and Prevention. Participants were selected if they were 40 years of age or older and did not meet exclusion criteria such as being blind, having eye infections, or using bilateral eye patches. A human subject review board approved the NHANES protocol. All participants provided written consent.

Tsugawa et al. (2012) found that the existence of retinopathy starts to increase at a lower HbA1c level in Blacks than in Whites. In addition, these researchers added that diabetic retinopathy is elevated for Blacks at any given HbA1c level from 5.0% through 7.0% and that the "risk for retinopathy at an HbA1c level of 5.5% to 5.9% for blacks was similar to the risk at an HbA1c level of 6.0% to 6.4% among whites" (p. 157). Based on their findings, Tsugawa et al. (2012) are not in favor of increasing the HbA1c diagnostic threshold for blacks.

Limitations of this study included: cross-sectional design did not allow for HbA1c duration effect; no statistically significant interaction between HbA1c level and

(continued)

EBP 11.1 *(continued)*

race; and inability to determine reason for differences between HbA1c and diabetic retinopathy. Tsugawa et al. (2012) suggested a longitudinal study with
larger participants to determine if a lower threshold of HbA1c is warranted for
Blacks.

Applications to Practice

- Recall your classroom and clinical experiences learning about diabetes mellitus. Have you had opportunities to apply your didactic learning about diabetes
  when caring for diverse clients?
- Now that you have read these studies, will you be in favor of increasing the
  HbA1c diagnostic threshold for Blacks? Explain your reason.
- Analyze the course you are taking/teaching. Is there integration of cultural
  concepts about ethnicity and incidence of illnesses? If yes, in what course? If
  not, in which course would you include this content?
- If you were to replicate this study, how would you conduct it? What would
  you change in terms of conceptual framework, sampling, and analysis of
  findings?

Sources: Herman (2009, July); and Tsugawa, Mukamal, Davis, Taylor, & Wee (2012).

COMMUNICATION

Communication patterns differ between and among cultures. Communication may present as a barrier between nurses and patients, especially if they are from different cultures
(Giger & Davidhizar, 2008; Muñoz & Luckmann, 2005). In health care, casual first name
basis has become common; however, this is inappropriate in some cultures (Boyle, 2012).
For example, in some cultures, titles of "Mr." or "Mrs." are preferred. Among Filipinos, for
example, an honorific title such as "ate" or older sister may be used, or titles such as "po",
or "opo."

When looking at communication, it is important to examine what it achieves. In
health care, does it allow for accurate assessment, planning, intervention, and evaluation
of client outcomes? Does it make the client and the family or significant other feel that they
have been heard and treated the same as other clients? In the process of cultural assessment, the health care provider must also consider the client's level of **acculturation**, degree
of assimilation with the dominant culture, and biculturalism, the maintenance of values of
an individual's own and dominant culture (Muñoz & Luckmann, 2005).

Every client is entitled to culturally and linguistically appropriate care from all health
care providers. All institutions need to follow the enhanced culturally and linguistically
appropriate services ([CLAS], USDHHS, OMH, 2013b) standards. The latest copy of these
standards must be in the policies and procedure manual for every institution. All other
communication policies must be congruent with these standards. The availability of language access services (LAS) must be prominently displayed at strategic places in the institution in languages commonly used in the community.

ENVIRONMENTAL CONTROL

Environmental control, the belief of being able to control events, is very important when looking at how the client and his family view health and illness; this perception of control affects how the client and his family or significant other will follow the therapeutic regimen of western medicine. Giger and Davidhizar (2008, 2013) clarified that the environment is comprised of systems and processes affecting the individual; therefore, environmental control could be simply stated as maintaining balance with the environment.

To this effect, individuals employ generic folk practices to maintain well-being and to prevent and treat illnesses. Health care professionals must assess these healing and alternative modalities to effectively bridge the generic folk and professional health care systems, a key to culturally congruent care (Leininger, 2006).

SPACE

The concept of **space,** the area that encloses an individual's body (Giger & Davidhizar, 2008), may be seen as a segregating mechanism. For example, Muslim men and women have separate parties. In India, there is segregation by upper and lower castes, between secular and religious, and between males and females (Giger & Davidhizar, 2008). An individual from a largely populated, overcrowded nation may experience discomfort in another place where there is no overcrowding, and vice versa.

Territoriality denotes the individual's jurisdiction, possessiveness, and control of a spatial area as well as the need to establish rules for that area (Giger & Davidhizar, 2008, 2013). Making modifications for visiting hours is one way to respect the client's needs for territoriality; the nurse's creativity and organizational skills are at play here in balancing culturally congruent care and prioritization of care.

Citing Oland (1978), Giger and Davidhizar (2008, 2013) specified that the need for space calls for cultural diversity and congruent behaviors with regards to the following four functions: security, privacy, autonomy, and self-identity (pp. 61–62). **Safety** is inclusive of physical protection as well as the feeling of being safe. A 50-year-old Vietnamese client who has limited English proficiency (LEP) who may think that hospitals are for people who are dying will need an appropriate interpreter to explain this. Clients have the right to **privacy** of space and communication. The Health Insurance Portability and Accountability Act (HIPAA) and the Health Information Technology for Economic and Clinical Health Act (HITECH) contain "national standards for the privacy of protected health information, the security of electronic protected health information, and breach notification to consumers laws" (USDHHS, 2013a, para 1).

It is important that clients retain **autonomy**, or control of what occurs, such as the time of treatment, room arrangement, or the freedom to consult extended family members for opinions. When a client is admitted to the hospital, bringing a bedspread from home, a prayer rug, a rosary, and pictures of saints may enhance one's **self-identity** or self-expression.

TIME ORIENTATION

With regards to time, behaviors of persons from different cultures indicate the primary ordering of past, present, and future (Giger & Davidhizar, 2008). Accepting that there are differences in time perception between people from diverse cultures is the initial step in developing tolerance for time-related cultural behaviors such as assisting clients with treatment and meals. The melding of tradition and **past orientation** puts more emphasis in the past, such as reverence for ancestors or older members of society. In **future orientation**, there is dominance of the future in the present behavior (Giger & Davidhizar, 2008). For example, a family with future orientation may postpone buying a home or an expensive car in favor of saving for their two children's educations.

For individuals with **present orientation**, the present is more important than the past or the future. Patient education on preventive care, one of the most powerful tools in improving health outcomes, needs the utmost creativity in the inclusion of culturally congruent teaching strategies for people with present orientation.

SOCIAL ORGANIZATION

The nature of the family has evolved over the years. Despite these changes, it is still the basic unit of society (Giger & Davidhizar, 2008). To be able to partner with families in planning, implementing, and evaluating care, health care professionals must be able to work with the family on **social organization**. Some concepts to consider for integration in planning care are roles, family organization, kinship, and religion, among others. In the TAM, the family may be viewed as the environment whereby the individual, physical, and psychosocial needs of each member are taken into account. Viewed as clients, the nurse must assess for essential factors affecting family structure and organization. For example, when caring for a diabetic client, the nurse must thoroughly assess the family's needs: dietary patterns, available resources, knowledge about diabetes, support of the ill member, and coping abilities (Giger & Davidhizar, 2008). Caring for aging parents and relatives is another area of family responsibility and varies from culture to culture.

The care of aging parents presents many challenges for adults who are also dealing with child and grandchild care. There are cultural variations in the caregiving of aging parents. According to Boyle (2012), **caregiving** is the rendering of long-term care to family or friends. Caregiving to aging parents places additional stress on an already demanding schedule of being parents and grandparents in addition to work demands; this situation is referred to as being in the **sandwich generation**. In the area of caregiving, **respite,** or the interval for relief or a break, for the caregiver is important; the nurse needs to assess available community resources and make the appropriate referral.

CRITICAL THINKING EXERCISES 11.1

Undergraduate Student
1. You often hear faculty at your school say that you need to be prepared to care for culturally diverse clients as preparation for a complex health care system for an increasingly diverse nation. Has your confidence in providing culturally congruent care to adults increased?
2. Do you think there is enough content of cultural diversity and promotion of cultural competence integrated in your adult nursing classes (theory) and in clinical?
3. How often do you have opportunities to care for culturally diverse adult clients? Have you reflected on the learning that occurs with these encounters? Do you feel prepared to care for the client whose culture is other than your own? Why? Why not?

Graduate Student
1. How many adult health courses are in your master's/DIP program? Is TCN integrated in the rest of the courses in your program?
2. Is there a conceptual framework used for your graduate courses in TCN? Which theory or model is being used in your program?
3. If you were to apply a TCN theory or model, which one will you use? Discuss.
4. For research-focused doctoral students only: Does your dissertation focus on adult clients? Is there a diversity and cultural competence focus to your dissertation? Explain?

(continued)

CRITICAL THINKING EXERCISES 11.1 *(continued)*

Faculty in Academia
1. How many credits in adult health nursing do you have in the BS in Nursing program at your school?
2. Describe the concepts threaded or woven in to those courses. Are any concepts threaded vertically? Horizontally? Describe.
3. How do you critically appraise diversity and cultural competence content in your adult health courses?
4. Are there enough diverse clients in your affiliating agencies to meet objectives in adult health courses? Describe.

Staff Development Educator
1. Do you have students in adult health courses assigned to your health care facility for clinical rotation? Is a module or class in cultural diversity and promotion of cultural competence part of the required orientation packet?
2. Do you have ethnically diverse clients? Do students have opportunities to provide care, alongside staff nurses and instructors, to these culturally diverse clients?
3. Are you familiar with the enhanced culturally and linguistically appropriate services (CLAS) standards? Do you have language access services (LAS)? How much orientation time do staff and affiliates get for the LAS? Do the health care and ancillary staff use the LAS?
4. If you have diverse clientele, does the institution's decor, furniture, and artifacts celebrate diversity? Is signage in languages other than English visible and readable and is it posted at strategic places?

SUMMARY

Adult health courses, also referred to as medical–surgical courses in programs with a medical model, carry a heavy weight in undergraduate nursing programs such as associate, diploma, and baccalaureate programs. The concepts discussed in this chapter will also apply among graduate programs preparing adult health nurse practitioners or people in other clinical tracks. The six concepts of the Giger and Davidhizar TAM, namely biological variations, communication, environmental control, time orientation, space, and social orientation, lend themselves effectively into planning, implementing, and evaluating culturally congruent care for adult populations.

REFERENCES

Andrews, M. M. (2012). Cultural competence in the health history and physical examination. In M. M. Andrews & J. S. Boyle, *Transcultural concepts in nursing care* (6th ed., pp. 38–72). Philadelphia, PA: Walters Lower Health /Lippincott Williams & Wilkins.

Boyle, J. S. (2012). Transcultural perspectives in the nursing care of adults. In M. M. Andrews & J. S. Boyle (Eds.), *Transcultural concepts in nursing care* (6th ed., pp. 157–181). Philadelphia, PA: Walters Kluwer/Lippincott Williams & Wilkins.

Davidhizar, R. E., & Giger, J. N. (2001). Teaching culture within the nursing curriculum using the Giger–Davidhizar model of transcultural nursing assessment. *Journal of Nursing Education, 40*(6), 282–284.

Dowd, S. B., Giger, J. N., & Davidhizar, R. E. (1998). Use of Giger and Davidhizar's transcultural assessment model by health professions. *International Nursing Review, 5*(4), 119–122, 128.

Giger, J. N., & Davidhizar, R. E. (2008). *Transcultural nursing: Assessment and intervention* (5th ed.). St. Louis, MO: Mosby Elsevier.

Giger, J. N., & Davidhizar, R. E. (2013). *Transcultural nursing: Assessment and intervention* (6th ed.). St. Louis, MO: Elsevier Mosby.

Herman, W. (2009, July). Do race and ethnicity impact hemoglobin A1c independent of glycemia? *Journal of Diabetes Science and Technology, 3*(4), 656–660. Retrieved August 8, 2013, from www. ncbi.nlm.nih.gov/pmc/articles/PMC2769981

Leininger, M. M. (2006). Culture care diversity and universality and evolution of the ethnonursing method. In M. Leininger & M. McFarland (Eds.), *Culture care diversity and universality: A worldwide nursing theory* (pp. 1–41). Sudbury, MA: Jones & Bartlett.

Muñoz, C., & Luckmann, J. (2005). *Transcultural communication in nursing* (2nd ed.). Clifton Park, NY: Thomson Delmar Learning.

Ryan, M., Carlton, K. H., & Ali, N. (2000). Transcultural nursing concepts and experiences in nursing curricula. *Journal of Transcultural Nursing, 11*(4), 300–307.

Sagar, P. L. (2012). *Transcultural nursing theory and models: Application in nursing education, practice, and administration.* New York, NY: Springer Publishing.

Schwecke, L. H. (2003). Models for working with psychiatric patients. In L. N. Keltner, L. H. Schwecke, & C. E. Bostrom (Eds.), *Psychiatric nursing* (4th ed., pp. 20–35). St. Louis, MO: Mosby/Elsevier.

Spector, R. E. (2013). *Cultural diversity in health and illness* (8th ed.). Boston, MA: Pearson Education.

Tsugawa, Y., Mukamal, K. J., Davis, R. B., Taylor, W. C., & Wee, C. C. (2012). Should the Hemoglobin A1c diagnostic cutoff differ between Blacks and Whites? A cross-sectional study. *Annals of Internal Medicine, 157*(3), 153–159.

United States Department of Health and Human Services, Office of Civil Rights. (2013a). *HIPAA privacy, security, and breach notification audit program.* Retrieved August 16, 2013 from www.hhs. gov/ocr/privacy/hipaa/enforcement/audit/index.html

United States Department of Health and Human Services, Office of Minority Health. (2013b). *Enhanced national CLAS standards.* Retrieved August 16, 2013, from https://www.thinkculturalhealth.hhs.gov/Content/clas.asp

TCN Concepts in Caring for Older Adults Courses

Priscilla Limbo Sagar

KEY TERMS

Caregiving
End-of-life issues
Ethnopharmacology
Familism
Gerontology
Integrity versus despair

Obligations
Reciprocity
Sandwich generation
Spirituality
Subjective burden (SB)

LEARNING OBJECTIVES

At the completion of this chapter, the learner will be able to

1. Discuss the importance of integrating transcultural concepts when planning courses in the care for older adults.
2. Analyze activities to promote cultural sensitivity among students when caring for older adults.
3. Compare and contrast care of the older adults in diverse cultures.
4. Develop culturally and linguistically appropriate nursing interventions for older adults.
5. Apply Leininger's Cultural Care Theory in caring for older adults.

OVERVIEW

According to the World Health Organization (WHO, 2012), between 2000 and 2050, the percentage of the global population over 60 years old will double from approximately 11% to 22%; that is an increase from 605 million to 2 billion older people. In addition, the WHO predicted that the number of people aged 80 years will nearly quadruple to 395 million between 2012 and 2050. By 2017, the number of adults 65 years and over will outnumber children under the age of 5 (WHO, 2012).

Nationally, in addition to getting more diverse, the population is likewise getting older. The U.S. Census Bureau (2012) anticipated that between 2012 and 2060, the number of people 65 years and older will more than double, from 43.1 million to 92 million—that is one in five people. Furthermore, the U.S. Census Bureau also projected that individuals 85 years or older will increase over three times from today's 5.9 million to 18.2 million at the end of 2060. Globally and nationally, the aging trend has tremendous implications to nursing and health care.

Culture strongly influences how people view the aging process, coping behavior, associated health-seeking behaviors, and family caring practices (McKenna, 2012). Immigration and acculturation may affect expectations across generations. Caregiving for older family members have been documented in literature. Nurses and health care professionals need to exercise caution, however it is important to remember that there are variations within as well as between cultural groups. With this in mind, nurses provide about 80% of health care globally; migration trends and distribution of registered nurses (RNs) will greatly impact health care (International Council of Nurses [ICN], 2007), especially in light of the global aging trends.

Integration of TCN Concepts

When planning for integration of TCN concepts in an existing course or a new **gerontology** course, the following areas are suggested for inclusion: developmental stage, disparities in access and quality of care, caregiving for family members, **ethnopharmacology**, and views about the end of life, among others. When nurses are mindful of the client's cultural background, they are more likely to plan and implement care that is individualized for the client (McKenna, 2012). Leininger's (2006) Cultural Care Theory (CCT) is highly applicable in the assessment, planning, implementation, and evaluation of care of the older client. The CCT, along with the enhanced culturally and linguistically appropriate services (CLAS) standards (United States Department of Health and Human Services, Office of Minority Health, 2013), will guide the provision of culturally congruent care for the older adult client in all settings of practice.

Developmental Stage: Integrity Versus Despair

Development and adaptation occur throughout life; this has been recognized both in research and clinical practice (Melillo, 2011). Building on the work of Freud, Erik Erikson's (1963, 1968, as cited in Schwecke, 2003) developmental model covers the life cycle from birth to death. Erikson proposed that in his eight developmental stages, there are opportunities to grow, including the acceptance of one's own death in the eighth stage of life.

In this stage, 65 years to the point of death, the task is **integrity versus despair.** According to Schwecke and Wood (2001), as illustrated in Schwecke (2003), some positive manifestations at this stage include self-acceptance, dignity, worth, and importance; negative feelings include helplessness, hopelessness, uselessness, and meaninglessness (p. 28).

Disparities in Access and Quality of Care

The Agency for Healthcare Research and Quality (AHRQ, 2012) indicated that health care quality and access are suboptimal, particularly for minority and low-income groups. In the area of quality of care, the following groups received worse care than Whites: Blacks, Hispanics, American Indians (AI)/Alaska natives (AN), and Asians. The AHRQ also reported the existence of common disparities in access to care, especially among AI/ANs, Hispanics, Blacks, Asians, and poor people.

The poverty rate for Americans 65 years and above in 2008 was 9.7%; the rates were much higher among minorities: Blacks (20%), Hispanics (19.3%), and Asians, (12.1%) (Administration on Aging [AOA], 2010a, 2010b, n.d.-b). Being a minority and being poor present double the risk for poorer health outcomes.

Disparities in access and quality of care among older adults have been well-documented in the literature. Older members of some racial and ethnic groups have higher rates of illness compared to the White population: hypertension in Blacks (AOA, 2010a), diabetes in AIs/ANs and Mexicans (AOA, n.d.-b McKenna, 2012), and higher rates of inpatient heart attack mortality among Asians and Pacific Islanders ([APIs], AHRQ, 2011).

The prevalence of depression and mental health issues is high among the older population, yet only half of those who admit to mental health problems receive treatment (Melillo, 2010). In many cultures, there is still a high stigma placed on being mentally ill. Many believe that there is underreporting of mental health problems among the elderly (Melillo, 2010).

Disparities in the care of older adult residents in nursing homes have likewise been reported. The study by Li, Yin, Cai, Temkin-Greener, & Mukamel (2011) reveals that while there is reduced pressure ulcer rates among chronic residents of nursing homes, there are continuing disparities between Black and White residents (EBP 12.1).

EBP 12.1

Li et al. (2011) performed a cohort study of the rates of pressure ulcers (PU) among 2.1 million White and 346,808 Black residents in 12,473 certified nursing homes in the United States. This study was conducted from 2003 through 2008 among nursing homes that employed Centers for Medicare and Medicaid Services (CMS) resident assessment; online survey, certification, and reporting files; and area resource files. The institutional review boards of the University of Iowa and the University of California at Irvine approved this study.

The inclusion criteria for this study was the requirement for extensive or total dependence on staff assistance for bed mobility, being in a coma, or having malnutrition. Li et al. (2011) obtained nursing home characteristics from the CMS online survey, certification, and reporting facility database. Black residents (average age = 76) were generally 6 years younger than their White counterparts (average age = 82) and more likely to be male, be diabetic, and have a history of stroke.

Overall, PU rates are down from 2003 to 2008, from 16.8% to 14.6% for Black residents and from 11.4% to 9.6% for White residents. However, this shows continued higher PU rates for Black residents of nursing homes. Li et al. reiterated that the risk-adjusted disparity between Black and White residents in pressure ulcer rates occurred between rather than within sites. In addition, the researchers pointed

(continued)

EBP 12.1 *(continued)*

out that nursing homes with more Black residents were inclined to have fewer registered nurses (RNs) and certified nurse assistants (CNAs), to be for-profit, and to be urban facilities.

Li et al. (2011) acknowledged the following limitations of this study: (1) analyses focusing on prevalence and (2) limited availability in multivariate risk adjustment in terms of differences in the characteristics of residents and sites of care. The researchers suggest initiatives to reduce disparity reduction among nursing home residents.

Applications to Practice

■ Investigate the incidence and prevalence of pressure ulcers in a local nursing home. Is it congruent with the findings in this study?

■ Analyze the content of the gerontology course you are taking/teaching. Have you included disparities in care among the elderly? How are concepts in disparities integrated in the course?

■ If you were to replicate this study, how would you conduct it? What would you change in terms of conceptual framework, sampling, and analysis of findings?

Source: Li, Yin, Cai, Temkin-Greener, & Mukamel (2011).

Caregiving for Family Members

Caregiving—the process whereby a family provides care for its members—differs from culture to culture, as well as within cultures. **Familism** refers to the individual's allegiance, dedication, and reciprocity to family members (Knight & Sayegh, 2010). Neufeld and Harrison (1998, as cited in del-Pino-Casado, Frias-Osuna, & Palomino-Moral, 2011) defined **reciprocity** as a two-way exchange of resources and "can be motivated by altruism, reciprocation from the past, the wish to be cared for in the future, the elder's gratitude, a satisfactory affect exchange, or the exchange of support" (p. 284). Employing analysis of 1,284 informal caregivers of older adults, del-Pino-Casado et al. (2011) investigated obligation and reciprocity as motives for caregiving and its relationship to **subjective burden (SB)** of caregivers of disabled older people in Spain. The researchers found that (1) **obligations** and reciprocity were higher in spouses than in other relatives, (2) balanced reciprocity was higher in men, (3) obligations were not related with SB, and (4) balanced reciprocity was positively related to SB. Findings from the del-Pino-Casado et al. (2011) study can be used in the prevention and intervention of SB in informal caregivers of older adults.

As many as 30% of older Asian women live with other relatives (AOA, n.d.a); this can influence access to health care and resources. For example, among older Filipino immigrants in the United States, health care access is influenced by the availability of working adult children (Purnell, 2013). Some older people are members of the **sandwich generation— people** simultaneously caring for their own children as well as for aging parents—thereby carrying added burden. Another source of stress is migration and acculturation.

Ethnopharmacology

In a given week, four out of five adults in the United States take prescribed medications, over-the-counter drugs (OTC), or food supplements; one-third of these adults use five or more separate medications (Institute of Medicine [IOM], 2006). Among older adults, the most frequent physician intervention is the issuance of a prescription (Vestal & Gurwitz, 2000). Vestal and Gurwitz further added, citing Nelson and Knapp (1997), that ambulatory patients 75 years or older are prescribed 70% more medications than clients 25 to 44 years of age.

Older adults' ability to metabolize drugs are compromised by their gastrointestinal (GI) functioning, diminished excretory functions, and nutritional status, to name just a few. Some of these examples of altered GI functioning include decline in acid production, thereby increasing pH and altering lipid solubility; decrease in gastric emptying and delivery of the drug to the small intestine for absorption; and decreased GI motility that may impair drug absorption (Vestal & Gurwitz, 2000). The age-related reduction in elimination rate of drugs by the kidneys is related to both glomerular and tubular functions (Vestal & Gurwitz, 2000). Considering that the nation is getting intensely more diverse in addition to having one out of five older adults, the magnitude of this problem is overwhelming. There has been increasing interest in the relationship between biological variations and pharmacogenetics in the last two decades. The genetic makeup of the individual can alter drug action in many ways. Within the often considered "standard" dosage, deficiencies in enzymes can delay drug inactivation and ensuing excretion, resulting in toxic concentrations (Meyer, 2000, p. 1180). Additional information about biological variations affecting drug metabolism can be reviewed in Chapter 14.

Health professionals who are willing to spend more time performing a culturally and linguistically appropriate health history and physical examination will contribute more to preventing adverse drug events for elderly clients. Campinha-Bacote (2007) urged providers to perform a thorough assessment for clients on herbal supplements and psychotropic medications. This reminder is quite important, considering the high incidence of depression among the elderly. In addition to finding out the use of herbal supplementation, providers need to assess older adults for use of OTC, food supplements, and complementary alternative therapies. The use of CAMs is discussed in Chapter 14.

Views About the End of Life

Culture and religion influence **end-of-life issues** such as how death is viewed, spirituality, care of the body, grieving, and beliefs in the afterlife. Death and bereavement practices are not easy topics. Indeed, even reference to death takes on phrases such as "passed away" and "left us" instead of mentioning the word "death." Many cultures perceive death other than as a failure in western medicine, whereby life prolongation is usually the main goal.

Spirituality provides inner strength and gives meaning to one's life (Purnell, 2013). Some people's inner strength may come from faith in a higher being or from remaining in harmony with the environment; for others, strength may flow from a combination of these two factors (Purnell, 2013). Thoroughly assessing the client's spiritual life and well-being (Melillo, 2011) will guide individuals in planning culturally congruent care for clients and their families.

There is a wide variation in the process of grief among individuals from different cultures, as well as between individuals from the same culture (Muñoz & Luckmann, 2005); it is not appropriate to pass judgment on people with overt expressions of grief such as loud crying, wailing, or passing out. In addition, neither is it fair to assume that a person is not grieving if there are no visible expressions of grief; in some people, grieving is expressed not only covertly but with stoicism. Respect for clients is paramount; their active participation in decision making should guide the planning, implementation, and evaluation of care (Muñoz & Luckmann, 2005; Purnell, 2013).

The method of caring for the body after death varies from culture to culture. It is of utmost importance to follow the client's wishes and those of the family. Health care workers must accept and respect culturally specific bereavement customs and traditions.

APPLICATION

The CCT (Leininger, 2006) is an applicable framework in assessing older adults and planning culturally congruent care using three modes of action: preservation/maintenance, accommodation/negotiation, and repatterning/restructuring. All seven, or a few of the seven, factors of the CCT may be used. Table 12.1 illustrates the integration of Leininger's (2006) seven factors that influence care when assessing and planning culturally congruent care of older adults.

TABLE 12.1 Using Factors From Leininger's Cultural Care Theory

Factors	Assessment	Mode of Actions
Kinship and social	What is the composition of the client's family or significant other? What are the roles of family members in health and illness? Is there conformity to traditional gender roles?	Preservation/maintenance of family assistance in care, such as bathing and feeding if offered. Accommodation/negotiation for visits from extended family.
Economic	Who is the main wage earner and what is the client's level of income? What is the client's insurance? What is the client's experience with cost, coverage, and reimbursement of health services?	Repatterning/restructuring for appropriate referral to social services, if necessary.
Educational	What is the client's educational level? What is the primary language? Any regional dialect? Is the client able to speak English? Does the client have LEP? Are translators and interpreters needed?	Accommodation/negotiation for language access services (LAS) as necessary. Repatterning/restructuring for use of interpreter; avoid using relatives even if offered by client.
Political and legal	How does the community perceive its diverse members? What is the legal status of the client?	Repatterning/restructuring in community education about diverse members. For example, educating the community about the adjacent Amish community. Assistance in applying for amnesty, refugee, or permanent residency, or acquiring citizenship status.

(continued)

TABLE 12.1   Using Factors From Leininger's Cultural Care Theory   (continued)

Factors	Assessment	Mode of Actions
Religious and philosophical	What is the client's religious affiliation? How does religion affect health and illness? Are there items needed for worship? Are fasting and abstinence required? Is there an exception for persons who are ill? Are there prescribed rites for the seriously ill? Are there necessary healing rituals? Who performs these rituals? Will there be required space and materials for these rituals?	Accommodation/negotiation for clergy, folk healer visit. Repatterning/restructuring of fasting/abstinence rules after consultation with clergy.
Cultural values, beliefs, and ways of life	What is the cultural view on aging? Is there respect for older persons' wisdom? What is the client's belief about health and illness? How does the client interact with persons outside of his or her own cultural group? What are the caregiving patterns in the family and in the cultural group? Are older persons cared for in the home or in institutions? If in the home, who are the caregivers? Is there a belief in respite for the caregiver?	Preservation/maintenance of respect. Accommodation/negotiation Repatterning/restructuring for appropriate referral
Technological	Is there a preference to have a television or phone line in the room? Does the client use technology such as a cell phone or personal computer? Does the client use the Internet for electronic mail, for health information, or for recreation?	Repatterning/restructuring in using community resources to learn computer use for communication, recreation, or accessing health resources.

Source: Adapted from Leininge (2006).

CRITICAL THINKING EXERCISES 12.1

Undergraduate Student
1. How comfortable are you when caring for a culturally diverse older adult?
2. How prepared are you in caring for older adult clients during your clinical rotations? What factors in your classes, clinical, or simulation contribute to this preparation?
3. Do you think there is enough content on the older adult and promotion of cultural competence integrated in your classes (theory) and in clinical?
4. Would you be in favor of including a 3-credit care of the older adult course in your current curriculum? If yes, which course would you be in favor of deleting from your BS in Nursing curriculum? Why?

(continued)

CRITICAL THINKING EXERCISES 12.1 *(continued)*

Graduate Student
1. Do you think there is enough content on the older adult and promotion of cultural competence integrated in your graduate curriculum classes?
2. Do you have opportunities to manage care for older clients in your clinical practice? Are the older adult clients you work with from culturally diverse groups? Describe.
3. If you are pursuing a master's in gerontology, do you plan to take certification in this specialty? Explain.
4. Would you be in favor of adding a 3-credit care of the older adult course in your current curriculum? If yes, which course would you be in favor of deleting from your masters/DNP program curriculum? Why?

Faculty in Academia
1. How many credits do you have in the BS in Nursing program at your school?
2. If you were to add a 3-credit care of the older adult course, which current course would you delete? Why?
3. Are TCN concepts woven or threaded into your older adult course(s) in the graduate and undergraduate curricula? Describe.
4. How do you critically appraise care of the older adult in your curricula?

Staff Development Educator
1. What continuing education credits (CEs) are offered face-to-face in the institution to develop culturally competent care of older adults? How often are they offered?
2. Are there CEs offered online to develop culturally competent care of older adults?
3. How long has it been since you attended a workshop/conference on cultural diversity and promotion of cultural competence in the care of older adults? When are you planning to attend a workshop/conference on this topic?

SUMMARY

In the future, nurses and allied health care professionals will be working with even more older adults in all phases of services and settings: acute, home, communities. There are marked disparities in the access and quality of care among minority older adults. This chapter discussed concepts integral to planning new courses or course revisions of existing courses for older adults. The suggestions are not all inclusive; concepts in other chapters could be added, depending on the particular need of the SON or staff development settings. The assessment and plan for culturally congruent care is illustrated with the use of Leininger's Cultural Care Theory.

REFERENCES

Administration on Aging. (2010a). *A statistical profile of Black older Americans aged 65+.* Retrieved July 11, 2013, from www.aoa.gov/AoARoot/Aging_Statistics/minority_aging/Facts-on-Black-Elderly-plain_format.aspx

Administration on Aging. (2010b). *A statistical profile of Hispanic older Americans aged 65+.* Retrieved July 11, 2013, from www.aoa.gov/AoARoot/Aging_Statistics/minority_aging/Facts-on-Hispanic-Elderly.aspx

Administration on Aging. (n.d.-a). *A statistical profile of American Indian and Native Alaskan older Americans aged 65+*. Retrieved July 11, 2013, from www.aoa.gov/AoARoot/Aging_Statistics/minority_aging/Facts-on-AINA-Elderly2008-plain_format.aspx

Administration on Aging. (n.d.-b). *A statistical profile of Asian older Americans aged 65+*. Retrieved July 11, 2013, from http://aoa.gov/AoARoot/Aging_Statistics/minority_aging/Facts-on-API-Elderly2008-plain_format.aspx

Agency for Healthcare Research and Quality. (2011). *AHRQ-funded research on health care for Asian Americans/Pacific Islanders*. Retrieved June 1, 2013, from www.ahrq.gov/research/findings/nhqrdr/nhdr12/nhdr12_prov.pdf

Agency for Healthcare Research and Quality. (2012). *National healthcare disparities report, 2012*. Retrieved June 1, 2013, from www.ahrq.gov/research/findings/nhqrdr/nhdr12/nhdr12_prov.pdf

Campinha-Bacote, J. (2007). Becoming culturally competent in ethnic psychopharmacology. *Journal of Psychosocial Nursing, 45*(9), 27–33.

del-Pino-Casado, R., Frias-Osuna, A., & Palomino-Moral, P. A. (2011). Subjective burden and cultural motives for caregiving in informal caregivers of older people. *Journal of Nursing Scholarship, 43*(3), 282–291.

Institute of Medicine. (2006). *Preventing medication errors*. Retrieved June 29, 2013, from www.iom.edu/~/media/Files/Report%20Files/2006/Preventing-Medication-Errors-Quality-Chasm-Series/medicationerrorsnew.pdf

International Council of Nurses. (2007). Nurse retention and migration. Retrieved July 11, 2013, from www.icn.ch/images/stories/documents/publications/position_statements/C06_Nurse_Retention_Migration.pdf

Knight, B. G., & Sayegh, P. (2010). Cultural values and caregiving: The updated sociocultural stress and coping model. *Journals of Gerontology. Series B. Psychological Sciences and Social Sciences, 65B*(1), 5–13.

Leininger, M. M. (2006). Culture care diversity and universality theory and evolution of the ethno-nursing method. In M. M. Leininger & M. R. McFarland (Eds.), *Culture care diversity and universality: A worldwide nursing theory* (2nd ed., pp. 1–41). Sudbury, MA: Jones & Bartlett.

Li, Y., Yin, J., Cai, X., Temkin-Greener, H., & Mukamel, D. (2011). Association of race and sites of care with pressure ulcers in high-risk nursing home residents. *Journal of the American Medical Association, 306*(2), 179–186.

McKenna, M. A. (2012). Transcultural perspectives in the nursing care of older adults. In M. M. Andrews & J. S. Boyle (Eds.), *Transcultural concepts in nursing care* (6th ed., pp. 182–207). Philadelphia, PA: Wolters Kluwer/Lippincott Williams & Wilkins.

Melillo, K. D. (2011). Introduction and overview of aging and older adulthood. In K. D. Melillo & H. C. Houde (Eds.), *Geropsychiatric and mental health nursing* (2nd ed., pp. 3–30). Sudbury, MA: Jones & Bartlett Learning.

Meyer, U. A. (2000). Core topics in clinical pharmacology: Pharmacogenetics. In S. G. Carruthers, B. B. Hoffmann, K. L. Melmon, & D. W. Nierenberg (Eds.), *Melmon and Morelli's clinical pharmacology* (4th ed., pp. 1179–1205). New York, NY: McGraw-Hill Medical.

Muñoz, C., & Luckmann, J. (2005). *Transcultural communication in nursing*. Clifton Park, NY: Thompson/Delmar Learning.

Purnell, L. D. (2013). The Purnell model for cultural competence. In L. D. Purnell (Ed.), *Transcultural healthcare: A culturally competent approach* (4th ed., pp. 15–44). Philadelphia: F. A. Davis.

Schwecke, L. H. (2003). Models for working with psychiatric patients. In L. N. Keltner, L. H. Schwecke, & C. E. Bostrom (Eds.), *Psychiatric nursing* (4th ed., pp. 20–35). St. Louis, MO: Mosby/Elsevier.

U.S. Census Bureau. (2012). *U.S. Census Bureau projections show a slower growing, older, more diverse nation a half century from now*. Retrieved August 3, 2013, from www.census.gov/newsroom/releases/archives/population/cb12–243.html

U.S. Department of Health and Human Services, Office of Minority Health. (2013). *Enhanced national CLAS standards*. Retrieved August 16, 2013, from https://www.thinkculturalhealth.hhs.gov/Content/clas.asp

Vestal, R. E., & Gurwitz, J. H. (2000). Core topics in clinical pharmacology: Geriatric pharmacology. In S. G. Carruthers, B. B. Hoffmann, K. L. Melmon, & D. W. Nierenberg (Eds.), *Melmon and Morelli's clinical pharmacology* (4th ed., pp. 1151–1177). New York, NY: McGraw-Hill Medical.

World Health Organization. (2012). *Are you ready? What you need to know about ageing*. Retrieved July 7, 2013, from www.who.int/world-health-day/2012/toolkit/background/en

CHAPTER

TCN Concepts in Mental Health and Psychiatric Nursing Courses

13

Drew Y. Sagar and Priscilla Limbo Sagar

KEY TERMS

Acculturation
Assimilation
Avoidance
Culture-bound syndrome (CBS)
Community mental health centers
Cultural shock
De-institutionalization
Depression
Enculturation
Folk diseases

Folk illnesses
Hyperarousal
Integration
Marginalization
Mental health
Posttraumatic stress disorder
Psychopharmacology
Reexperiencing
Stigma

LEARNING OBJECTIVES

At the completion of this chapter, the learner will be able to

1. Analyze concepts of mental health and mental illness in various cultures.
2. Provide culturally congruent care to clients with mental illness.
3. Collaborate with the interprofessional team in the safe administration of psychopharmacologic medications.
4. Critique community-based mental health centers for clients with mental illness.
5. Develop a plan of care for clients with post-traumatic stress syndrome.

OVERVIEW

The concepts of **mental health** and mental illness are regarded differently within and among cultures. Across cultures, there is **stigma**—a trait that brings "a stain or reproach" on a person's reputation (Giger et al., 2007, p. 214)—attached to mental illness. Henceforth, some individuals may express their anxiety with somatic problems such as headaches or backaches. Nurses need to pay close attention to two trends that are vital to meet the needs of clients with mental illness: the increase in cultural diversity and the rising of community-based treatment centers (Ehrmin, 2012). These two trends have profound implications in the education of allied health care professionals such as nurses, physicians, pharmacists, physical therapists, and social workers. The trend for increased community-based treatment in mental health care was greatly facilitated by the creation of the Substance Abuse and Mental Health Services Administration (SAMHSA, 2013a), a branch of the United States Department of Health and Human Services (USDHHS), in 1992. SAMHSA (2013a) aims to improve access to information, care, and treatment resources; its mission is to decrease the effect of mental illness and drug abuse on communities.

SAMHSA (2013b) highlighted the provision and support for good mental health as a public health issue, an issue as important as ensuring safe quality of drinking water or the prevention and management of infectious diseases. According to SAMHSA (2013b), mental health problems affect one in five Americans; of those with mental health problems, slightly more than one out of three will obtain mental health services. In regards to cost to human lives, SAMHSA (2013b) noted that suicide claimed the lives of more than 3,800 people—more than double the number who died by homicide—in 2010 alone. In 2012, it is estimated that the cost of serious mental illnesses in terms of lost earnings reached $193.2 billion in the United States (SAMHSA, 2013b). Indeed, the cost of mental health problems is staggering.

De-institutionalization, or the movement to close state mental hospitals and discharge people with mental afflictions began in 1963 with the passage of the Community Mental Health Centers Act (Townsend, 2012). A **community mental health center (CMHC)** is a community-based center whose main goal is to improve coping and prevent episodes of acute exacerbations among individuals with serious and unrelenting mental illnesses (Townsend, 2012, p. 899). Over the years, lack of state funding and the eventual termination of federal funding for CMHCs continue to challenge the much needed provision of community-based services for the mentally ill.

Between the years 2002 and 2007, the Bush administration increased federal expenditures to expand services provided by community-based health treatment centers (CHTCs) from $1 billion to $2 billion, with over $7 million awarded specifically to mental health care at 50 community-based treatment centers (Wells, Morrisey, Lee, & Radford, 2010). Furthermore, in 2008 the Obama administration signed into effect the Mental Health Parity Act, which requires health insurance carriers that provide coverage for mental health care to do so on a parity with coverage for medical illness (SAMHSA, 2011, 2013a), helping to assure greater access to adequate mental health care in the United States.

Integration of TCN Concepts

The need to address our increasing cultural diversity through cultural awareness and sensitivity when providing health care is now being recognized as more colleges and universities adapt existing curricula to meet the demands of increasingly diverse populations in their respective communities, the country, and the world. Ndiwane et al. (2004) noted the modification to the curriculum of one such program for advance practice nursing (APNS) in Massachusetts. The following concepts may be integrated to existing or developing courses: acculturation, culture-bound syndromes, depression, and psychopharmacology.

THE PROCESS OF ACCULTURATION

The **acculturation** process is a process by which an individual or group from one culture takes on the values and ways of life of another from another culture, which is generally presumed to be a host culture (Leininger, 1995). **Enculturation** is a somewhat different process that involves comprehensive learning about a culture's attributes of beliefs, values, and traditions in order to prepare children and adults to live and function within that culture (Leininger, 1995).

The process of acculturation is thought to occur through different mechanisms of either **assimilation,** in which the individual or group abandons heritage cultures either voluntarily or because they are coerced to do so. Another means of acculturation is the process of **integration,** in which the host culture's values and ways of life are accepted, while heritage ways of life and values are selectively retained (Kunst & Sam, 2013).

In a meta-analytical study of literature addressing issues of acculturation, enculturation, and marginalization, Yoon et al. (2013) explored these phenomenon and found that acculturation is associated with both positive mental health outcomes such as self-esteem, positive affect, and satisfaction with life, and negative mental health outcomes of anxiety, depression, and negative affect. However, enculturation, while associated with anxiety, demonstrated a greater association with positive mental health outcomes. This is ostensibly because enculturation— along with associated support of those from similar backgrounds—is important in helping to solve many day to day problem situations and to provide a strong foundation in life.

The most positive mental health outcomes are associated with both effective external acculturation such as language and dress, and internal enculturation that relates to a sense of identity (Yoon et al., 2013). The concept of **marginalization** is associated with failed acculturation in which a sense of connection to a dominant culture is absent. In this sense, the phenomenon of marginalization may occur voluntarily, as certain groups may choose it as an option because its ideology differs from the mainstream (Ray, 2010). Marginalization generally possesses negative connotations due to inherent implied discrimination and ostracization by mainstream society (Ray, 2010). In another context, marginalization may refer to the rejection of both heritage and host cultures and is generally associated with the least favorable mental health outcomes (Yoon et al., 2013).

CULTURE-BOUND SYNDROMES

Culture-bound syndrome (CBS) may be alternately known as **folk illnesses** or **folk diseases** and disorders limited to a specific culture or group of cultures (Andrews, 2012) in certain geographical regions of the globe (Basuray, 2013). CBS are generally locality specific, abnormal, and often disturbing behaviors that recur intermittently (American Psychiatric Association [APA], 2000). Some CBS do not affect health while some are quite serious and oftentimes fatal (Basuray, 2013). To assist practitioners with culturally congruent care, a glossary of CBS was developed by the APA (2000) in its *Diagnostic and Statistical Manual of Mental Disorders (DSM-IV-TR)*. In recognition of the vital role that culture plays in diagnostic assessment and clinical management of illnesses, the *DSM-5* (APA, 2013) contains an updated cultural formulation (CI). The CI contains a framework for the assessment of the cultural manifestations of an individual's mental health problem and how it correlates with social and cultural history (APA, 2013). For listing of CBS, refer to Chapter 8, Table 8.2.

DEPRESSION

The experience of depression is perhaps a universal phenomenon in which the individual may experience many feelings in common. Sadock and Sadock (2007) provided a description of **depression** as a state of mind in which an individual may experience feelings of sadness and/or loneliness. Additionally, depressed individuals often report feelings of poor self-esteem and experience a sense of guilt. It is understood that the process of acculturation is a stressful process among immigrant families, and that response to this process may contribute to symptoms of depression and subsequent associated behaviors including attempted and completed suicide. Goldston, Mollock, Murakami, Zayas, and Nagayama (2008) reported that the stress of maintaining a dual role as a member in a traditional family and an individual western society might increase the risk of suicidal thoughts and behaviors.

In a Canadian study of depressive symptoms experienced by adolescents and young adults of recent immigrant backgrounds, Nguyen, Rawana, and Flora (2011) identified several factors including self-esteem, optimism, and maternal cohesion that are associated with lower levels of depression in children and young adults of immigrant families. Additional findings from the Nguyen et al. (2011) study indicate that children of immigrants or second-generation immigrants have higher levels of depressive symptoms than first generation immigrants. Furthermore, the greater proficiency in a host language such as English or French correlates to greater predicted levels of depression later in life. The implications being that increased acculturation among second generation immigrants decreases the cohesion between parents and their children as well as increasing the gap between them and the heritage culture. This appears to demonstrate that acculturation—while associated with certain mainstream lifestyle benefits—may result in subsequent loss of the protective influences associated with identification with the heritage culture (Nguyen et al., 2011).

PSYCHOPHARMACOLOGY

The term **psychopharmacology** generally refers to the study of how medication affects the brain (Stahl, 2008). This is a rapidly developing area in the treatment of psychiatric illness that needs to be systematically reviewed and organized according to methods of psychiatric care in order to continue to advance the practice of ethnic psychopharmacology. Research in the past decades indicated important differences in metabolism and clinical efficacy of some medications (Campinha-Bacote, 2007).

EBP 13.1

Chandra and Batada (2007) used mixed methods to explore stress and coping among African American adolescents from East Baltimore, Maryland. The Johns Hopkins Committee on Human Research approved the study. In addition, the Johns Hopkins Center for Adolescent Health Youth Advisory Committee (CAHYAC) reviewed the research design and instruments. A total of 26 teens, all in ninth grade, participated in the study. Nineteen of the 26 participants were female. The average age for participants was 14.5 years, representing nine high schools in East Baltimore.

The researchers used questionnaires, audio-taped journals, pile-sorting activities, and illustrations of personal–social support networks. The 16-page questionnaire asked about demographics, symptoms of stress, conflicts in the family, strategies used to cope with stress, and racial discrimination. Participants answered questions daily in the audio journal for 30 days; only every 3 days were questions related to

(continued)

EBP 13.1 (*continued*)

the study—the rest were fillers. In the pile-sort activities, the teens sorted the stress cards according (1) to the ways that made sense to them; (2) to the frequency of stress in their lives; and (3) to their level of worry about the stress. After receiving instructions from the researchers, the participants illustrated personal network maps of the persons and places they use as support when handling their stress.

Chandra and Batada (2006) used the SPSS version 11.5 to analyze the quantitative data from the questionnaire. Texts from the audio journal were coded in Atlas.ti version 4.2. The researchers also spent a day and interacted with each participant in the study; the researchers found this interaction useful in data analysis.

Findings indicate that teen participants utilized a variety of both avoidant and active coping strategies. The majority of teens stayed away from the problem in order to avoid conflict. Many participants admitted talking to a friend or an adult about problems and how to devise ways to cope with stress. There were important differences in coping styles between boys and girls: 24% of boys reported frequent use of avoidance compared to girls at 20%; a higher percentage of boys (25%) used distraction coping strategies than girls (14%).

In addition, the analysis of variance tests showed that boys used fewer strategies to seek support (2.43) than girls (4.05) and employed fewer active strategies (4.71) than girls (8.10). None of the boys reported thinking about a problem in order to handle the situation, whereas nearly half of the girls did. Furthermore, about a third of the girls reported use of preventive strategies such as avoidance of problems before they developed; none of the boys stated that they prevent problems in a similar manner.

Chandra and Batada (2006) acknowledged the following as limitations of this study: small sample; possibility of selection bias; and sample size with unequal number of boys and girls. In addition, the stress categorization from the initial focus groups may have prevented teens from discussing stress not included in the groupings.

To apply the Chandra and Batada (2006) research findings in Baltimore city, three interventions resulted: creation of a health promotion video about teen stress by participants and other youth; documentation of the development of the youth-created video for researchers wishing to engage youth participation; and collaboration between the CAHYAC and the community to produce a practical guide for adults in working with teens in stress.

Applications to Practice

■ Investigate your psychiatric and mental health nursing course. Are stress and coping covered in depth in that course? If your answer is "No," is stress and coping covered in other course(s)? Explain.

■ Analyze the psychiatric and mental health nursing course that you are taking/ teaching. How are cultural concepts integrated?

■ If you were to replicate this study, how would you conduct it? What would you change in terms of conceptual framework, sampling, and analysis of findings?

Source: Chandra & Batada (2006).

Before prescribing medications, the health care provider needs to be aware of factors including pharmacogenetics, as well as pharmacodynamics and the correlated implications of administering or withholding medication based on that knowledge (Sadock & Sadock, 2005). Additionally, the health care provider needs to solicit information from the client— inquiring in as nonthreatening and nonjudgmental manner as possible—about what the illness means to him or her. Furthermore, the health care provider needs to assess client expectations for getting well as well as other medications, herbal preparations, tobacco, alcohol, and illicit drugs that clients may be using (Sadock & Sadock, 2005). Further coverage of biological variations, drug interactions, and metabolism is provided in Chapter 14.

The use of self-learning modules (SLMs) is an effective way to present important concepts in academic or staff development settings. In other sources, SLMs may be presented with or without pre- and posttests. In this book, SLMs are provided with pre- and posttests as aids to learner's mastery of content. A review of Chapter 3 is suggested prior to undertaking Self-Learning Module 13.1.

SELF-LEARNING MODULE 13.1 POSTTRAUMATIC STRESS DISORDER (PTSD) IN WOMEN

Toni Ann Cervone, BS, RN
Staff Nurse, Sing Sing Correctional Facility
Fishkill, New York

Take Pretest (Appendix 14)

OVERVIEW

This module focuses on promoting awareness about the risk for **posttraumatic stress disorder (PTSD)** in women to facilitate symptom reduction and mental health wellness. The educational information in this module is intended to help professional nurses involved in caring for women, in staff development, and in academic settings to develop appropriate care programs for women with PTSD. Women of all cultures are susceptible for developing PTSD.

OBJECTIVES

At the completion of this module, the learner will

1. Identify risk factors for PTSD.
2. Enumerate and explain symptoms of PTSD.
3. Discuss treatments for PTSD.
4. Analyze nursing intervention for women with PTSD.

CONTENT OUTLINE

Definition: According to the American Psychiatric Association (APA, 2000), posttraumatic stress disorder (PTSD) is a psychiatric disorder which may follow as a result of the person being exposed to a traumatic event. The traumatic event involves both of the following: (1) experiencing, witnessing, or confronting an event or events that involved actual or threatened death or serious injury, or a threat to the physical integrity of self or others; and (2) response involving intense fear, helplessness, or horror (APA, 2000, p. 467). The person's response involves intense fear, helplessness, or horror (p. 467).

(continued)

SELF-LEARNING MODULE 13.1   POSTTRAUMATIC STRESS DISORDER (PTSD) IN WOMEN *(continued)*

Statistics: A 1-year survey conducted in 2010 revealed there were 1.3 million women raped in 1 year and one in five women raped within their lifetime; among these women, 63% experienced symptoms of PTSD (Centers for Disease Control and Prevention, 2010). Women have a 10% higher risk for being diagnosed with PTSD versus men, who have a 5% risk. Furthermore, 23% of women veterans are sexually assaulted (National Center for PTSD, 2012a). Intimate partner violence (IVP) is also experienced by 23% of women.

Risk Factors: Risk factors for PTSD in women include homelessness, low income, witnessing violence, IVP, multiple assaults (Glass, Perrin, Campbell, & Soeken, 2007), childhood physical/sexual abuse, adult physical/sexual assault, and veteran status (National Center for PTSD, 2012c). Violence is accepted and used as a means of conflict resolution by husbands to discipline their wives in countries such as Mexico, Zimbabwe, Pakistan, Tanzania, India, Bangladesh, Papua New Guinea, and Cambodia. Women of these cultures are at high risk for developing PTSD (Carretta, 2008). Traumatic childbirth such as emergency caesarean section and vaginal forceps/vacuum delivery (Gamble & Creedy, 2005) is another risk factor for women to develop PTSD. In the Latina culture, pregnancy is considered a happy and a positive family event, so Latina women may not be willing to admit to negative feelings related to childbirth (Anderson, 2010).

Manifestations: The PTSD symptoms cluster consists of reexperiencing, avoidance, and hyperarousal. Nightmares, flashbacks, intrusive memories (National Center for PTSD, 2012d), and maternal fear of a baby dying (Bailham & Joseph, 2003) are examples of **reexperiencing**. Avoiding reminders of the trauma, emotional numbness, detachment, difficulty remembering important details, negativity toward others, loss of interest (National Center for PTSD, 2012d), maternal–infant attachment issues, sexual evasion, and fear of childbirth (Bailham & Joseph, 2003) are examples of **avoidance**. Manifestations of **hyperarousal** include hypervigilance, jitteriness, outburst of anger and irritability, difficulty concentrating and sleeping, and being startled (National Center for PTSD, 2012d). Symptoms appear in 1 to 3 months after trauma (Guess, 2006).

Treatment: Counseling treatment for PTSD includes cognitive behavioral therapy (CBT; National Alliance on Mental Illness, 2012), cognitive processing therapy (CPT), prolonged exposure (PE) therapy, and eye movement desensitization and reprocessing (EMDR; National Center for PTSD, 2012c). Antidepressants such as sertraline, paroxetine, and fluoxetine treat depression and anxiety associated with PTSD. Alpha-adrenergic agents such as clonidine, propranolol, and prazosin promote sleep and decrease nightmares (Blizzard, Kemppainen, & Taylor, 2009).

Nursing Interventions: Nursing interventions include establishing trust and assessing a woman for risk factors of PTSD. Incorporating the *Primary Care PTSD Screen (PC-PTSD)* as part of the regular assessment process is a helpful tool to assist nurses in determining if a woman has experienced exposure to trauma, so appropriate mental health referrals can be made (National Center for PTSD, 2012b). It is important for the nurse to be sensitive and aware of different cultural beliefs about men having the

(continued)

accepted right to use violence against women as a disciplinary measure (Carretta, 2008). In regards to childbirth experiences, open-ended questions should be asked (Stone, 2009) and cultural beliefs related to pregnancy should be considered (Anderson, 2010). Provide emotional support, such as encouraging the woman to talk about the trauma and her feelings, along with educating the woman, family, and friends that repeating the story of the trauma promotes healing. It is important to educate women, family, and friends about the risk factors, symptoms, and treatment for PTSD (Guess, 2006). Providing a community resource pamphlet containing information for PTSD treatment and supportive services is important to facilitate the healing process.

Learning Resources

READINGS

1. Anderson, C. (2010). Impact of traumatic birth experience on Latina adolescent mothers. *Issues in Mental Health Nursing, 31*(11), 700–707. doi:10.3109/0161284 0.2010.518784
2. Gamble, J., & Creedy, D. (2005). Psychological trauma symptoms of operative birth. *British Journal of Midwifery, 13*(4), 218–224.
3. Glass, N., Perrin, N., Campbell, J., & Soeken, K. (2007). The protective role of tangible support on post-traumatic stress disorder symptoms in urban women survivors of violence. *Research in Nursing & Health, 30*(5), 558–568.
4. National Center for PTSD Website: www.ptsd.va.gov
5. Postpartum Support International Website: www.postpartum.net
6. Primary Care PTSD Screen (PC-PTSD) Website: www.ptsd.va.gov/professional/pages/assessments/pc-ptsd.asp

Learning Activities*

1. You are encouraged to assess the needs of the particular population of women you provide care for and research appropriate community resources available for PTSD treatment and support to promote healing.
2. If you were to create a community resource pamphlet of treatment and support for women with PTSD, what information would you include? Why?

Self-Assessment*

1. Were you aware of the statistics and risk factors for women developing PTSD prior to taking this module?
2. Do you feel more competent assessing and recognizing women at risk for or who may have PTSD?
3. Would you feel comfortable using the Primary Care PTSD Screen (PC-PTSD) as a tool to assess women as potential victims of trauma and provide a referral to mental health services for appropriate diagnosing and treatment of PTSD? Explain.

---

*If a module has an online component or is offered totally online, these may be used as discussion questions (DQs).

(continued)

SELF-LEARNING MODULE 13.1   POSTTRAUMATIC STRESS DISORDER (PTSD) IN WOMEN   *(continued)*

Take Posttest (Appendix 15; the key to pretest and posttest is available in Appendix 16.)

LESSON EVALUATION

1. Complete Module Evaluation Form (Appendix 3)
2. Analyze your learning experience by comparing your pretest and posttest answers.

Sources:

American Psychiatric Association. (2000). *Diagnostic and statistical manual of mental disorders* (4th ed., text rev.). Washington, DC: Author.

Anderson, C. (2010). Impact of traumatic birth experience on Latina adolescent mothers. *Issues in Mental Health Nursing, 31*(11), 700–707. doi:10.3109/01612840.2010.518784

Bailham, D., & Joseph, S. (2003). Post-traumatic stress following childbirth: A review of the emerging literature and directions for research and practice. *Psychology, Health & Medicine, 8*(2), 159–168.

Blizzard, S., Kemppainen, J., & Taylor, J. (2009). Post-traumatic stress disorder and community violence: An update for nurse practitioners. *Journal of the American Academy of Nurse Practitioners, 21*(10), 535–541. doi: http://dx.doi.org/10.1111/j.1745–7599.2009.00442.x

Carretta, C. (2008). Domestic violence: A worldwide exploration. *Journal of Psychosocial Nursing & Mental Health Services, 46*(3), 26–35.

Centers for Disease Control and Prevention. (2010). *The National intimate partner and sexual violence survey fact sheet.* Retrieved March 09, 2013, from www.cdc.gov/ViolencePrevention/pdf/NISVS_FactSheet-a.pdf

Centers for Disease Control and Prevention. (2012). *Intimate partner violence: Consequences.* Retrieved January 29, 2013, from http://cdc.gov/ViolencePrevention/intimatepartnerviolence/consequences.html

Gamble, J., & Creedy, D. (2005). Psychological trauma symptoms of operative birth. *British Journal of Midwifery, 13*(4), 218–224.

Glass, N., Perrin, N., Campbell, J., & Soeken, K. (2007). The protective role of tangible support on post-traumatic stress disorder symptoms in urban women survivors of violence. *Research in Nursing & Health, 30*(5), 558–568.

Guess, K. (2006). Post-traumatic stress disorder: Early detection is key. *Nurse Practitioner, 31*(3), 26–32.

National Alliance on Mental Illness. (2012). *Cognitive behavioral therapy fact sheet.* Retrieved February 8, 2013, from www.nami.org/factsheets/CBT_factsheet.pdf

National Center for PTSD. (2012a). *How common is PTSD?* Retrieved January 20, 2013, from http://www.ptsd.va.gov/public/pages/how-common-is-ptsd.asp

National Center for PTSD. (2012b). *Primary care PTSD screen (PC-PTSD).* Retrieved January 20, 2013, from www.ptsd.va.gov/professional/pages/assessments/pc-ptsd.asp

National Center for PTSD. (2012c). *What is PTSD?* Retrieved January 20, 2013, from www.ptsd.va.gov/public/pages/what-is-ptsd.asp

National Center for PTSD. (2012d). *Symptoms of PTSD.* Retrieved January 20, 2013, from www.ptsd.va.gov/public/pages/symptoms_of_ptsd.asp

Stone, H. (2009). Post-traumatic stress disorder in postpartum patients: What nurses can do. *Nursing for Women's Health, 13*(4), 284–291. doi: http://dx.doi.org/10.1111/j.1751–486X.2009.01438.x

CRITICAL THINKING EXERCISES 13.1

Undergraduate Student
1. Do you feel prepared to care for mentally ill clients from diverse cultures and various sexual orientations?
2. Do you think there is enough content of cultural diversity and promotion of cultural competence integrated in your mental health and psychiatric nursing class (theory) and in clinical?
3. When caring for clients with mental illness, have you noticed the stigma attached to the illness? Describe. Do you find this stigma across cultures and sexual orientation? Describe.

Graduate Student
1. Is diversity and cultural competence integrated in your master's/DNP program? Describe.
2. If you are in the mental health psychiatric nursing track, how many separate courses do you have in diversity and cultural competence? If you have no separate courses, is diversity and cultural competence integrated in other courses? Describe.
3. How many clinical hours, both in institutions and in the community, are you required to complete when working with clients with mental illness?
4. In the above clinical practice, do you have opportunities to work with culturally diverse clients?

Faculty in Academia
1. How many credits are offered by the mental health and psychiatric nursing course that you teach? Is diversity and promotion of cultural competence integrated in this course?
2. How many clinical hours do students need to complete for mental health and psychiatric nursing? Do they have opportunities to care for clients from diverse cultures and sexual orientation?
3. How do you critically appraise diversity content in mental health and psychiatric nursing?
4. Are you planning to add more TCN concepts in this course? How?

Staff Development Educator
1. Do you have students on clinical rotation for mental health and psychiatric nursing courses?
2. Do you require a module in cultural diversity and promotion of cultural competence as part of their orientation to your facility?
3. What follow-up activities regarding diversity and cultural competence do you have for affiliating students? For nurses and ancillary staff?
4. How long has it been since you attended a workshop or conference on diversity and promotion of cultural competence? Are those conferences regarding caring for clients with mental illness?

SUMMARY

Although mental health is as essential as safe drinking water or treatment of infectious diseases, there is a continuing stigma to mental illness. Consequently, clients do not readily seek appropriate health care. The cost of mental illness is staggering in terms of medication, therapy, and lost productivity. However, when considering the pain and anguish of those afflicted and of their loved ones, the cost is not measurable. Immigration poses additional stress to individuals and families as they enculturate and assimilate—most times in the margins—to the mainstream society. Recognizing this painful process could help health care professionals to ease this transition. In acknowledgment of the prevalence of PTSD across cultures, this chapter contains a full-length module dedicated to the assessment, planning, implementation, and evaluation of care for women with PTSD. With budget cuts and the closing of many inpatient psychiatric facilities, community day hospitals provide the structure and follow-up care that mentally ill populations critically need.

REFERENCES

American Psychiatric Association (2000). *Diagnostic and statistical manual of mental disorders* (4th ed., text rev. Washington, DC: Author.

American Psychiatric Association. (2013). *Diagnostic and statistical manual of mental disorders* (5th ed.). Arlington, VA: American Psychiatric Publishing.

Anderson, C. (2010). Impact of traumatic birth experience on Latina adolescent mothers. *Issues in Mental Health Nursing, 31*(11), 700–707. doi:10.3109/01612840.2010.518784

Andrews, M. (2012). The influence of cultural and health belief systems on health care practices. In M. M. Andrews & J. S. Boyle (Eds.), *Transcultural concepts in nursing care* (6th ed., pp. 73–88). Philadelphia, PA: Wolters Kluwer/Lippincott Williams & Wilkins.

Bailham, D., & Joseph, S. (2003). Post-traumatic stress following childbirth: A review of the emerging literature and directions for research and practice. *Psychology, Health & Medicine, 8*(2), 159–168.

Basuray, J. M. (2013). Health beliefs across cultures: Understanding transcultural care. In J. M. Basuray (Eds.), *Culture & health: Concept and practice* (Rev ed., pp. 58–84). Ronkonkoma, NY: Linus.

Blizzard, S., Kemppainen, J., & Taylor, J. (2009). Post-traumatic stress disorder and community violence: An update for nurse practitioners. *Journal of the American Academy of Nurse Practitioners, 21*(10), 535–541. doi: http://dx.doi.org/10.1111/j.1745-7599.2009.00442.x

Campinha-Bacote, J. (2007). Becoming culturally competent in ethnic psychopharmacology. *Journal of Psychosoical Nursing, 45*(9), 27–33.

Carretta, C. (2008). Domestic violence: A worldwide exploration. *Journal of Psychosocial Nursing & Mental Health Services, 46*(3), 26–35.

Centers for Disease Control and Prevention. (2010). *The national intimate partner and sexual violence survey fact sheet*. Retrieved March 09, 2013, from www.cdc.gov/ViolencePrevention/pdf/NISVS_FactSheet-a.pdf

Centers for Disease Control and Prevention. (2012). *Intimate partner violence: Consequences*. Retrieved January 29, 2013, from http://cdc.gov/ViolencePrevention/intimatepartnerviolence/consequences.html

Chandra, A., & Batada, A. (2006). Exploring stress and coping among urban African American adolescents: The Shifting the Lens study. *Preventing Chronic Disease: Public Health Research and Policy, 3*(2), 1–10.

Ehrmin, J. T. (2012). Transcultural perspectives in mental health nursing. In M. M. Andrews & J. S. Boyle (Eds.), *Transcultural concepts in nursing care* (6th ed., pp. 243–276). Philadelphia, PA: Wolters Kluwer/Lippincott Williams & Wilkins.

Gamble, J., & Creedy, D. (2005). Psychological trauma symptoms of operative birth. *British Journal of Midwifery, 13*(4), 218–224.

Giger, J. N., Davidhizar, R., Purnell, L., Harden, J. T., Phillips, J., & Strickland, O. (2007). Understanding cultural language to enhance cultural competence. *Nursing Outlook, 55*(4), 212–214.

Glass, N., Perrin, N., Campbell, J., & Soeken, K. (2007). The protective role of tangible support on post-traumatic stress disorder symptoms in urban women survivors of violence. *Research in Nursing & Health, 30*(5), 558–568.

Goldston, D. B., Molock, S. D., Whitbeck, L. B., Murakami, J. L., Zayas, L. H., & Nagayama Hall, G. C. (2008). Cultural considerations in adolescent suicide prevention and psychosocial treatment. *American Psychology, 63*(1), 14–31. doi:10.1037/0003-066X.63.1.14

Guess, K. (2006). Post-traumatic stress disorder: Early detection is key. *Nurse Practitioner, 31*(3), 26–32.

Kunst, J. R., & Sam, D. L. (2013). Expanding the margins of identity: A critique of marginalization in a globalized world. *International Perspectives in Psychology: Research, Practice, Consultation.* Advance online publication. doi:10.1037/ipp0000008

Leininger, M. M. (1995). *Transcultural nursing: Concepts, theories, research and practices* (2nd ed.). New York, NY: McGraw-Hill.

National Alliance on Mental Illness. (2012). *Cognitive behavioral therapy fact sheet.* Retrieved February 8, 2013, from www.nami.org/factsheets/CBT_factsheet.pdf

National Center for PTSD. (2012a). How common is PTSD? Retrieved January 20, 2013, from www.ptsd.va.gov/public/pages/how-common-is-ptsd.asp

National Center for PTSD. (2012b). *Primary care PTSD screen (PC-PTSD).* Retrieved January 20, 2013, from www.ptsd.va.gov/professional/pages/assessments/pc-ptsd.asp

National Center for PTSD. (2012c). *What is PTSD?* Retrieved January 20, 2013, from www.ptsd.va.gov/public/pages/what-is-ptsd.asp

National Center for PTSD. (2012d). *Symptoms of PTSD.* Retrieved January 20, 2013, from www.ptsd.va.gov/public/pages/symptoms_of_ptsd.asp

Ndiwane, A., Miller, K., Bonner, A., Imperio, K., Matzo, M., McNeal, G,...Feldman, Z. (2004) Enhancing cultural competencies of advanced practice nurses: Health care challenges in the twenty first century. *Journal of Cultural Diversity, 11*(3), 118–121. Retrieved July 28, 2013, from http://0search.proquest.com.opac.acc.msmc.edu/docview/219313008/13F8C8A482A7A6C ABD4/9?accountid=28089

Nguyen, H., Rawana, J. S., & Flora, D. B. (2011). Risk and protective predictors of trajectories of depressive symptoms among adolescents from immigrant backgrounds. *Journal of Youth Adolescence, 44,* 1544–1558. doi:10.1007/s10964–011-9636–8.

Ray, M. A. (2010). *Transcultural caring dynamics in nursing and health care.* Philadelphia, PA: FA Davis.

Sadock, B. J., & Sadock, V. A. (2007). *Kaplan & Sadock's synopsis of psychiatry: Behavioral sciences/clinical psychiatry* (10th ed.). Philadelphia, PA: Wolters Kluwer/Lippincott Williams & Wilkins.

Stahl, S. M. (2008). *Stahl's essential psychopharmacology: Neuroscientific basis and practical applications* (3rd ed.). New York, NY: Cambridge University Press.

Stone, H. (2009). Post-traumatic stress disorder in postpartum patients: What nurses can do. *Nursing for Women's Health, 13*(4), 284–291. doi:http://dx.doi.org/10.1111/j.1751–486X.2009.01438.x

Substance Abuse and Mental Health Service Administration. (2011). *Understanding health reform: Understanding the federal parity law.* Retrieved August 4, 2013, from www.samhsa.gov/healthreform/docs/ConsumerTipSheetParity508.pdf

Substance Abuse and Mental Health Service Administration. (2013a). *About us: Who we are.* Retrieved July 27, 2013, from http://beta.samhsa.gov/about-us/who-we-are

Substance Abuse and Mental Health Service Administration. (2013b). *Community conversations about mental health information brief.* Retrieved August 4, 2013, from http://store.samhsa.gov/shin/content//SMA13–4763/SMA13–4763.pdf

Townsend, M. C. (2012). *Psychiatric mental health nursing: Concepts of care in evidence-based practice* (7th. ed.). Philadelphia, PA: F.A. Davis.

Wells, R., Morrisey, J., Lee, I., & Radford, A. (2010). Trends in behavioral health care service provision by community health centers, 1998–2007. *Psychiatric Services, 61*(8), 759–764. Retrieved July 27, 2013, from http://0-search.proquest.com.opac.acc.msmc.edu/docview/75034/9?accountid=28089

Yoon, E., Chang, C. T., Kim, S., Gomez, A. M., Clawson, A., Cleary, S. E.,...Chan, T. K. (2013). A meta-analysis of acculturation, enculturation, and mental health. *Counseling Psychology, 60*(1), 15–30.

TCN Concepts in Pharmacology Courses

Priscilla Limbo Sagar

Acupuncture
Adverse drug events
Alternative medicine
Biocultural ecology
Biological variations
Complementary and alternative medicine
Complementary medicine
Ethnopharmacology

Generic folk remedies
Herbal remedies
Meditation
Meridians
Moxa
Qi
Yoga

LEARNING OBJECTIVES

At the completion of this chapter, the learner will

1. Analyze biological variations in specific ethnocultural groups and safety in the administration of medications.
2. Compare drug interactions and metabolism in selected ethnic groups.
3. Assess use of generic folk remedies among peoples of diverse cultures.
4. Analyze use of complementary alternative healing modalities among diverse clients.
5. Collaborate with the interprofessional team for the safe administration of medications.

OVERVIEW

The Institute of Medicine ([IOM], 2006) estimates that in a given week, four out of five adults in the United States take prescribed medications, over-the-counter drugs, or food supplements; a third of these adults use five or more separate medications. According to the IOM (1999), approximately 44,000 to 98,000 deaths annually are attributed to medication errors. **Adverse drug events** (ADEs) or injuries secondary to medications fall under avoidable or unavoidable events (IOM, 2006). Injuries due to the drug itself are not preventable; those incurred in prescribing, administering, or taking the drugs are avoidable.

In a study of 108 nurses in a 735-bed tertiary academic medical center, Kehoane et al. (2008) established that 26.9% of nurses' time is spent on medication-related tasks. This is more than a quarter of the total percentage of nurses' responsibilities in client care. See EBP 14.1 for more details of this informative study. It is therefore essential to prepare future nurses for this very important responsibility of safe medication administration. The actual skills in administering medications are generally taught in fundamental skill courses. A separate pharmacology course is part of associate, diploma, and baccalaureate nursing programs, while an advanced pharmacology course is a requirement of master's curricula for advanced practice nursing (APN). Safety in medication administration is emphasized and integrated in all nursing, pharmacology, and nutrition courses.

EBP 14.1

Aiming to measure the proportion of time spent by nurses on different aspects of patient care, Keohane et al. (2008) conducted a time-motion observation of 108 nurses. The study was performed in a 735-bed tertiary academic medical center over a 6-month period.

Three master of science prepared educators and one doctorally prepared nurse educator with experience in conducting orientation to recently licensed nurses participated in the development of the time-motion observation instrument. Each educator prepared a list independently before the meeting, resolved initial differences in labeling and defining, and reached a consensus list of 112 tasks under 12 major categories. This classification was similar to the classification tools of Urden and Roode (1997) and Capuano, Bokovoy, Halkin, and Hitchings (2004), both cited in Kehoane et al. (2008).

With the use of Microsoft Access database software, the list was installed into a laptop computer and later into a tablet personal computer for easier portability. The researchers pilot tested the instrument by performing 10 observations on 4 units to assess (1) observer agreement, (2) instrument utility and comprehensiveness, and (3) ease of use. Data from observer examination and a user's field notes were used to develop the final task list. The final instrument is composed of 112 patient care tasks grouped into 12 major categories.

Two research assistant observers underwent training about the task categories, their definitions, and placement of observation instruments prior to performing any observations. The observers discussed their questions with experienced observers, designers of the tasks list, and the senior investigator. In addition, each observer conducted three 2-hour practice sessions.

This study was approved by the institutional review board of Brigham Women's Hospital. The study did not involve any patient data.

(continued)

One hundred eight (108) nurses voluntarily participated. The researchers assured participants of confidentiality of observations and deidentified all demographic information. Only the researchers had access to information; analysis of information was by aggregate only. Prior to each observation session, researchers met with staff nurses and unit managers to discuss the study's objectives. There was no mention of participants' ages nor of their educational preparations. To further maintain confidentiality, the researchers assigned random numbers for all participants.

The observations were completed in 23 medical, surgical, and medical–surgical units with approximately 15 beds each and in six intensive care units (ICUs) with 10 beds each. Every nurse participant was observed for about 2 hours; there was a total of 116 2-hour observations in all with seven nurses observed more than once. Nurses working in medical and surgical units generally care for two to five patients; those in the ICUs manage one to two patients. To capture medication administration activities and the impact of the bar code and electronic medication administration record (e-MAR), 50 of the 116 observation subjects (43%) were completed during times when medications were commonly administered (Keohane et al., 2008).

Findings indicate that nurses spent 24.7% of their time in medication-related activities such as obtaining and verifying medications (7.44%), medication administration (6.7%), information retrieval (3.87%), managing doctors' orders (3.86%), and documentation of medication given (2.83%). Nurses' nonmedication-type activities center on communication (22.6%), patients' physical care (14.5%), miscellaneous or task not fitting in any of the 12 categories (14%), paper documentation (10.1%), computer use (8.4%), and searching for items in care delivery (3.5%).

The researchers acknowledged these limitations of this study: performed in only one institution; potential observer errors in recording observations; and possible variations in activity categorizations. Despite these limitations, Keohane et al. were able to illuminate the proportion of time that nurses devote on various patient activities including medication-related functions.

Applications to Practice

■ Investigate the medication administration system that you have used. Do the medication-related activities that you performed relate to some of the activities from this study? Describe.

■ Analyze the pharmacology course that you are taking/teaching. Does this course include concepts described for safe medication management in this study? Explain.

■ If you were to replicate this time-motion study, how would you conduct it? What would you change in terms of conceptual framework, instruments, sampling, and analysis of findings?

Source: Keohane et al. (2008).

Safety in medication administration also calls for multidisciplinary (interdisciplinary) and interprofessional education early on for health care professionals (IOM, 2010). The disparities in health care in the United States according to the IOM (Smedley, Stith, & Nelson, 2002) are partly caused by health care providers. Hence, the IOM (2010) recommends cross-cultural education of health care providers to eradicate bias and prejudice and therefore close the gap in quality of care between minority and nonminority groups. Nursing, medicine, dentistry, and pharmacy education have all integrated diversity and cultural competence in their respective curricula. The continuing evaluation of outcomes of cultural competence education would need to be monitored among students, faculty, graduates, and clients.

Nursing education, spearheaded by the American Association of Colleges of Nursing ([AACN], 1999, 2008a, 2008b, 2009, 2011) and the National League for Nursing ([NLN], 2009a, 2009b), has begun to embrace the field of diversity, promotion of cultural competence, and elimination of health disparities. With funding from the California Endowment, the AACN (2008) developed *Cultural Competency in Baccalaureate Nursing Education: End-of-Program Competencies for Baccalaureate Nursing Program Graduates and Faculty Toolkit for Integrating These Competencies into Undergraduate Curriculum*. The AACN (2009, 2011) developed and later updated the master's and doctoral *Tool Kit for Cultural Competence in Master's and Doctoral Nursing Education*. The NLN (2009a) has promoted continuing dialogue in *A Commitment to Diversity in Nursing and Nursing Education*. Furthermore, the NLN (2009b) had likewise developed a *Diversity Toolkit* to guide teaching and integration of cultural competence in all levels of nursing curricula.

The development of *Promoting, Reinforcing, and Improving Medical Education (PRIME)* in 1998, a project of the U.S. Department of Health and Human Services (USDHHS), Health Resources and Services Administration (HRSA), and the Bureau of Health Professions' (BHPR) Division of Medicine and Dentistry (DUD) was a recognition of the vital part of culture and diversity in client care outcomes (Garrison & Bloom, 2004). PRIME's aim—among others—was to create a culturally competent curriculum that could be implemented in medical schools nationally; seven schools were selected for the pilot program as trial sites. The result was *Cultural Competency in Medical Education: A Guide for Schools*, a suggested curriculum outline that can be adapted to any medical school (Garrison & Bloom, 2004). The guide specifies core competencies for each of the five content areas in cultural competence education. The area of "cultural and traditional health care practices" calls for students' (1) recognition of cultural and traditional health care practices; (2) awareness of nonallopathic and nonosteopathic health care practices; and (3) assessment of traditional remedies and traditional healers (Garrison & Bloom, 2004).

The American Association of Colleges of Pharmacy uses *Caring for the Underserved: A Delineation of Educational Outcomes Organized Within the Clinical Prevention and Population Health Curriculum Framework for the Health Professions* as curricular guidelines (Patterson, 2008). This guide uses student outcomes in cultural competency, health literacy, and health disparities in pharmacy curriculum. In addition, the American Council for Pharmacy Education (ACPE) updated its accreditation standards in 2007 to include diversity and cultural issues. As an essential aspect of public health, cultural competence has gained prominence as a requisite part of pharmaceutical education (Patterson, 2008). To disseminate this new content of cultural competence, a train-the-trainer program was conducted for pharmacy faculty across the United States (Assemi, Mutha, & Hudmon, 2007).

Integration of TCN Concepts

BIOLOGICAL VARIATIONS

Both the *Cultural Competence Model* by Purnell (2013) and *Transcultural Assessment Model (TAM)* by Giger and Davidhizar (2008) contain domains regarding **biological variations** and **biocultural ecology**. People of different races metabolize drugs in different ways and at varying rates (Giger & Davidhizar, 2008). In the last few decades, research in pharmacology and genetics uncovered substantial differences among racial and ethnic groups in terms of metabolism and clinical efficacy of some important drugs (Campinha-Bacote, 2007; Warren, 2008). Information about drug metabolism among racial and ethnic groups as well as its implications in administering and prescribing medications are vital areas of learning among health care professionals (Purnell, 2013).

   Campinha-Bacote (2007) pointed out the importance of culturally and linguistically appropriate assessment of clients in regards to ethnic pharmacology. For example, a comprehensive dietary assessment is imperative when prescribing psychotropics. Malnutrition could delay the absorption of metabolic enzymes and change the body's ability to absorb or excrete psychotropic medications (Campinha-Bacote, 2007); as an example, health care providers need to keep this in mind when working with recent refugees from Somalia.

DRUG INTERACTIONS AND METABOLISM

There are racial variations in drug metabolism. The growing field of pharmacogenetics emerged from observations of significant ethnic differences in response to drugs (Sadock & Sadock, 2007). To illustrate, some variant reactions occur in the metabolism of isoniazid, succinylcholine, alcohol, and some antihypertensives.

   Individuals either metabolize isoniazid very slowly or very rapidly (Sadock & Sadock, 2007). People with very slow metabolism of isoniazid are at risk for emerging peripheral neuropathy (Giger & Davidhizar, 2008). Some groups quickly inactivate isoniazid; for example, Asians (85% to 90%), American Indians (60% to 90%), African Americans (60%), and Whites (40%). For individuals needing a gradual reaction, doses are given at longer intervals and administered with pyridoxine (Giger & Davidhizar, 2008).

   The muscle relaxant succinylcholine is inactivated by the enzyme pseudocholinesterase. Generally, most individuals readily inactivate succinylcholine; however, some individuals with an unusual form of the enzyme that slows that metabolism may suffer prolonged muscle paralysis and failure to breathe (Giger & Davidhizar, 2008). According to Kalow (1982, 1986, 1989), as cited in Giger and Davidhizar (2008), one out of 135 Alaskan Eskimos is unable to metabolize succinylcholine; some individuals of Jewish heritage may also be at greater risk.

   The metabolism of alcohol varies considerably by race. Two enzymes are at play in the metabolism of alcohol: alcohol dehydrogenase (ADH) and aldehyde dehydrogenase (ALDH) (Sadock & Sadock, 2007). The enzyme ADH converts alcohol to acetaldehyde and ALDH changes the toxic acetaldehyde to the nontoxic acetic acid. Among Whites who possess normal levels of ADH and ALDH, alcohol is metabolized effectively. In comparison, among American Indians and Asians, high-activity ADH converts alcohol to acetaldehyde, but the metabolism of acetaldehyde to acetic acid is delayed, resulting in facial flushing and other vasomotor manifestations (Giger & Davidhizar, 2008; Sadock & Sadock, 2007). Furthermore, Sadock and Sadock (2007) went on to elaborate that ADH and ALDH influence the development of alcoholism or its avoidance, citing as examples Asians with an atypical ALDH2 gene who are sensitive to alcohol and thus have a low risk for alcoholism.

Cytochrome P450, an important enzyme system, is key in the metabolism of drugs as well as environmental toxins; the genetic defect in this enzyme system is unequally distributed among diverse populations (Sadock & Sadock, 2007). Two cytochrome P450— CYP2D6 (debrisoquin hydroxylase) and CYP2Cmp (mephenytoin hydroxylase)—are poor metabolizers. CYP2D6 poor metabolizers are low for Asians (0.5% to 2.4%) and higher for Whites (2.9% to 10%); likewise, CYP2Cmp poor metabolizers are low among Whites (3%), intermediate for African Americans (18%), and increased in Asians, especially among Japanese (20%) (Sadock & Sadock, 2007).

COMPLEMENTARY AND ALTERNATIVE MEDICINE

There has been an increasing number of studies regarding the use of **complementary and alternative medicine** (CAM) in the United States for both health promotion and maintenance among the general population and as an adjunct to therapy in illness. **Complementary medicine** includes therapeutic modalities or products used in combination with biomedicine (western medicine), while **alternative medicine** denotes therapeutic modalities used in combination with biomedicine (Andrews, 2012b; Basuray, 2013).

To explore the relationships among gender, physical and psychological symptoms, and use of CAM, Fouladbakhsh and Stommel (2010) performed a secondary analysis of the 2002 National Health Interview Survey (NHIS) of 2,262 adults with cancer in the United States. Their findings revealed prevalent use of CAM in 2.1 million middle-aged, well-educated female cancer survivors (26%), with pain, depression, and insomnia as clear predictors for practice (Fouladbakhsh & Stommel, 2010). Comparatively, being a minority is connected to lower odds of CAM use.

The Fouladbakhsh and Stommel (2010) study showed an interesting trend of client contact with nurse practitioners (NPs), physician assistants (PAs), physical therapists, and mental health professionals as being associated with increased use of CAM. These researchers called attention to the "no cost" practice of deep breathing and **meditation** as invaluable for populations suffering from stress and hypertension related to lower socioeconomic status.

Herbal remedies. Since the dawn of history, peoples from different cultures have used herbs for health promotion, maintenance, and restoration and for treatment of maladies. Herbs and spices traditionally used as cooking ingredients are now topics of research for their healing properties (Basuray, 2013). Immigrants often preserve their devotion to **generic folk remedies** alongside western biomedicine (Sadock & Sadock, 2007). The use of herbal preparations is imbedded in the study of **ethnopharmacology** (Warren, 2008). However, health care providers must be vigilant to assess and monitor potential interactions between herbs, over-the-counter medications, and prescribed drugs. It is crucial, according to Basuray (2013), that health care providers identify herbal efficacy as well as their potential dangers.

Some examples of **herbal remedies** include *echinacea* for reduction of cold symptoms; *ginko* for enhancement of short-term memory and attention span; and *gotu kola* for improvement of memory (Andrews, 2012a). The root of the shrub American and Asian *ginseng* appears to be widely used. Asian ginseng is used as a remedy for physical and mental fatigue (Campinha-Bacote, 2007), as well as lack of appetite, shortness of breath, impotence in men (Basuray, 2013), lack of concentration, reduced work capacity, and improvement of sense of well-being (Andrews, 2012a). American ginseng has been traditionally used for anemia, edema, hypertension, colds, and inflammation (Andrews, 2012a).

Campinha-Bacote (2007) exhorted health care providers to perform a thorough cultural assessment for clients on herbal supplements while receiving psychotropic medications. The extract of *kava* root, known for treatment of anxiety, insomnia, and stress, is contraindicated for depressed clients due to its ability to potentiate actions of psychopharmacological agents (Campinha-Bacote, 2007). Asian ginseng is known to enhance the effects of monoamine oxidase inhibitors (Campinha-Bacote, 2007). Ginseng and glycyrrhiza may stimulate or inhibit cytochrome P450 (Sadock & Sadock, 2007).

Yoga. Yoga is an active internal experience that unites the body, the mind, and the spirit. A holistic system of mind–body practices for mental and physical health, yoga integrates several techniques such as meditation, breathing, and postures that increase strength and flexibility (Khalsa, Shorter, Cope, Wyshak, & Sklar, 2009). Yoga is effective in pain control (McGonigal, 2009); in lowering stress, anxiety and mood disturbance (Khalsa et al., 2009; Smith, Hancock, Blake-Mortimer, & Eckert, 2007); and in mild depression (Woolery, Myers, Sternlieb, & Zeltzer, 2004). While many positive effects are attributed to yoga, it is of utmost importance to warn people—at every level of practice—about safety when practicing yoga and the need to avoid injury. Lasater (2003) reminded people about wearing comfortable, clean clothing; avoiding eating for at least 3 hours prior to practice; and honoring oneself and acknowledging one's own limitations. Modest loose clothing is best; this prevents exposing body parts as the person goes into yoga poses.

Several studies attest to the effectiveness of yoga. Khalsa et al. (2009) conducted a controlled study of 45 young adult professional musicians. The musicians were randomly placed in yoga lifestyle intervention (*n* = 15), in yoga and meditation practice only (*n* = 15), and in a no practice control group (*n* = 15). Both groups in yoga attended three Kripalu yoga sessions each week; in addition, the musicians in the yoga lifestyle intervention had weekly group practice and discussions. All participants completed self-report questionnaires at baseline and at the end of the program regarding anxiety, mood, performance-related musculoskeletal disorders (PRMDs), stress, and quality of sleep (Khalsa et al., 2009). With results being comparable in the two yoga groups, Khalsa et al. (2009) concluded that yoga and meditation can lessen performance anxiety and mood problems among young professional musicians.

Woolery et al. (2004) examined the effects of yoga among 18 to 29 young adults with mild levels of depression, as indicated by scores of 10 through 15 in the Beck Depression Inventory (BDI; Beck, 1972, as cited in Woolery et al., 2004) and the *State Trait Personality Inventory* (STPI; Spielberger, Gorshuch, & Lushene, 1970, as cited in Woolery et al., 2004). The Human Subjects Protection Committee approved the study. There were two random group assignments: yoga group (*n* = 13) and control group (*n* = 15). The participants completed the BDI and STPI before the initial class, after the fifth class, and after the last class; the participants also provided cortisol samples as pretest, midcourse, and posttest. Woolery et al. (2004) reported significant reduction of depression and anxiety midway and throughout the end of the course as well as slight elevation in cortisol levels—associated with self-esteem, resilience, and lower levels of depression—among the yoga group.

Meditation. As noted in the previous section on yoga, meditation is usually used in yoga practice. In Australia, Smith et al. (2007) conducted a study comparing hatha yoga with the progressive relaxation method. The 131 participants had moderate levels of stress and anxiety prior to the study. The participants—with ages between 18 and 65 years and 89% of which were women—were randomly assigned to the yoga group (*n* = 68) and relaxation group (*n* = 63) and were required to attend ten 1-hour classes of 10 to 15 participants per class. Smith et al. (2007) administered the STPI (Spielberger, Gorshuk, & Lushene, 1983, as cited in Smith et al., 2007) questionnaire to determine anxiety levels. To measure psychological stress, the researchers used the *General Health Questionnaire 12* (GHQ-12; Goldberg & Williams, 1991, as cited in Smith et al., 2007). Participants completed the instruments prior to the study, at the end of the 10-week intervention, and at 16 weeks. No difference was noted between the two groups; however, the participants in the relaxation group showed higher scores in social functioning, mental health, and vitality (Smith et al., 2007).

Acupuncture. Acupuncture is a modality centering on the concept of **"qi,"** or energy or life force, and inserting needles into **meridians** or points where energy accumulates; this is believed to stimulate the body's own healing reaction, thus restoring balance of energy (Sobel, 2013, p. 67). In good health, qi moves freely and efficiently. Physical factors, such as inadequate nutrition, infections, and trauma, and emotional factors, such as stress, anxiety, and grief, could interrupt the flow.

"Will the needles hurt?" is the most common question that clients ask when contemplating the use of acupuncture. Acupuncture needles are solid, finer, and much smaller than needles for injections and other medical procedures; clients may have sensations of tingling or a dull ache (Sobel, 2013). Sobel (2013) acknowledged that only about 100 points of stimulation out of 500 known points are commonly utilized; stimulating a point can influence the function of a certain organ. The use of **moxa**, or heat, may also be used with acupuncture (Andrews, 2012b); heat can be in the form of a lighted stick near the needle, laser therapy, or small electrical current to the point of the needle (Sobel, 2013).

CRITICAL THINKING EXERCISES 14.1

Undergraduate Student
1. How would you assess your multicultural clients as part of safety in medication administration?
2. What additional knowledge do you need to plan care for multicultural clients?
3. Have you taken pharmacology as an interprofessional course?
4. What are your perceptions of interprofessional course(s)? Are you in favor of interprofessional courses in your nursing program?

Graduate Student
1. As a future advanced practice nurse (APN), what assessment parameters will you need to include to effectively manage the medications of your clients?
2. Have you reflected on the use of CAM among clients? What type of clients use CAM?
3. How do you integrate CAM in planning, implementation, and evaluation of care among your clients? Discuss.
4. Is holism part of your master's curriculum? Explain.

Faculty in Academia
1. What are the areas included in the current pharmacology course that you are teaching?
2. Is CAM included among the concepts in your pharmacology course? If not, will you be adding it?
3. Are electronic medical records (EMR) and e-MARs covered in your curriculum? Do students' clinical programs include experience in using these, including bar codes?
4. Do you teach in a multidisciplinary course that involves safety in medication administration? Describe.

Staff Development Educator
1. How is medication assessed and administered in your institution? Do you have a tool in place to reconcile medications from home or from another institution?
2. How much of the current admission tool pertains to medication administration in multicultural patients?
3. When revising the current tool, which model would you use?
4. What modality of CAM does your institution use? Describe.

SUMMARY

This chapter discussed important TCN concepts to include in pharmacology courses: biological variations, drug interactions and metabolism, and some selected complementary and alternative medicine (CAM). A brief overview of interprofessional education was provided. A section on CAM discussed commonly used health maintenance and healing modalities such as yoga, meditation, and acupuncture. There is growing emphasis on the role of the nurse and other health professionals in integrating ethnopharmacology in the care of culturally and ethnically diverse clients. The innovative time-motion study by Kehoane et al. (2008) has significant implications in nursing and health care, especially with the persistent nursing shortage. Nurses are urged to replicate this pioneering study.

REFERENCES

Accreditation Council for Pharmacy Education. (2007). *Accreditation standards for continuing pharmacy education.* Chicago, IL: Author. Retrieved July 19, 2003, from https://www.acpe-accredit.org/pdf/CPE_Standards_Final.pdf

American Association of Colleges of Nursing. (1999). *Nursing education's agenda for the 21st century.* Washington, DC: Author.

American Association of Colleges of Nursing. (2008a). *The essentials of baccalaureate education for professional nursing practice.* Washington, DC: Author.

American Association of Colleges of Nursing. (2008b). *Cultural competency in baccalaureate nursing education.* Washington, DC: Author.

American Association of Colleges of Nursing. (2009). *Tool kit for cultural competence in master's and doctoral nursing education.* Washington, DC: Author.

American Association of Colleges of Nursing. (2011). *Tool kit for cultural competence in master's and doctoral nursing education.* Washington, DC: Author.

Andrews, M. M. (2012a). Cultural competence in the health history and physical examination. In M. M. Andrews & J. S. Boyle (Eds.), *Transcultural concepts in nursing care* (6th ed., pp. 38–72). Philadelphia, PA: Wolters Kluwer Health/Lippincott Williams & Wilkins.

Andrews, M. M. (2012b). The influence of cultural and health belief systems on health care practices. In M. M. Andrews & J. S. Boyle (Eds.), *Transcultural concepts in nursing care* (6th ed., pp. 73–88). Philadelphia, PA: Wolters Kluwer/Lippincott Williams & Wilkins.

Assemi, M., Mutha, S., & Hudmon, K. S. (2007). Evaluation of a train-the-trainer program for cultural competence. *American Journal of Pharmaceutical Education, 71*(6), 1–8.

Basuray, J. M. (2013). Health beliefs across cultures: Understanding transcultural care. In J. M. Basuray (Ed.), *Culture & health: Concept and practice* (Rev ed., pp. 57–84). Ronkonkoma, NY: Linus.

Campinha-Bacote, J. (2007). Becoming culturally competent in ethnic psychopharmacology. *Journal of Psychosocial Nursing, 45*(9), 27–33.

Fouladbakhsh, J. M., & Stommel, M. (2010). Gender, symptom experience, and use of complementary and alternative medicine practices among cancer survivors in the US cancer population. *Oncology Nursing Forum, 37*(1), E7–15.

Garrison, S., & Bloom, S. (2004). *Cultural competency in medical education: A guide for schools.* United States Department of Health and Human Services, Health Resources Services Administration. Retrieved July 12, 2013, from www.hrsa.gov/culturalcompetence/cultcomp.pdf

Giger, J. N., & Davidhizar, R. E. (2008). *Transcultural nursing: Assessment and intervention* (5th ed.). St. Louis, MO: Mosby Elsevier.

Institute of Medicine. (1999). *To err is human: Building a safer health system.* Washington, DC: National Academy Press.

Institute of Medicine. (2006). *Preventing medication errors.* Retrieved June 29, 2013, from www.iom.edu/~/media/Files/Report%20Files/2006/Preventing-Medication-Errors-Quality-Chasm-Series/medicationerrorsnew.pdf

Institute of Medicine. (2010). *The future of nursing: Focus on education.* Washington, DC: National Academy of Sciences.

Keohane, C. A, Bane, D. A., Featherstone, E., Hayes, J., Woolf, S., Hurley, A,...Poon, E. (2008). Quantifying nursing workflow in medication administration. *Journal of Nursing Administration, 38*(1), 19–26.

Khalsa, S. B. S., Shorter, S. M., Cope, S., Wyshak, G., & Sklar, E. (2009). Yoga ameliorates performance anxiety and mood disturbance in young professional musicians. *Applied Psychophysiological Biofeedback, 34*, 279–289. doi:10.1007/s10484–009-9103–4

Lasater, J. (2003). *30 essential yoga poses for beginning students and their teachers.* Berkeley, CA: Rodmell.

McGonigal, K. (2009). *Yoga for pain relief: Simple practices to calm your mind & heal your chronic pain.* Oakland, CA: New Harbinger.

National League for Nursing. (2009a). *A commitment to diversity in nursing and nursing education.* Retrieved July 10, 2013, from www.nln.org/aboutnln/reflection_dialogue/refl_dial_3 .htm

National League for Nursing. (2009b). *Diversity toolkit.* Retrieved July 10, 2013, from www.nln.org/ facultyprograms/Diversity_Toolkit/diversity_toolkit.pdf

Patterson, B. Y. (2008). An advanced pharmacy practice experience in public health. *American Journal of Pharmaceutical Education, 72*(5), 1–8.

Purnell, L. D. (2013). The Purnell model for cultural competence. In L. D. Purnell (Ed.), *Transcultural health care: A culturally competent approach* (4th ed., pp. 15–44). Philadelphia, PA: F.A. Davis.

Sadock, B. J., & Sadock, V. A. (2007). *Kaplan & Sadock's synopsis of psychiatry: Behavioral sciences/clinical psychiatry* (10th ed.). Philadelphia, PA: Wolters Kluwer/Lippincott Williams & Wilkins.

Smedley, B. D., Stith, A. Y., & Nelson, A. R. (Eds.). (2002). *Unequal treatment: Confronting racial and ethnic disparities in health.* Washington, DC: National Academies Press.

Smith, C., Hancock, H., Blake-Mortimer, J., & Eckert, K. (2007). A randomised comparative trial of yoga and relaxation to reduce stress and anxiety. *Complementary Therapies in Medicine, 15*, 77–83.

Sobel, R. (2013). Detailed description on the theory and art of acupuncture. In J. M. Basuray (Ed.), *Culture & health: Concept and practice* (Rev ed., pp. 67–75). Ronkonkoma, NY: Linus.

Warren, B. J. (2008). Ethnopharmacology: The effect on patients, health care professionals, and systems. *Urologic Nursing, 38*(4), 292–295.

Woolery, A., Myers, H., Sternlieb, B., & Zeltzer, L. (2004). A yoga intervention for young adults with elevated symptoms of depression. *Alternative Therapies, 10*(2), 60–63.

TCN Concepts in Nutrition Courses

Priscilla Limbo Sagar

Abstinence
Body mass index (BMI)
"Comfort food"
Fasting
"Freshman 15"
Fusion food
Generic care
Geophagy
Halal
Heritage

Kashrut
Kosher
Lactose intolerance
Melting pot
Nutrition
Obesity
Pica
Salad
Traditional foods
Vegetarian

At the completion of this chapter, the learner will be able to

1. Integrate nutritional factors that are influenced by culture when planning a nutrition course.
2. Compare and contrast the meaning of food in different cultures.
3. Examine different dietary guidelines as influenced by diverse cultures and religious practices.
4. Analyze nutritional assessment tools in a given institution.
5. Explore research studies addressing obesity.
6. Devise health education strategies for specific cultural groups.

OVERVIEW

Food, the essence for survival, is vital in every culture. **Nutrition,** as a cultural domain, encompasses the meaning of food, common food items, associated rituals, nutritional deficiencies, and food limitations (Purnell, 2013). Nutrition plays an important role in health promotion, maintenance, and restoration. Peoples' cultural values and beliefs and the availability of food items influence what they eat. It is heart-rending to see food wasting in some wealthy nations while hunger takes place on the opposite end of the spectrum in poor communities and nations. It is a paradox that, in some cultures, the problem is malnutrition and the dire scarcity of food, whereas in most industrialized nations epidemics of **obesity** are urgent national health problems.

Globally and in the United States, obesity has taken central prominence as an epidemic and as a tremendous health issue due to its consequent risk for cardiovascular diseases, stroke, type 2 diabetes, and some cancers (Centers for Disease Control and Prevention [CDC], 2012a, 2012b, 2012c; Edberg, 2012; Fung et al., 2012; Gores, 2008). Childhood obesity has tripled in the past few decades; recent statistics indicate that 16.2%, or one in six children and adolescents in the United States are obese (U.S. Department of Health and Human Services [USDHHS], 2013). In Canada, an approximate 8.6% of Canadian children are also obese (Fung et al., 2012). Obesity among adults in the United States is calculated at 34.0%; this means one in every three adults is obese (USDHHS, 2013). In addition to the above serious health aftermaths, overweight and obesity significantly escalate costs and create an added burden to the health care delivery system. Among the leading health indicators of *Healthy People 2020* are nutrition, physical activity, and obesity (USDHHS, 2013).

The CDC (2012c) defines obesity in adults as a **body mass index** (BMI) of 30 or higher; in most people, the BMI is associated with their amount of body fat. An adult with a BMI between 25 and 29.9 is considered overweight (CDC, 2012c). In a different manner, the CDC (2012c) classifies obese children as those at BMI belonging to the 95th percentile of children of the same age and sex; overweight children's BMI are at the 85th percentile. Obese children are liable to have high blood pressure and cholesterol; they have a high risk for type 2 diabetes, joint difficulties, and breathing problems. In addition, obese children tend to become obese adults.

Schools are not only implementing programs to prevent obesity but also to measure outcomes of such programs. The study by Fung et al. (2012) in EBP 15.1 shows the effects of a comprehensive health program in fifth-grade students' diets, activity level, and body weights.

The current guidelines for MyPlate, *Dietary Guidelines Consumer Brochure: Let's Eat for the Health of It!,* is a good resource. Other resources are available from the United States Department of Agriculture ([USDA], 2011a). The brochure is colorful, portable, and easy to read; this is an excellent, yet simple tool to bring along for health education sessions with clients, groups, and the community. Currently, the brochure is available in English, Spanish, French, and Vietnamese (USDA, 2011b).

Oldways (n.d.) is a nonprofit continuing professional education (CPE) accredited provider with the Commission on Dietetic Registration of the Academy of Nutrition and Dietetics. Founded by K. Dun Gifford in 1990, Oldways (n.d.) seeks to promote healthy eating and drinking through various programs that help consumers "improve their food and drink choices..." and to "encourage traditional sustainable food choices" (para 1), among others. Oldways (2000, 2009, 2011) adapted the USDA pyramid into ethnic cultural pyramids such as African American (Figure 15.1), Asian (Figure 15.2), and Hispanic (Figure 15.3). Each traditional pyramid aims to illustrate the balance of real foods that are supportive of good health (Oldways, n.d.). The Mediterranean and **vegetarian** diet

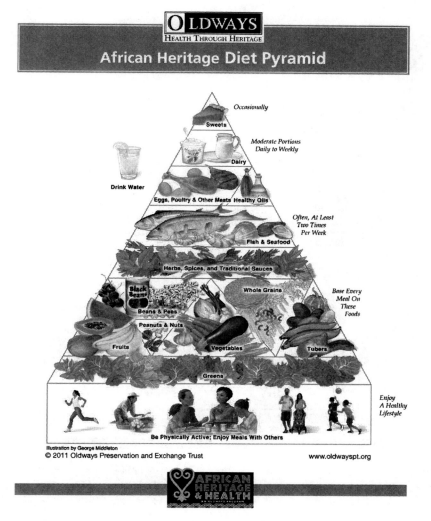

FIGURE 15.1 African American food pyramid. *Source:* Oldways (2011). Reprinted with permission. Copyright © 2009 Oldways Preservation & Exchange Trust.

pyramids are also available. Several other ethnic cultural food pyramids such as Japanese and Indian are available from the USDA website (USDA, 2011b).

Food also exemplifies trends in cultural identity. For example, the early immigrants made an effort to shed remnants of their old countries. For example, in terms of communication, they tried to lose their accents and speaking more English, then eventually lost their native tongues. Some names were anglicized in order to sound more mainstream. The proverbial **melting pot** signifies this; ingredients in a stew are blended and not readily recognizable. In the past few decades, however, cultural identity has been stronger, more exemplified by a **salad**; even mixed and tossed, individual ingredients retain their properties and are readily recognizable.

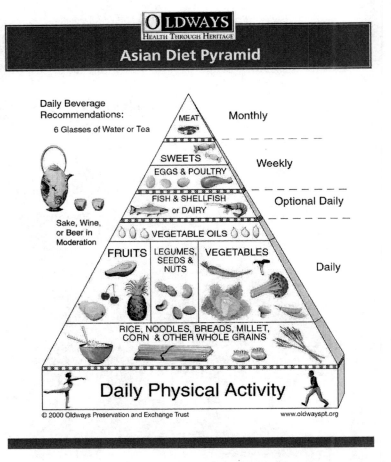

FIGURE 15.2 Asian food pyramid. *Source:* Oldways (2000). Reprinted with permission. Copyright © 2009 Oldways Preservation & Exchange Trust.

Integration of TCN Concepts

When planning a nutrition course or revising an existing course, the Boyle/Andrews Transcultural Nursing Assessment Guide for Individual and Families (Boyle & Andrews, 2012), the Purnell Model of Cultural Competence ([PMCC], Purnell, 2013), or the Giger and Davidhizar Transcultural Assessment Model ([TAM], Giger & Davidhizar, 2008) are all handy tools to consult. The PMCC includes separate sections on nutrition while the TAM integrates nutrition under *biological variations.* Some important points to include in syllabus preparation or updating of a syllabus may include meaning of food, religious beliefs and practices, nutritional deficiencies and limitations, home and folk remedies, and selected groups at risk.

Meaning of Food

Railey (2009) made a strong argument about food practices among cultures, illustrating ancestral traditions, teaching, and habits. Food is equated with celebrations and rituals of

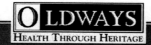

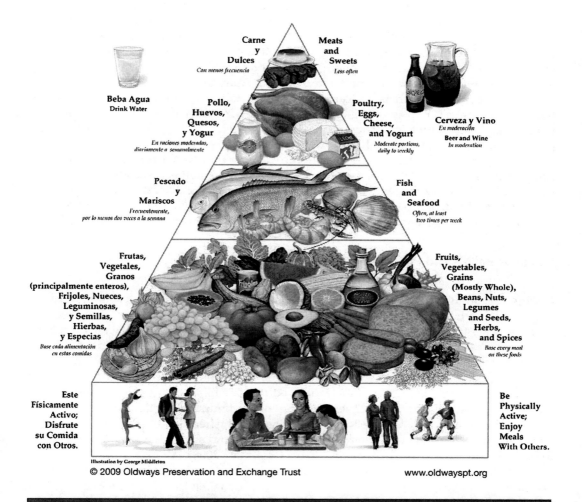

FIGURE 15.3 Latino diet and food pyramid. *Source:* Oldways (20009). Reprinted with permission. Copyright © 2009 Oldways Preservation & Exchange Trust.

birth, marriage, and death; of milestone events and other happy occasions; and of gathering for feasts, holy days, and other festivities. Cultural values and beliefs influence what is prepared, served, and eaten. For example, among people in the Appalachian region, there is an effort to cut down on the use of lard in cooking food, even though many of the recipes still call for lard and salted meats (Huttlinger, 2013).

Railey (2009) pointed out that African American slaves' sustenance used to come from scraps from the masters' dining table, imperfect crops, and pork. Consequently, the slaves became very creative in preparing pork and its organ meats such as pig snoots, pig feet, chitterlings, and tripe, along with greens; these were mostly fried and seasoned with a generous amount of salt (Railey, 2009). At the end of the day, the slaves gathered and enjoyed a communal meal. This has been a long-term exposure to social factors and cultural norms; thus, eating particular foods became a statement for self-identification, fulfillment, and liberation (Railey, 2009). This type of diet in part can be attributed to the poor health outcomes of African Americans (Rose, 2011) and the high prevalence of hypertension, diabetes, and cardiovascular diseases.

These ethnocultural types of foods are becoming increasingly available in groceries of many U.S. towns and cities. Sometimes within a few blocks—with the sampling and array of food from all continents—it is not difficult to pile and stock up on food items from the old countries and satisfy that longing to revisit tastes of childhood. There is great comfort in the familiar taste, smell, and texture of food. Adaptations of the food pyramid into ethnic food pyramids such as African, Asian, Latin, and Mediterranean, as well as other **heritage** pyramids (Oldways, 2000, 2009, 2011; USDA, 2011b), will be of utmost assistance in planning health education programs on diet and activity. In recognition of religious and personal preference, Oldways also has a vegetarian food pyramid.

Comfort food, which may also be referred to as **traditional foods,** are items long associated with childhood; their familiar taste, sight, and smell is associated with memories of growing up. As the United States undergoes continuing diversification of its population, **fusion food,** or mixtures and amalgams of different styles of formulation of cooking and/or preparation, are increasingly available in many restaurants and eating places.

Religious Beliefs and Practices

Fasting (abstaining from all or certain foods or drink) and **abstinence** (voluntary doing without) (Guralnik, 1984) are practiced in diverse cultures. The health care provider may ask: If you are fasting or in abstention, is this a religious requirement? When do you need to fast or abstain? Are there exceptions to fasting and abstinence such as in times of illness, pregnancy, or lactation? If unsure of exemptions, is there someone we can ask to clarify? These are very important questions to ask in planning, implementation, and evaluation of culturally congruent care, including patient education. Table 15.1 presents selected religious dietary prohibitions, guidelines, exemptions, and nursing implications.

Jewish. Orthodox and observant Jews adhere to **kosher** diet; this signifies discipline and reverence for life in addition to satisfying hunger and sustaining life. For food items to be kosher—-state of being acceptable to eat (Hoffman, 2008)—there are strict guidelines to follow in the process of slaughtering, preparation, and consumption (Selekman, 2013). The laws pertaining to allowed food is **kashrut** and are taken from the books of Leviticus and Deuteronomy (Selekman, 2013). Observant Jews, in compliance with dietary laws, do not mix milk and meat—hence, they use separate utensils and dishes in the preparation of food and cooking, for serving, and for eating. The health care professionals' awareness, knowledge, and acceptance of these practices will be helpful in planning, implementing, and evaluating culturally appropriate care for diverse groups.

Nutritional Deficiencies and Limitations

Immigrants may come in to the host country with existing nutritional deficiencies. Limitations for immigrants may include the lack of food availability in the new country,

TABLE 15.1   Selected Religious Dietary Prohibitions and Guidelines

Selected Religious Groups	Fasting and Abstinence	Exceptions	Nursing Implications
Judaism (Orthodox, observant) Slaughter has to be kosher; animals are killed fast with the least possible pain. Do not mix milk and meat in preparation, cooking, serving, and eating. No pork. Pigs do have split hooves but do not chew cud. Eggs from non-Kosher birds (grab prey).	Yom Kippur (Day of Atonement). Early dinner the night before; fast until sunset the following day. Passover. No bread or product with yeast; unleavened bread eaten. Seder around dining table during first 2 nights; recounting Moses and exodus from Egypt, singing.	Sick, pregnant, lactating, physically incapacitated individuals are exempted. Consult rabbi if unsure.	Monitor for potential nonadherence to treatment.
Islam (practicing, Devout) Alcohol is forbidden. No pork. "**Halal**," Islamic form of slaughter. Lamb and chicken are important meats. Beverages may not be served until the end of the meal. Food is eaten with the right hand (clean hand).	Ramadan is month of fasting. Abstinence from food, drink, smoking, and marital intercourse during daylight hours.	Sick, pregnant, lactating, and elderly persons are not required to fast; some devout Muslims may still fast while hospitalized.	Monitor for potential nonadherence to treatment, especially to drugs requiring certain blood levels, or antibiotics that may crystallize in the kidneys.
Catholicism, Roman Alcohol and tobacco in moderation.	Ash Wednesday, Good Friday, and all Fridays of Lent. Healthy persons between age 18 and 62 are obliged to fast and abstain from meat and meat products.	Sick exempted.	Patient education regarding deleterious effects of fasting and abstinence.

(continued)

TABLE 15.1 Selected Religious Dietary Prohibitions and Guidelines *(continued)*

Selected Religious Groups	Fasting and Abstinence	Exceptions	Nursing Implications
Seventh Day Adventists Encourages a vegetarian diet; some eat meat and poultry. Poultry such as chicken and turkey are permitted. Fish with fins and scales are acceptable. Fermented beverages are prohibited.	Fasting or abstention, involving both food and liquids, may be required by some churches.	Discouraged if likely to harm an individual.	Patient education regarding deleterious effects of fasting and abstinence.

Sources: Developed from Hanson & Andrews (2012); Kulwicki & Ballout (2013); Selekman (2013); and Wehbe-Alamah (2008).

or they may not be knowledgeable about comparable food items for substitution (Purnell, 2013). Socioeconomic status may restrict food choices. In some poor neighborhoods, fast food restaurants may be plentiful but access to fresh fruits and vegetables is not. In these places, the availability of farmers' markets is a welcome opportunity to get fresh produce.

Lactose intolerance, or intolerance to milk and dairy products, is caused by an insufficient amount of lactase, the enzyme that converts the nonabsorbable lactose into the absorbable glucose and galactose (Giger & Davidhizar, 2008). The cramps, flatulence, bloating, and diarrhea result from the undigested lactose, which eventually draws water and combines with acetic acid and hydrogen gas in the colon. Lactose intolerance is prevalent among adult African Blacks (90%) and among African Americans, Asians, and Native Americans (79%); this problem is least common among Whites at about 5% to 15% (Giger & Davidhizar, 2008). Health care providers must be knowledgeable about milk substitutes such as soy milk and aged cheese of more than 60 days; the aging process in cheese changes lactase to lactic acid (Giger & Davidhizar, 2008).

Some cultural and ethnic groups may have unusual cravings for nonfood items such as clay or dirt. This practice, **geophagy** or **pica**, has been documented mainly among pregnant African American women of lower economic status and was thought to be due to their insufficient calcium, iron, and other mineral intake (Giger & Davidhizar, 2008). When clay is not available, laundry starch may be consumed. Basuray (2013) estimated that eating clay may be more widespread globally, with more than 200 cultures practicing it daily. This calls for culturally sensitive client education, including the harmful effects of consuming nonfood substances.

Home and Folk Remedies

Generic care refers to the indigenous or folk practices in a cultural group (Leininger & McFarland, 2006). The use of home and folk remedies is widespread in many cultures. The discussion in this chapter will be limited to food and drinks used in health promotion, in treatment of illnesses, and in health restoration. For herb supplementation, see Chapter 14.

African Americans. The use of folk medicine continues among Blacks or African Americans. Poultices are placed on inflamed or painful body parts to draw out the cause of affliction; among substances used as poultices are grated potatoes, cornmeal, peach leaves, and onions (Spector, 2013). Several remedies are cited for colds: (1) hot lemon water with honey; (2) hot toddies with tea, honey, lemon, peppermint, and a dash of brandy for congestion; and (3) chopped raw garlic, onion, fresh parsley, and water mixed in a blender as expectorant (Spector, 2013). For cuts and wounds, Spector cited the use of either (1) spoiled milk lathered on stale bread and wrapped in a cloth or (2) salt pork laid on a rag and applied on the cut or wound.

Filipinos. Many traditional Filipinos still observe the theory of hot and cold. A person with a cold may not drink cold drinks. While recovering from illness, many eat *arroz caldo*—chicken and rice soup. *Malunggay,* a type of dark leafy greens added to chicken soup, is alleged to cleanse the blood (Muñoz, 2013). Garlic and onions are also used as blood thinners; garlic is also believed to have antihypertensive properties. Ginger root boiled in water and served as a beverage called *salabat* is a popular folk remedy for sore throat and for enhancement of digestion. Malunggay and *ampalaya* (bitter melon) leaves, when added to stews, are used to foster recovery from loss of stamina and fatigue, from anemia, and to deal with stresses (Muñoz, 2013).

High-Risk Groups

Some ethnic or cultural groups have a higher risk of developing illness or altered nutrition. Some of those included in these high-risk groups are the vulnerable population, college age clients, and the elderly, among others. Identification and awareness of these groups will assist health care providers to assess, plan, implement, and evaluate culturally congruent care.

High risk for diabetes. Native Americans have a higher risk for diabetes than the general population. Aiming to estimate the prevalence and incidence of diabetes, clinical characteristics, and risk factors for chronic complications among Navajo youth, Dabelea et al. (2009) conducted a population-based study using data from the SEARCH for Diabetes in Youth Study. The population denominators used were (1) below 20 years of age, (2) self-identified as Navajo, and (3) had at least one visit during the preceding 3 years to any of the six Indian Health Services (IHS) care facilities. Potential participants had one or more diabetes-related ICD-9 codes, were diagnosed in 2002–2005, and were less than 20 years old in December 31 of the year of diagnosis. The study included youth diagnosed with type 1 and type 2 diabetes, excluding those with a hybrid or unknown type of diabetes.

College age clients. College age clients are one of the target groups for interventions against obesity. When college students leave home and have freedom to be on their own, there is a high risk for unhealthy eating habits (Gores, 2008). While a weight gain of 15 pounds, the so-called "**freshman 15**," may be an exaggerated amount, gaining a few pounds in the initial year in college may be the beginning of a persistent weight gain. Promotion of healthy lifestyles is one of the foremost goals of *Healthy People 2020* (USDHHS, 2013). College students, in allied health and in other fields, are in vantage positions to influence the community as role models in clinical, field, and service learning experiences.

Elderly people. Elderly people, especially those who live alone, generally do not eat balanced meals. People who are sick or disabled need referral to Meals on Wheels; usually this entails one hot meal for the day, a cold meal for later, and food for breakfast on the following day (Purnell, 2013). Thorough patient education—in a culturally and linguistically appropriate manner—must be provided for the elderly regarding balanced meals, thorough checking of food labels, reduction of sugar and salt intakes, and safety when preparing, cooking, and storing food. Most of these people have chronic diseases such as diabetes and cardiovascular diseases. Many examples of comfort food are also high in sugar, fat, and salt.

EBP 15.1

Fung et al. (2012) surveyed grade 5 students from approximately 150 schools in Alberta, a province of Canada, in 2008 and 2010. The surveys were conducted to measure the effectiveness of comprehensive school health (CSH) implemented in 2005 in the areas of improvement of diets, activity level, and body weights. The

(continued)

CSH became a "best practice" and inspired the formation of the Alberta Project Promoting Active Living and Healthy Eating (APPLE) in 10 schools, mostly located in disadvantaged areas.

The APPLE schools project, initially started in 2008, is a 3-year intervention by the School of Public Health at the University of Alberta in 10 schools in the province of Alberta. The participating schools decided to support healthy eating and an active lifestyle among students. From 2008 through 2010, 8 of the 10 schools adopted a nutrition policy. In addition, all 10 schools adopted policies to ensure that all students had a minimum of 30 minutes of activity every school day. Community and parent involvement in all schools include community and parent activities such as community gardens, walking to school days, breakfast and lunch programs, and other activities led by parents.

In 2008, 3,421 students with written consent forms from their parents participated in the survey. When the surveys were again conducted in 2010, 3,656 students completed the surveys.

The survey tools consisted of the Harvard Youth Adolescent Food Frequency Questionnaire (FFQ) and the Physical Activity Questionnaire for Older Children (PAQ-C). The FFQ has been widely used as a valid tool in nutrition research among children (Rockett et al., 1997, as cited in Fung et al., 2012). The PAQ-C has proven to be a valid and reliable tool to measure physical activity (Crocker et al., as cited in Fung et al., 2012). The body mass index (BMI) was used for assessment of obesity.

Findings indicated that students in APPLE schools (1) had increased intake of fruits and vegetables; (2) had lower caloric intakes, (3) were more physically active, and (4) were less likely to be obese (Fung et al., 2012, p. 4). Limitations of the study include nonrandom selection of 10 APPLE schools; possible reporting error and subjectivity with self-reporting; and lack of precision of the FFQ. Despite these limitations, the researchers concluded that CSH improves health behaviors, showing that "best practice" may result in success in another setting.

Applications to Practice

■ Investigate the abilities of dietary services in your practice setting.
■ Analyze your own assessment tool when admitting a new patient. What areas are included in terms of nutritional assessment? Do these areas have implications in terms of findings from this study?
■ If you were to replicate this study, what would you change in terms of participants, method, and analysis of data? Explain.

Source: Fung, Kuhle, Lu, Purcell, Schwartz, Storey, & Veugelers (2012).

CRITICAL THINKING EXERCISES 15.1

Undergraduate Student

1. How would you assess the nutritional needs of your multicultural clients?
2. What additional knowledge do you need to plan care for multicultural clients?
3. Examine the Oldways ethnic heritage food pyramids for African, Asian, and Latin Americans. Do you think that the food distribution adequately reflects food groups in those ethnic groups? Explain.

Graduate Student

1. As a future advanced practice nurse (APN), what are assessment parameters that you need to include to manage the nutritional needs of your clients?
2. Examine the Oldways ethnic heritage food pyramids for African, Asian, and Latin Americans and other pyramids. How would you integrate this in your client education?
3. Review your institutional admission tool. Pay close attention to the nutritional assessment portion.
4. If you will be asked to revise the nutrition assessment portion of your admission tool, what would you add? What would you delete. Explain.

Faculty in Academia

1. What are the TCN areas already included in the current nutrition course that you teach?
2. What other areas, based on EBP, could you integrate?
3. Do you use ethnic food pyramids when teaching students? What are the advantages of ethnic food pyramids?
4. What nutritional assessment tool do students use for their assigned clients? If you have the leeway, what areas would you add to this tool? Why?

Staff Development Educator

1. How is nutrition assessed among your clients, both for initial intake and for continuing monitoring?
2. How much of the current admission tool pertains to nutrition in multicultural patients?
3. When revising the current tool, which model would you use to introduce a broader nutritional assessment?

SUMMARY

Food, the essence for survival, is vital in every culture. When planning health promotion programs, examine the meaning of food for diverse groups of people. This examination could be key to unlocking practices that predispose people to problems related to nutrition.

Obesity is an alarming problem, both in adults and among children and adolescents. It is presented along with its aftermath of cardiovascular diseases, stroke, type 2 diabetes, and even some cancers. One way of combating obesity is with school-based interventions; a synopsis of a research study is included in this chapter as evidence of effective health promotion intervention. As the United States becomes more diverse, there is burgeoning availability of ethnic food markets and restaurants in most cities and towns in the United States, increasing the availability of familiar food to immigrants. As evidence of acculturation, fusion food is increasingly becoming more popular.

REFERENCES

Basuray, J. M. (2013). Health beliefs across cultures: Understanding transcultural care. In J. M. Basuray (Eds.), *Culture & health: Concept and practice* (Rev ed., pp. 57–84). Ronkonkoma, NY: Linus.

Boyle, J. S., & Andrews, M. M. (2012). Andrews/Boyle transcultural nursing assessment guide for individuals and families. In M. M. Andrews & J. S. Boyle (Eds.), *Transcultural concepts in nursing care* (6th ed., pp. 451–455). Philadelphia, PA: Wolters Kluwer/Lippincott Williams & Wilkins.

Centers for Disease Control and Prevention. (2012a). *Nutrition and obesity.* Retrieved February 15, 2013, from www.cdc.gov/obesity/index.html

Centers for Disease Control and Prevention. (2012b). *Nutrition resources for health professionals.* Retrieved February 15, 2013, from www.cdc.gov/nutrition/professionals/index.html

Centers for Disease Control and Prevention. (2012c). *Overweight and obesity.* Retrieved June 27, 2013, from www.cdc.gov/obesity/adult/defining.html

Dabelea, D., DeGroat, J., Sorrellman, C., Glass, M., Percy, C. A., Avery, C., ... Hamman, R. (2009). Diabetes in Navajo youth: Prevalence, incidence, and clinical characteristics: The SEARCH for Diabetes in Youth Study. *Diabetes Care, 32*(S.2), S141–147. doi:10.2337/dc09-S206

Edberg, M. (2012). *Essential of health, culture, and diversity: Understanding people, reducing disparities.* Burlington, MA: Jones & Bartlett Learning.

Fung, C., Kuhle, S., Lu, C., Purcell, M., Schwartz, M., Storey, K., & Veugelers, P. J. (2012). From "best practice" to "next practice": The effectiveness of school-based health promotion in improving healthy eating and physical activity and preventing childhood obesity. *International Journal of Behavioral Nutrition and Physical Activity, 27,* 1–9. Retrieved July 23, 2013, from www.ijbnpa. org/content/pdf/1479–5868-9-27.pdf

Giger, J. N., & Davidhizar, R. E. (2008). *Transcultural nursing: Assessment and intervention* (5th ed.). St. Louis, MO: Mosby Elsevier.

Gores, S. E. (2008). Addressing nutritional issues in the college-aged client: Strategies for the nurse practitioner. *Journal of the American Academy of Nurse Practitioners, 20,* 5–10.

Guralnik, D. B. (Ed.). (1984). *Webster's new world dictionary* (2nd college ed.). New York, NY: Simon & Schuster.

Hanson, P. A., & Andrews, M. M. (2012). Religion, culture, and nursing. In M. M. Andrews & J. S. Boyle (Eds.), *Transcultural concepts in nursing care* (6th ed., pp. 351–402). Philadelphia, PA: Wolters Kluwer/Lippincott Williams & Wilkins.

Hoffman, C. (2008). *Judaism.* London, UK: McGraw-Hill.

Huttlinger, K. W. (2013). People of Appalachian heritage. In L. D. Purnell (Ed.), *Transcultural healthcare: A culturally competent approach* (4th ed., pp. 137–158). Philadelphia: F. A. Davis.

Kulwicki, A. D., & Ballout, S. (2013). People of Arab heritage. In L. D. Purnell (Ed.), *Transcultural healthcare: A culturally competent approach* (4th ed., pp. 159–177). Philadelphia: F. A. Davis Co.

Leininger, M. M., & McFarland, M. M. (2006). *Culture care diversity and universality: A worldwide nursing theory* (2nd ed.). Sudbury, MA: Jones & Bartlett.

Muñoz, C. C. (2013). People of Filipino heritage. In L. D. Purnell (Ed.), *Transcultural healthcare: A culturally competent approach* (4th ed., pp. 228–249). Philadelphia: F. A. Davis.

Oldways. (n.d.). *About us: Founder and history.* Retrieved June 25, 2013, from http://oldwayspt.org/about-us/founder-history. Boston, MA: Author.

Oldways. (2000). *Asian diet and pyramid.* Retrieved June 25, 2013, from http://oldwayspt.org/resources/heritage-pyramids/asian-diet-pyramid. Boston, MA: Author.

Oldways. (2009). *Latino diet and pyramid.* Retrieved June 25, 2013, from http://oldwayspt.org/resources/heritage-pyramids/latino-diet-pyramid. Boston, MA: Author.

Oldways. (2011). *African heritage diet pyramid.* Retrieved June 25, 2013, from http://oldwayspt.org/resources/heritage-pyramids/african-diet-pyramid/overview. Boston, MA: Author.

Purnell, L. D. (2013). The Purnell model for cultural competence. In L. D. Purnell (Ed.), *Transcultural healthcare: A culturally competent approach* (4th ed., pp. 15–44). Philadelphia: F. A. Davis.

Railey, M. T. (2009). Cultural proficiency and health disparity: The St. Louis, Missouri, perspective. In S. Kosoko-Lasaki, C. T. Cook, & R. L. O'Brien (Eds.), *Cultural proficiency in addressing health disparities* (pp. 331–356). Boston, MA: Jones & Bartlett Learning.

Rose, P. R. (2011). *Cultural competency for health administration and public health.* Boston, MA: Jones & Bartlett Learning.

Selekman, J. (2013). People of Jewish heritage. In L. D. Purnell (Ed.), *Transcultural healthcare: A culturally competent approach* (4th ed., pp. 339–356). Philadelphia: F.A. Davis.

Spector, R. E. (2013). *Cultural diversity in health and illness* (8th ed.). Boston, MA: Pearson.

United States Department of Agriculture. (2011a). *Dietary guidelines consumer brochure: Let's eat for the health of it!* Retrieved June 27, 2013, from www.choosemyplate.gov/print-materials-ordering/dietary-guidelines.html

United States Department of Agriculture. (2011b). *Ethnic/cultural food pyramids*. Retrieved June 27, 2013, from http://fnic.nal.usda.gov/dietary-guidance/myplatefood-pyramid-resources/ethniccultural-food-pyramids

United States Department of Health and Human Services. (2013). *Healthy People 2020: Leading health indicators: Nutrition, physical activity, and obesity*. Retrieved July 23, 2013, from www.healthy-people.gov/2020/LHI/nutrition.aspx

Wehbe-Alamah, H. (2008). Bridging generic and professional care practices for Muslim patients through use of Leininger's culture care modes. *Contemporary Nurse, 28*(1), 83–97.

TCN Concepts in Nursing Research Courses

Priscilla Limbo Sagar

Back translation
Ethnonursing method
Emic
Etic
Fatigue severity syndrome
General informants
Interpretation
Interpreters
Key informants

Observation-participation-reflection method
Qualitative design
Quantitative design
Research
Research utilization
Stranger–friend model
Translation
Translators

At the completion of this chapter, the learner will be able to

1. Differentiate between quantitative and qualitative research methods.
2. Investigate the use of the ethnonursing method in generating a transcultural body of knowledge.
3. Analyze the steps of data analyses in ethnonursing research.
4. Examine the steps of translation and back translation of research instruments.
5. Propose two areas of research priorities in reducing health disparities.

OVERVIEW

The International Council of Nurses (ICN, 2007) maintains that practice duly based on research "is a hallmark of professional nursing" (p. 1). **Research** is a rigorous, scientific process of inquiry whereby new knowledge is generated. Flowing from the ICN definition, the American Association of Colleges of Nursing ([AACN], 2006) position statement on nursing research states: "Nursing research worldwide is committed to rigorous scientific inquiry that provides a significant body of knowledge to advance nursing practice, shape health policy, and impact the health of people in all countries" (p. 1). The ICN (2007) added that qualitative and quantitative nursing research are equally imperative in achieving quality, cost-effective health care. These statements truly underscore the equal importance of qualitative and quantitative methods in adding to the body of knowledge in professional nursing.

Many nurses contend that nursing research began with Florence Nightingale. Her *Notes on Nursing*, published in 1859, revealed meticulous analysis of influences of soldier morbidity and mortality during the Crimean War (Polit & Beck, 2010) as well as outcomes of her interventions. A landmark report, the Goldmark Report, *Nursing and Nursing Education in the US*, advocated for university-based schools of nursing "to train nursing leaders" (Lundy, 2014, p. 27). The first doctoral program in nursing was founded at Columbia University in 1923; in time, more doctorally prepared nursing studies emerged, mainly focused on nursing students' characteristics, difficulties, and satisfactions (Polit & Beck, 2010).

There were two foci of nursing research during World War II: (1) supply of nurses and (2) amount of time necessary to complete specific nursing activities (Polit & Beck, 2010). The establishment of the National Center for Nursing Research (NCNR) at the National Institutes of Health (NIH) in 1985 was an important milestone in nursing research (National Institute of Nursing Research [NINR], 2010). In 1993, the NCNR was promoted to NINR, a full institute within the NIH (NINR, 2010). Notably, funding for the NINR grew from $16 million in 1986 to $70 million in 1999 (Polit & Beck, 2010).

For a number of years, quantitative and qualitative researchers created a polarity; some believe that this schism was destructive to knowledge advancement in nursing (DiCenso, Ciliska, & Guyatt, 2005). However, there is now a recognition that both quantitative and qualitative methods are not only crucial to nursing, but also complementary to each other (Dicenso et al., 2005; ICN, 2007; Polit & Beck, 2010). Polit and Beck (2010) explain that **quantitative designs** are suited for evaluation of safety and efficacy of interventions and strength of causal relationships, whereas **qualitative designs** lend themselves well to understanding the meaning of attitudes and beliefs as well as lived experiences (pp. 10–11). In the last 50 years, nurse researchers in the 1950s and nurse theorists in the 1960s and the 1970s added to the growing body of knowledge with their studies and development of models and theories. It is not within the scope of this chapter to discuss theories; rather, the chapter's focus is on Leininger's Culture Care Theory (CCT) and the development of one widely used qualitative method: the ethnonursing method.

The CCT, developed in the 1950s with the primary goal of providing *culturally congruent care*, was one of the earliest nursing theories (Leininger, 2002, 2006a). The sunrise model symbolizes the CCT's goal "to discover new ... knowledge, that could markedly raise nursing to a bright sunrise of knowing" (Leininger, 1995, p. 107). Leininger's (1970) pioneering book, *Anthropology and Nursing: Two Worlds to Blend*, laid the groundwork for transcultural nursing (TCN). Dr. Leininger developed the ethnonursing method to study nursing phenomena in depth; she was concerned about nursing's heavy use of research tools and instruments from other disciplines and its concomitant missing of nursing insights and meanings.

The ethnonursing method, as well as other qualitative methods such as grounded theory and phenomenology, are best employed to study lived experiences, cultural values, beliefs, and attitudes. Quantitative methods may be employed to help tap the vast areas of research gaps and health care disparities in access and health outcomes among minority populations, such as Africans, Native Americans, Hispanics (Sullivan Commission, 2004), and Asian. Americans (Agency for Health Research and Quality [AHRQ], 2012). The Institute of Medicine (IOM) report *Unequal Treatment: Confronting Racial and Ethnic*

Disparities in Health Care (Smedley, Stith, & Nelson, 2003) had a compelling impact on disparities as a national problem and urged various stakeholders to tackle this problem. The IOM report called for research both to identify reasons for racial and ethnic disparities and to develop intervention strategies (Smedley et al., 2003).

Research showed that minority medical health care professionals often elect to practice in minority communities (Keith, Bell, Swanson, & Williams, 1985; Davidson & Montoya, 1996, both cited in Wilson & Gamble, 2009). There is some evidence in nursing that most of its minority graduates go back to their own communities to care for their own people (Katz, O'Neill, Strickland, & Doutrich, 2010; Paquiao, 2007; Williams, 2008). Although this shows correlation between increasing the number of diverse graduates and reducing disparities in health care, this is still a high-priority area for research to move toward eliminating disparities in health care access and quality.

Integration of TCN Concepts

Some TCN concepts that need to be integrated in research courses include the continuing disparities in health care access and quality; Leininger's (1995, 2002, 2006a) ethnonursing method; translation and back translation of instruments or tools from one language to another; and gaining access and retention of minority participants. Minority populations regard health care establishments with distrust and are unwilling to participate in research (Kosoko-Lasaki & Cook, 2009). A sample syllabus for nursing research is included in the online Ancillary Package.

Continuing Health Care Disparities

There are continuing disparities of quality of care and access among minority populations (AHRQ, 2012; Sullivan Commission, 2004). When looking at quality of care, the following receive worse care than Whites: Blacks and Hispanics for 40% of measures; American Indians and Alaska natives (ANs) for 33.3% of measures; and Asians for 25% of quality measures (AHRQ, 2012). Poor people and those with low income received worse care than high-income people for approximately 60% of quality measures.

In terms of disparate access, these groups had worse access to care than Whites with corresponding measures: Hispanics compared to non-Hispanic Whites, 70%; AI/ANs, 40%; Blacks, 33.3%; Asians, 20% (AHRQ, 2012). Poor people had worse access than high-income people on 80% of measures, and worse access than middle-income people on 70% of measures. Asian Americans (AA), and Pacific Islanders (PI) had 74.5% more heart attacks compared with 67.5% for Whites; receive worse care than Whites for 20% of measures, and only 87.6% compared to Whites at 90.7% receive recommended hospital care (AHRQ, 2011).

Moreover, there is paucity of research conducted among Native Americans due to lack of data infrastructure, barriers related to culture, and lack of knowledge regarding Native cultures (Jaiyeola & Stabler, 2009). Jaiyeola and Stabler (2009) credited the training of more Native researchers and increase in knowledge of Native cultures and spirituality; these are making it possible for researchers to progress toward culturally appropriate studies that honor and respect Native culture, values, and ways of life. Disparate areas such as cardiovascular diseases, diabetes, malignancy, maternal and infant mortality, injuries, and other health hazards, to name a few, and the efficacy of solutions to current Native American problems such as community partnerships, telemedicine, and telepharmacy all are priority areas for research. There is also a glaring need to increase the number of Native

American health professionals who serve their own communities (Jaiyeola & Stabler, 2009; Sullivan Commission, 2004). Research is likewise imperative on the recruitment, engagement, and retention of Native American nursing and other health care disciplines, such as students and their subsequent choice of areas to practice after graduation.

Leininger's Ethnonursing Method

The word *ethno* pertains to people or specific cultures with a focus on their "worldview, ideas, and cultural practices related to nursing phenomena" (Leininger, 2006a, p. 47). Thus evolved the **ethnonursing method**, a unique qualitative method that includes ethnography, attesting to the richness of Leininger's preparation in nursing and anthropology. There are more than 400 research studies with the ethnonursing method conducted by Dr. Leininger and those who followed her (Glittenberg, 2004).

The pivotal purpose of the ethnonursing method was to foster a naturalistic, **emic** (insider's view) inquiry into nursing phenomena, especially in relation to the CCT (Leininger & McFarland, 2006). *Etic* refers to an outsider's view. Leininger and McFarland (2002, 2006) emphasize the importance of key and general informant selection when using the ethnonursing method. Key informants are participants deemed most knowledgeable regarding the culture and domain of interest; general informants possess general knowledge about the culture and are likely to provide reflections and insights (Leininger & McFarland, 2002, 2006)

It was imperative—the mother of TCN eloquently exhorted—that nursing needed rigorous and scientific research methods that will establish itself as a scholarly, well-grounded discipline focused on human care. Leininger's dual preparation in nursing and anthropology assisted her in developing the ethnonursing method. In the 1960s, Leininger (2006a) found herself very much alone and without mentors in her study of human care from a transcultural nursing viewpoint; however, she began mentoring graduate students in the ethnonursing method. Leininger (2006a, 2012) realized the interest in TCN from both undergraduate and graduate students and credited them for making it a reality. The CCT was an important guide researchers used to directly learn from people about their culture.

According to Leininger (2006a), there are four general and philosophical features of the ethnonursing method

- Moving into familiar and naturalistic people settings;
- Reflecting detailed observations, reflections..., and data from unstructured open-ended inquiries;
- Withholding, suspending, and controlling researcher's biases, prejudices...;
- Requiring that the researcher focus on the cultural context of...phenomena being studied (pp. 53–55).

Three enabling guides. Leininger (2002, 2006a) developed three enabling guides when using the ethnonursing method: *stranger–friend model, observation–participation–reflection method*, and four phases of data analysis. In Leininger's (2006a) **stranger–friend model**, the researcher moves from being a stranger to a *trusted friend* and enters people's world with its rich and meaningful data. This model can also be used by clinicians to gain people's trust and achieve better patient outcomes (Leininger, 2006a).

The **observation–participation–reflection** method (Leininger, 2006a) serves as a guide in "entering and remaining with the people to study their ways of life in relation to nursing care phenomena" (p. 50). When using this enabler, the researcher moves into phases such as primarily observing and actively listening; primarily observing with limited participation; primarily participating with continued observations; and primarily reflecting and reconfirming findings with informants (Leininger, 2006a).

Data analysis guide. Leininger (2006a) also developed a four-phase data analysis guide as the third set of enablers: (1) collection, description, and documentation of raw data; (2) identification and categorization of "descriptors and components" (p. 62) including coding of data and similarities and differences in emic and etic descriptors; (3) examining patterns and contextual analysis for "saturation of ideas and patterns" (p. 62); and (4) synthesizing, interpreting, and analyzing "major themes, research findings, theoretical formulations, and recommendations" (p. 62). Analysis of data in the ethnonursing method, indeed, is a detailed and rigorous process. In so doing, the research meets the criteria of "credibility, recurrent patterning, confirmability, and meaning in context, saturation, and transferability"; each criteria is in accordance with the purposes and philosophy of qualitative research (Leininger, 2006a, pp. 22–23),

There is a wide range of areas to use the ethnonursing method in nursing education, practice, and administration. The list here is merely a sampling; the studies are numerous. In nursing education, the ethnonursing method was utilized to explore recruitment, engagement, and retention of culturally diverse, financially and educationally disadvantaged nursing students (McFarland, Mixer, Lewis & Easley, 2006) and to discover nursing faculty care expressions, patterns, and practices when teaching culture care (Mixer, 2008, 2011).

In nursing practice, the CCT was used to study the care expressions and patterns of the Gadsup Akuna of the eastern highlands of New Guinea in 1960 (Leininger, 2006b), German American elders in a nursing home (McFarland & Zhender, 2006), experience of violence among Potawatomi Native Americans (Farrell, 2006), and the generic care of Lebanese women (Wehbe-Alamah, 2006). In nursing administration, the CCT was used as a framework to study ethical, moral, and legal dimensions of TCN (Cameron-Traub, 1996) as well as politics and care (Miller, 1996). These samplings of researchers' use of the CCT attest to the wide variety of its use in nursing education, practice, and administration

Translation and Back Translation of Instruments

The appropriateness of instruments or tools to be used needs to be evaluated early on when planning research among a multicultural population. Both **interpreters** and **translators** work with a concept communicated from one language to another (Muñoz & Luckmann, 2005). Difference lies in the format of that language. **Translation** is defined as the "process of translating [written] words or text from one language into another" (Oxford Dictionaries, 2013, para 1): translation differs from interpretation; that is, interpretation deals with the *spoken* word. **Back translation** involves translating back to the original language; this iensures that none of the content is lost during the translation process. For example, a tool that is originally written in English, such as the **Fatigue severity syndrome** (Laranjeira, 2012), is translated into Portuguese. Back translation into English is necessary to be able to validate that the accuracy of the original material is intact and is relaying the original meaning of the words.

The process of translation and back translation can be expensive; researchers may want to explore the availability of funding opportunities through specialty and international organizations such as the TCNS, the Sigma Theta Tau International (STTI) Honor Society of Nursing, or their respective chapters to defray this cost. Laranjeira (2012) conducted a study to translate and examine the reliability and validity of the Portuguese version of Fatigue Severity Syndrome (FSS). He administered the FSS to 4,204 Portuguese nurses, along with the Portuguese versions of the Maslach Burnout Inventory (MBI),

Depression Anxiety scale (DASS), and the Visual Analog Scale (VAS). (See EBP 25.1 for more details of this study.)

Tools to Measure Cultural Competence

Many tools have been developed to measure cultural competence among health profession-als, students, and faculty. For professionals, some of the tools being used are the *Inventory for Assessing the Process of Cultural Competence Among Healthcare Professionals—Revised (IAPCC-R)* by Campinha-Bacote (2007) and the *Cultural Competence Clinical Evaluation Tool—(CCET)* by Jeffreys (2010). Specifically designed for nursing students are the *IAPCC-SV* by Campinha-Bacote (2007) and the student version, *CCET-SV* by Jeffreys (2010).

Specific for data collection of diverse client populations (Part I) and clinical problems directed at the 28 *Healthy People 2010* core areas (Part II), Jeffreys (2010) developed the *Clinical Setting Assessment Tool-Diversity and Disparity (CSAT-DD)*. The public–private pro-gram spearheaded by the AHRQ and the Consumer Assessment of Healthcare Providers and Systems (CAHPS) has developed a family of surveys to measure cultural compe-tence from the clients' perspectives (Clancy, Brach, & Abrams, 2012; Weech-Maldonado et al., 2012). The CAHPS, aimed beyond patient satisfaction, anticipates obtaining patient reports of their experiences with health care services. Chapter 2 has more discussion about the CAHPS survey.

The availability of valid and reliable tools is essential to the current and future agenda for research in diversity, cultural competence, and elimination of health dispari-ties. New tools need to be developed as research in measuring cultural competence in education, practice, and administration gain more momentum. To develop and test the Cultural Awareness Scale (CAS), Rew, Baker, Cookston, Khosropour, and Martinez (2003) conducted a two-phased study at the University of Texas at Austin. The synopsis of this study is in **EBP 16.1.**

Increasing Minority Participation in Research

Gaining knowledge from some cultural groups is sometimes difficult. It is challenging for nursing to obtain that knowledge in order to deliver culturally congruent care. One such group is the Amish, who deliberately separates from the mainstream culture.

Over a 3-year period of participation observation in the Amish community, Fisher (2002) and a team of nurse researchers from the Pennsylvania State University collaborated with a clinic in the community and an organization for farm safety. A product of their collabora-tion is the development of an interactive educational board game for Amish children, *Amos and Sadie's Farm: A Pathway to Safety;* this board game, used with picture cards, is intended to prevent farm-related injuries (Fisher, 2002). Some topics included were refraining from climbing into a grain silo's access window since this may cause suffocation due to the low level of oxygen and avoidance of potential dangerous pitchfork and hay holes in the hayloft. This health promotion board game is culturally sensitive and acknowledged the health care beliefs and practices of the Amish. Fisher (2002) emphasized the necessity of bringing health care programs to a community like the Amish. This form of outreach would dispel their notion that the outside community is not interested in them (Wenger & Wenger, 2013).

Among the lessons learned in her 3 years spent conducting research as a participant observer with the Amish, Fisher (2002) emphasized the value of building trust with com-munity members, accepting the Amish for who they are, and tailoring approaches to health

EBP 16.1

Aimed at developing and testing the Cultural Awareness Scale (CAS), Rew et al. (2003) conducted a two-phased study. The Departmental Review Committee (DRC) for protecting human subjects approved both phases of this study. In *phase 1*, the researchers developed a 37-item CAS scale from a review of literature regarding *cultural awareness, sensitivity,* and *competence* (p. 249).

The pilot group consisted of 72 students; these participants clarified ambiguous items and assisted the researchers to construct a scale that correctly represented the students' experiences. The cronbach alpha reliability coefficient of the survey was 0.91.

In *phase 2*, Rew et al. invited a panel of experts on culture, consisting of faculty from diverse backgrounds and ethnicity, to establish content validity of the CAS. Every faculty was mailed a copy of the CAS. Of the 10 invited, 7 returned the survey with useful data. The expert panel was composed of one man and six women who self-identified as White (4), Asian or Pacific Islander (2), and African American (1). The expert panel eliminated an item—resulting in 36 items—and revised the wording of some items. The content validity of the CAS was 0.88.

Continuing the second phase, the revised CAS was administered to students from various classes at the University of Texas at Austin, obtaining 118 utilizable surveys. Phase 1 and 2 samples were then combined for ensuing analysis. The combined cronbach alpha of the two samples was 0.82.

The combination of participants had 168 women and 18 men; the participants self-identified as European Americans (76%), Hispanic Americans (10%), Asian Americans (9%), African Americans (4%), or American Indian (1%). Baccalaureate, including RN-BS students, made-up most of the participants (143); the rest were master's (32) and PhD (15) students. Overall, participants had high mean scores on the five dimensions of CAS.

Five factors emerged: general educational experiences; awareness of attitudes; classroom and clinical instruction; research issues; and clinical practice. These factors were conceptualized in phase 1 and validated by the panel of experts in phase 2.

The researchers acknowledged the small number of participants and those participants representing a single university as limitations of this study.

Applications to Practice

■ Investigate your nursing program in terms of diversity and cultural competence. Do you use a tool to measure student cultural awareness? What tool do you use?

■ In the event that you decide to measure cultural awareness among students in your nursing programs, which tool would you use? Why?

■ If you were to replicate this study, how would you conduct it? What would you change in terms of conceptual framework, sampling, content validity, and analysis of findings?

Source: Rew, Baker, Cookston, Khosropour, & Martinez (2003).

care that are acceptable to them. The Amish avoid technology for personal use but may allow use of a telephone or computers for work purposes (Fisher, 2002) or if necessary for promoting health (Wenger & Wenger, 2013). Most important, Fisher reminded us that in health care, we are "students of our patients" (p. 28). This 3-year collaborative work with the Amish illustrated active participation if research was conducted in a culturally congruent, sensitive, and respectful manner. Some strategies are needed when interviewing informants in order to fully grasp the emic (insider) point of view (DeSantis, 2005).

Current and Future Research Agenda

The current and future research agenda includes disparities in health care access and quality among Blacks, American Indians/Alaska natives, Hispanics, and Asians/Pacific Islanders. Core measures that need follow-up and gaps in knowledge need to be pursued.

The CLAS agenda for research needs to include culturally inclusive initiatives; staff diversity at various levels; language assistance services; staff cultural competence training; and individual and organizational cultural competence (Fortier & Bishop, 2003). Research implementing the use of tools and instruments to measure client satisfaction of CLAS are imperative. Further studies to explore specialty certification and continuing competence in nursing are important.

Continuing research in nursing and allied health education must be pursued, including measurement of cultural competence among students, faculty, and practitioners; adherence to CLAS; role of multicultural centers in colleges and universities in enhancing cultural awareness on campus; and formal integration of diversity and cultural competence in curricula. Ongoing faculty development in cultural competence education and training including certification in TCN—the very group that needs to model and teach cultural competence to students—must be encouraged and compensated.

CRITICAL THINKING EXERCISES 16.1

Undergraduate Student
1. Do you have a separate research course? If you were to add a 3-credit research course, which current course would you delete from your BS in Nursing curriculum? Why?
2. Are you planning to pursue a master's degree in nursing? Are you aware that undergraduate research is a requirement in most master's program?
3. Do you think there is enough content on evidence-based practice integrated in your classes (theory) and in clinical?

Graduate Student
1. How many research courses do you have in your master's program? Do you need to complete a research project or a **research utilization** (RU) in your last research course? Describe.
2. What topic are you pursuing in your clinical practice dissertation? Discuss your interest in this area.
3. What topic are you pursuing in your research-focused dissertation? Discuss your interest in this area.
4. What other research areas do you think should be included in a future research agenda? Why?

(continued)

CRITICAL THINKING EXERCISES 16.1 *(continued)*

Faculty in Academia

1. When developing a content outline for a research course, how would you include disparity in health care access and quality?
2. How would you include the delivery of culturally and linguistically appropriate services in this content outline?
3. Do you have a separate research course? If you were to add a 3-credit research course, which current course would you delete? Why?
4. How do you integrate EBP in the courses that you teach, both in didactic and clinical classes? Explain.

Staff Development Educator

1. Do you have a Journal Club in your hospital or institution? If yes, how often does it meet? Who moderates it?
2. What follow-up activities that embrace EBP do you have for the nurses and ancillary staff? How often are these activities held?
3. How long has it been since you attended a workshop/conference on EBP? When are you planning to attend a workshop/conference on this topic?
4. Is there an incentive for nurses at your institution, such as participation in research or dissemination of findings through a poster or paper presentation at conferences? Does your institution pay the nurse for the day, pay for the conference, or award other incentives? Describe.

SUMMARY

Nursing research has been appropriately referred to as the hallmark of professional nursing practice. Despite an earlier preference for quantitative research, it is now recognized that both qualitative and quantitative types of research are complementary and are essential to nursing knowledge. However, disparities in health care access and quality persist. Research must concentrate on this issue and pursue ways to close the gaps of knowledge on this.

Leininger founded the CCT and the ethnonursing method and pioneered its use in building what is now a vast knowledge in TCN. The history and process of the ethnonursing method has been thoroughly discussed. The current and future research agenda are selected from health disparities and measurement of cultural competence among health professionals, faculty, and students. Valid and reliable tools are available to measure cultural competence among students, faculty, and other health professionals. Emerging tools to measure client satisfaction are promising. These areas offer hope for increasing use of research and evidence-based practice.

REFERENCES

Agency for Healthcare Research and Quality. (2011). *AHRQ funded research on healthcare for Asian Americans/Pacific Islander.* Retrieved July 5, 2013, from www.ahrq.gov/research/findings/fact-sheets/minority/aapifact/aapifact.pdf

Agency for Healthcare Research and Quality. (2012). *National healthcare disparities report, 2012.* Retrieved June 1, 2013, from www.ahrq.gov/research/findings/nhqrdr/nhdr12/nhdr12_prov.pdf

American Association of Colleges of Nursing. (2006). *AACN position statement on nursing research.* Retrieved July 11, 2013, from www.aacn.nche.edu/publications/position/NsgResearch.pdf

Cameron-Traub, J. (1996). Politics and care: A study of Czech Americans with Leininger's theory of culture care diversity and universality. *Journal of Transcultural Competence in Nursing, 9*(1), 3–13.

Campinha-Bacote, J. (2007). *The process of cultural competence in the delivery of healthcare services: The journey continues.* Cincinnati, OH: Transcultural C.A.R.E. Associates.

Clancy, C., Brach, C., & Abrams, M. (2012). Assessing patient experiences of providers' cultural competence and health literacy practices: CAHPS item sets. *Medical Care, 50*(9), S1-S2. Retrieved July 25, 2013, from www.lwww-medicalcare.com

Desantis, L. (2005). Exploring transcultural communication as a participant-observer. In C. C. Muñoz & J. Luckmann (Eds.), *Transcultural communication in nursing.* Clifton Park, NY: Thompson/ Delmar Learning.

DiCenso, A., Ciliska, D., & Guyatt, G. (2005). Introduction to evidence-based nursing. In A. DiCenso, G. Guyatt, & D. Ciliska (Eds.), *Evidence-based nursing: A guide to clinical practice* (pp. 3–19). St. Louis, MO: Elsevier Mosby.

Farrell, L. S. (2006). Culture care of the potawatomi Native Americans who have experienced violence. In M. M. Leininger & M. R. McFarland (Eds.), *Culture care diversity and universality: A worldwide nursing theory* (2nd ed., pp. 207–238). Sudbury, MA: Jones & Bartlett.

Fisher, K. (2002). Lessons learned while conducting research within an Amish community. *The Journal of Multicultural Nursing Research & Health, 8*(3), 21–28.

Fortier, J. P., & Bishop, D. (2003). *Setting the agenda for research on cultural competence in health care: Final report.* Edited by C. Brach. Rockville, MD: U.S. Department of Health and Human Services, Office of Minority Health and Agency for Healthcare Research and Quality. Retrieved September 1, 2013, from www.ahrq.gov/research/findings/factsheets/literacy/cultural/cultural.pdf

Glittenberg, J. (2004). A transdisciplinary, transcultural model for health care. *Journal of Transcultural Nursing, 15*(1), 6–10.

International Council of Nurses. (2007). Position statement: Nursing research. Retrieved July 11, 2013, from www.icn.ch/images/stories/documents/publications/position_statements/B05_Nsg_Research.pdf

Jaiyeola, A. O., & Stabler, W. (2009). Health disparities among Native American people of the United States. In S. Kosoko-Lasaki, C. T. Cook, & R. L. O'Brien (Eds.), *Cultural proficiency in addressing health disparities* (pp. 225–246). Boston, MA: Jones & Bartlett.

Jeffreys, M. R. (2010). Academic settings: General overview, inquiry, action, and innovation. In M. R. Jeffreys (Eds.), *Teaching cultural competence in nursing and health care* (2nd ed., pp. 117–181). New York, NY: Springer Publishing.

Katz, J. R., O'Neil, G., Strickland, C. J., & Doutrich, D. (2010). Retention of Native American nurses working in their communities. *Journal of Transcultural Nursing, 21*(4), 393–401.

Kosoko-Lasaki, S., & Cook, C. T. (2009). Cultural competency research: Description of a methodology. Part 1. In S. Kosoko-Lasaki, C. T. Cook, & R. L. O'Brien (Eds.), *Cultural proficiency in addressing health disparities* (pp. 129–148). Boston, MA: Jones & Bartlett.

Laranjeira, C. A. (2012). Translation and adaptation of the Fatigue Severity Scale for use in Portugal. *Applied Nursing Research, 25*, 212–217.

Leininger, M. M. (1970). *Anthropology and nursing: Two worlds to blend.* New York, NY: John Wiley and Sons.

Leininger, M. M. (1995). *Transcultural nursing: Concepts, theories, research, and practices.* New York, NY: McGraw-Hill.

Leininger, M. M. (2002). The theory of culture care and the ethnonursing method. In M. M. Leininger & M. R. McFarland (Eds.), *Transcultural nursing: Concepts, theories, research, and practice* (3rd ed., pp. 71–98). New York, NY: McGraw-Hill.

Leininger, M. M. (2006a). Ethnonursing: A research method to study the theory of culture care. In M. M. Leininger & M. R. McFarland (Eds.), *Culture care diversity and universality: A worldwide nursing theory* (2nd ed., pp. 43–81). Sudbury, MA: Jones & Bartlett.

Leininger, M. M. (2006b). Culture care of the Gadsup Akuna of the eastern highlands of New Guinea. In M. M. Leininger & M. R. McFarland (Eds.), *Culture care diversity and universality: A worldwide nursing theory* (2nd ed., pp. 115–157). Sudbury, MA: Jones & Bartlett.

Leininger, M. M., & McFarland, M. R. (Eds.). (2002). *Transcultural nursing: Concepts, theories, research, and practice* (3rd ed.). New York, NY: McGraw-Hill.

Leininger, M. M., & McFarland, M. R. (Eds.). (2006). *Culture care diversity and universality: A worldwide nursing theory* (2nd ed.). Sudbury, MA: Jones & Bartlett.

Leininger, M. M. (2012). Foreword. In P. L. Sagar (Ed.), *Transcultural nursing theory and models: Application in nursing education, practice, and administration.* New York, NY: Springer Publishing.

Lundy, K. S. (2014). A history of health care and nursing. In K. Masters (Ed.), *Role development in professional nursing practice* (3rd ed., pp. 3–46). Burlington, MA: Jones & Bartlett Learning.

McFarland, M., Mixer, S., Lewis, A. E., & Easley, C. (2006). Use of the culture care theory as a framework for the recruitment, engagement, and retention of culturally diverse nursing students in a traditionally European American baccalaureate nursing program. In M. Leininger & M. McFarland (Eds.), *Culture care diversity and universality: A worldwide nursing theory* (2nd ed., pp. 239–254). Boston, MA: Jones & Bartlett.

McFarland, M., & Zehnder, C. (2006). Culture care of German American elders in a nursing home context. In M. Leininger & M. McFarland (Eds.), *Culture care diversity and universality: A worldwide nursing theory* (2nd ed., pp. 181–205). Boston, MA: Jones & Bartlett.

Miller, J. (1996). Politics and care: A study of Czech Americans with Leininger's theory of culture care diversity and universality. *Journal of Transcultural Competence in Nursing, 9*(1), 3–13.

Mixer, S. J. (2008). Use of the culture care theory and ethnonursing method to discover how nursing faculty teach culture care. *Contemporary Nurse, 28*, 23–36.

Mixer, S. (2011). Use of the culture care theory to discover nursing faculty care expressions, patterns, and practices related to teaching culture care. *Online Journal of Cultural Competence in Nursing and Healthcare, 1*(1), 3–14. Retrieved January 18, 2013, from www.ojccnh.org/1/1/index.shtml

Muñoz, C. C., & Luckmann, J. (2005). *Transcultural communication in nursing.* Clifton Park, NY: Thompson/Delmar Learning.

National Institute of Nursing Research. (2010). *NINR: Bringing science to life.* Retrieved October 12, 2013, from www.ninr.nih.gov/sites/www.ninr.nih.gov/files/NINR_History_Book_508.pdf

Oxford Dictionaries. (2013). "Translation." In oxforddictionaries.com. Retrieved February 18, 2014, from http://www.oxforddictionaries.com/us/definition/american_english/translation?q=translation

Paquiao, D. (2007). The relationship between cultural competence education and increasing diversity in nursing schools and practice settings. *Journal of Transcultural Nursing, 18*(1), 28S–37S.

Polit, D. F., & Beck, C. T. (2010). *Essentials of nursing research: Appraising evidence for nursing practice* (7th ed.). Philadelphia, PA: Wolters Kluwer/Lippincott, Williams, & Wilkins.

Rew, L., Baker, H., Cookston, J., Khosropour, S., & Martinez, S. (2003). Measuring cultural awareness in nursing students. *Journal of Nursing Education, 42*(6), 249–257.

Sagar, P. L. (2012). *Transcultural nursing theory and models: Application in nursing education, practice, and administration.* New York, NY: Springer Publishing.

Smedley, B. D., Stith, A. Y., & Nelson, A. R. (2003). *Unequal treatment: Confronting racial and ethnic disparities in health care* (Committee on Understanding and Eliminating Racial and Ethnic Disparities in Health Care, Institute of Medicine). Washington, DC: National Academies Press.

Sullivan Commission. (2004). *Missing persons: Minorities in the health professions: A report of the Sullivan Commission on diversity in the healthcare workforce.* Retrieved January 6, 2013, from www.jointcenter.org/healthpolicy/docs/Sullivan.pdf

Weech-Maldonado, R., Carle, A., Weidmer, B., Hurtado, M., Ngo-Metzger, Q., & Hays, R. D. (2012). The consumer assessment of healthcare providers and systems (CAHPS) cultural competence (CC) item set. *Medical Care, 50*(9), S2, S22–S31. Retrieved July 25, 2013, from www.lwww-medicalcare.com

Wehbe-Alamah, H. (2006). Generic care of Lebanese Muslim women in the midwestern USA. In M. M. Leininger & M. R. McFarland (Eds.), *Culture care diversity and universality: A worldwide nursing theory* (2nd ed., pp. 307–325). Sudbury, MA: Jones & Bartlett.

Wenger, A. F. Z., & Wenger, M. R. (2013). The Amish. In L. D. Purnell (Ed.), *Transcultural healthcare: A culturally competent approach* (4th ed., pp. 115–136). Philadelphia, PA: F.A. Davis.

Williams, S. (2008). Lessons from my father. *Minority Nurse*, Fall, 40–44.

Wilson, R., & Gamble, V. (2009). The role of academic medical centers in the elimination of racial and ethnic disparities. In S. Kosoko-Lasaki, C. T. Cook, & R. L. O'Brien (Eds.), *Cultural proficiency in addressing health disparities* (pp. 73–85). Boston, MA: Jones & Bartlett.

TCN Concepts in Community Health Nursing Courses

Priscilla Limbo Sagar, Nancy Spear Owen, and Elizabeth Simon

KEY TERMS

Community
Gatekeeper
Globalization
Health disparity
Healthy People 2020
Migrant workers

Multiservice centers or one-stop shopping
Public health nursing
Purnell Model for Cultural Competence
Stereotyping
Vulnerable populations

LEARNING OBJECTIVES

At the completion of this chapter, the learner will be able to

1. Discuss teaching strategies to develop cultural competence in community health nursing students.
2. Explore the application of the *Purnell Model for Cultural Competence* into a community health nursing (CHN) course.
3. Engage students to reflect on strategies to reduce disparity in health care access and quality.
4. Integrate culturally and linguistically appropriate care in a CHN course.
5. Maximize individual, family, community, and population health promotion activities in accordance with *Healthy People 2020*.

OVERVIEW

As a starting point for CHN, it is imperative to highlight the pioneering works of nurses worldwide in health promotion and disease prevention. Florence Nightingale embarked to the Crimean War in 1854 and, finding deplorable conditions and a soldier mortality rate of up to 73%, immediately demanded they receive strict sanitation, proper nutrition, and fresh air (Lundy, 2013). In 1893, Lillian Wald and Mary Brewster established the Henry Street Settlement in New York City; this later evolved into the Visiting Nurses of New York ([VNANY], Stanhope & Lancaster, 2010). Another pioneering work was the founding of the Frontier Nursing Service (FNS) by Myra Breckinridge in the rural highlands of Kentucky (Stanhope & Lancaster, 2010).

In these historical works, nurses were powerful visionary change agents. Nightingale demonstrated with detailed statistics that improved environmental conditions drastically reduced mortality among the soldiers in Scutari from between 42% and 73% to 2% (Lundy, 2013). Wald and Brewster worked with poor immigrants of New York City while Breckinridge made possible care to the poor, disadvantaged, and underserved population of the Kentucky highlands. Many more undocumented endeavors of other nurses made a difference in improving the health care of individuals, communities, and populations.

Nightingale, Wald, Brewster, and Breckinridge's pioneering endeavors in CHN illustrated early on how nursing could make a vast difference in health promotion, illness prevention, and bridging gaps in access to health care. This concept, more than ever, is timely as the United States gets increasingly diverse and is spending more in health care yet showing continuing disparities in access and quality of care, especially among Hispanics, African Americans, Native Americans (Edberg, 2013; Rose, 2011), and Asians and Pacific Islanders (Agency for Healthcare Policy and Research [AHRQ], 2012).

One of the overarching goals of *Healthy People 2020*, the health promotion and disease prevention effort for all Americans since 1979, is the elimination of health disparities (U.S. Department of Health and Human Services [USDHHS], Office of Minority Health [OMH], 2010). Factors that contribute to disparities include education, insurance status, segregation, and immigration status (Pamies & Nsiah-Kumi, 2009); these issues need to be woven into CHN courses. There are disparities in health care quality and access among **vulnerable populations**. Vulnerability characterizes a population or group with the added risk of developing adverse outcomes (Edberg, 2013; Sebastian, 2010).

According to Edberg (2013), **globalization** points to not only the combination of economic production and markets but also to the social and political aftermath of this trend. In addition to making it possible for rapid routes of transmission of infectious diseases around the world, primarily due to faster transports of people and goods, globalization places the folk healing system alongside the medical health system (Edberg, 2013). This juxtaposition of folk healing and medical systems creates conflicts; it is imperative that nursing bridge these two systems and promote health among individuals and communities. It is not by chance that Leininger (2006) and her Culture Care Theory is right and fitting in health care in the 21st century, the answer to conflict management when folk care clashes with medical care. Cultural clashes can be tragic, as in the case of Lia Lee and her family in *The Spirit Catches You and You Fall Down* (Fadiman, 1997). Being a visionary, Leininger—as her life's work—developed and refined her theory since the 1950s. "The essence of nursing is caring," Leininger emphasized; in the CCT, the nurse sits at a vantage point, bridging generic folk care and the professional care systems.

Integration of TCN Concepts

This chapter will focus on CHN as a senior level course in a baccalaureate program. It is an expectation that the course will integrate knowledge from earlier courses into **community** experiences including transcultural concepts. A smooth progression is best developed throughout a nursing curriculum in the nursing program. TCN knowledge and skill will build upon previous knowledge and skill and enhance additional dimensions of to the CHN course. Some concepts that need to be included when planning the development or revision of an existing CHN course, and are expected content of both didactic and clinical experiences, include health disparities, community partnerships, vulnerability, and globalization.

Health Disparities

Rose (2011) defines **health disparity** as a "healthcare inequality or gaps in the quality of health and health care across racial, ethnic, and socioeconomic groups and population specific differences in the presence of disease, health outcomes, or access to health care" (p. 158). The National Health Disparities Report (NHDR) indicates that health care quality and access are "suboptimal, especially for minority and low-income groups" (AHRQ, 2012, p. 2). The AHRQ cited these groups as recipients of worse care than Whites: Blacks; American Indians (AI) and Alaska Natives (AN); Hispanics; Asians; poor people; and those with low income.

Disparities in access and quality of care among older adults, the largest growing population in the United States, have been documented in the literature. Older Americans 65 years and over had a poverty rate in 2008 of 9.7%; the rates are much greater among minorities: Blacks (20%), Hispanics (19.3%), and Asians (12.1%) (Administration on Aging [AOA], 2010a, n. d. a 2010b, n.d.b). To be a minority and to be poor present double the risk for poorer health outcomes.

Vulnerable Populations

Vulnerability characterizes a population or group with an added risk of developing adverse outcomes (Edberg, 2013; Sebastian, 2010). Vulnerable population groups include individuals belonging to these categories: poor and homeless, migrant workers and immigrants, severely ill mentally, victims of violence, and those afflicted with communicable diseases, among others (Sebastian, 2010). The cumulative, or additive, biological, environmental, personal, and social risks predispose the individuals to various illnesses.

Planning and implementing care for vulnerable populations entail much creativity, organization, and compassion. Fostering trust, respect, and concern is vital with a focus on navigating the health delivery system. One action proven effective is the use of **multiservice centers** or **"one-stop shopping"** whereby health care, social services, drug and alcohol rehabilitation, day care, and case managing are available in a central location at convenient times (Sebastian, 2010) such as before and after work or during work breaks. Neighborhood clinics and health care mobile vans are also valuable. When vulnerable populations are unable to access services—whether because of lack of belongingness, communication, knowledge, or transportation—services should come to them.

Globalization

Globalization has provided enormous opportunities as well as challenges to nursing education. There are various cultural and ethnic groups located in close proximities of urban life. Among the cultural and ethnic groups are **migrant workers,** or individuals employed on a seasonal basis, in that employment within the last 2 years, and living in a temporary home (Bushy & Napolitano, 2010). Migrant workers and their special needs are among the many challenges related to globalization and migration. For example, in the Northeast United States, there are many migrant workers in agriculture, dairy farming, and even horse-racing (Jenkins, Stack, May, & Earle-Richardson, 2009). In addition to lack of health insurance, migrant workers face language and cultural barriers, privacy issues posed when employers interpret for workers, lack of transportation, long working hours, and fear of losing their jobs. All these difficulties prevent migrant workers from seeking health care (Jenkins et al., 2009). In addition to integrating migrant workers among the vulnerable populations, there are various clinical practicum opportunities for nursing education among migrant workers.

The United States has 3 million migrant workers in various localities and types of occupations. They work and live in areas that are socially and physically isolated from mainstream American life. Apart from physical problems, there are psychological problems connected to lack of health care and social issues. The loneliness of new migrant workers compels them to seek social support from sexual workers, dance clubs, and bar acquaintances, and eventually to engage in risky sexual behaviors. Human immunodeficiency virus (HIV) is prevalent among migrant workers as a result of this condition. However, new migrants who go to Catholic churches do not encounter these risky behaviors (Munoz-Laboy, Hirsch, & Quispe-Lazaro, 2009; Persichino & Ibarra, 2012). Other health problems that migrant workers encounter include fungal infections, poor nutrition, diabetes, asthma, skin diseases, eye disorders, and sexually transmitted diseases (STDs).

In addition to these acute and chronic problems are periodic outbreaks of communicable diseases that are common to dormitory living. The lack of hygienic conditions, use of public toilets, poor nutrition, and lack of psychological ties make this population very vulnerable to various maladies. Horse-riding stable workers are housed in dormitories without separate kitchens or toilets, located between or above the stalls. Many of these temporary men and women workers have children, and the poor living conditions and long working hours endured by their parents pose many problems for the children as their parents move from job to job (Hawkes et al., 2007; Nevarez-La Torre, 2012). Social isolation drives many men to depression.

Community Partnerships and Collaborations

Migrant farm workers have caught the attention of many politicians; some academic medical centers and community agencies have developed projects that provide periodic health care to migrant workers. However, a horse-riding "backstretch" community of workers and their families has yet to get much attention from the outside "motor-riding world" (Lesniewski & Martone, 2011). A sustainable and longitudinal community partnership may be developed and maintained by schools of nursing (SON), with nursing students and faculty members providing health services and opening up doors for effective clinical education and transcultural nursing education.

Community collaboration with employers, community stakeholders, health care providers, and academic health centers is possible and in turn can provide occupational safety, health care awareness, empowerment, and access to care (Connor, Rainer, Simcox, & Thomisee, 2007). Such community partnership also increases interprofessional collaboration and cooperation, enhances awareness of the connection between environment and health, provides advocacy for an at-risk population, and establishes a foundation for future partnership.

Interprofessional education and partnership may be pursued for health care students with students in social work, in English as a second language (ESL), and in intercultural studies. Social responsibility and leadership skills of the health care and other students are augmented in a transcultural environment (Connor, Layne, & Thomisee, 2010). Social worker students can educate this community about how to obtain resources and access, enabling the community to recognize and deal with its own health care needs. In return, health care students will benefit from their experience in the migrant community by understanding specific health care problems and developing communication skills as they work with clients whose language is different from their own. Many opportunities for health care education arise in a collaborative learning environment to enhance clinical vigilance in dealing with common health issues such as occupational hazards related to farm products and pesticides, musculoskeletal injuries, problems of group living, elevated risks for different cancers, and parasite infestations (Mills, Dodge, & Yang, 2009).

Accurate data about the number of migrant workers and their health problems are not available since this population is always mobile and its vulnerability makes gathering research data difficult. Community projects provide opportunities for medical and nursing students to develop social responsibility and increase their commitment to work in needy areas. Community projects also recruit future health professionals to shortage areas and provide the impetus to initiate new community partnership models (Connor, Layne, et al., 2010; Pysklywec, McLaughlin, Tew, & Haines, 2011). "One-stop shopping centers" for health care (Sebastian, 2010) have been suggested in literature.

When working with the community, it is invaluable to first assess the community's needs as specified by the community and by data available. Second, identify the **gatekeeper** to the community or the person controlling access to the group (Onega & Barbero, 2010) as health care workers lay the foundation for trust between the two parties. The gatekeeper may invite health care workers after the determination of mutual benefits. Gatekeepers are well-respected in the community; however, they may not be the formal community leaders.

TCN concepts are of special importance in CHN because these affect not only how individuals, families, communities, and populations view health and illness but also how they access health care. In one community, there are many cultures, subcultures, and family cultures. Furthermore, the care takes place in another's home, in community facilities, or within the cultural context of their community as opposed to acute care or long-term settings where the nurse has more control over the environment. Unlike in acute or long-term care— where the health care professionals are in a familiar environment and the clients are in a foreign territory—in the community setting, the clients are in the more familiar environment.

SOME TEACHING AND LEARNING STRATEGIES

In a senior-level CHN course, it is essential to teach TCN concepts and develop students' cultural competence. With a focus on diverse families, groups, and populations, CHN affords an opportunity to immerse students into homes, neighborhoods, and cultures other than their own. Didactic and clinical teaching strategies may take cognitive, psychomotor, and affective aspects of learning development into consideration. Educators are fortunate to have many resources and toolkits available to assist with planning, implementing, and evaluating effective and innovative TCN teaching strategies. As research evidence in the area of teaching strategies to develop students' cultural competence in CHN courses builds, decisions on most effective methods should be integrated. TCN concepts, as in other nursing courses in the curriculum, are an expected part of both didactic and clinical experiences.

One of the best ways to attend to each student's diverse learning needs is to make the TCN assignments student-centered. Student-centered learning refers to a teaching/learning process that involves active student engagement in acquiring knowledge rather than acting as passive recipients of information from teachers (Young & Paterson, 2007). The following teaching–learning strategies are also student-centered: health education project, reflective journals, role plays, and unfolding case scenarios.

Health Education Project

Students in CHN at Mount Saint Mary College are required to complete an individual Healthy People Project (HPP). The whole premise of the HPP is to assist in creating healthy communities, a goal of *HP 2020* (U.S. Department of Health and Human Services, HRSA, 2012). The HPP includes both a teaching and a paper component and deals with a priority need of the agency or population in the community. Some HPPs that students have implemented in communities are health education regarding activity, bullying, dental care, disaster preparedness, hand washing, lead poisoning, nutrition, and many, many others.

Students in CHN are assigned in the neighboring counties in public and private schools with students from prekindergarten to college; departments of health; community health centers; home care agencies; college health services; employee health services; and other similar community agencies. Students also visit homeless shelters and other local community resources in Newburgh, New York. Newburgh is a very diverse, underserved community.

Reflective Journaling

Journaling in CHN will further aim to hone students' critical thinking and clinical judgment. One approach is to initially require reflective journals in the first nursing course and adopt a programmatic value attached to journaling, as in the consistent weight in grading journals across nursing courses (Emerson, 2007). Some guide questions will help students to further deepen their critical thinking skills and enhance their road into becoming reflective practitioners.

Many students in CHN reflect upon their surprise at discovering the poverty in "a country of plenty" such as the United States. In addition, students usually comment about finding homes without heat, running water, and necessities; students equate these conditions with developing countries rather than one of the most industrialized of countries, a country also recognized as a world leader. The study by Schuessler, Wilder, and Byrd (2012), conducted over four semesters, reveals increasing cultural awareness and cultural humility among students (EBP 17.1). (See Chapter 2 for more information about reflective journaling.)

Role Playing

Role playing is widely used in nursing education. According to Shearer and Davidhizar (2003), role plays not only increase students' cultural awareness but also challenge their

EBP 17.1

Schuessler et al. (2012) conducted a qualitative, descriptive study among students assigned at a local housing authority. This study was approved by the Internal Review Board of Auburn University. The study reports on 200 journal entries made over a 2-year period from 50 students as they moved through four semesters of a nursing program. Three faculty members reviewed the journal entries and analyzed developing themes. The journals were not graded and student names were removed prior to the analyses.

Students attended community clinical experiences at a local housing authority serving low-income residents. The students reflected on a semistructured interview question each semester. The primary question explored in the study was, "What does reflective journaling reveal about the experience of cultural humility in nursing students participating in the community partnership clinical?" (Schuessler et al., 2012, p. 96).

Findings revealed themes of increasing cultural humility emerging over four semesters. The first semester elicited three broad themes: (1) development of psychomotor skills; (2) beginning of understanding of the importance of culture in patients' lives; and (3) students began to understand the value of community nursing. The second and third semester entries revealed a deeper cultural understanding including: (4) student awareness of health disparities for those experiencing poverty; (5) critical examination of health teaching and learning to tailor the teaching to the audience; (6) importance of trust in CHN; and (7) value of encouragement, support, and being nonjudgmental when working with clients. The fourth semester themes illustrated that interaction with patients in order to meet their health care needs included: (8) gaining confidence interacting with clients; (9) the importance of health promotion and disease prevention; and (10) change in the students' thinking and feelings about people from different cultures.

Schuessler et al. (2012) conclude that combining reflective thinking and journaling over a period of time is an effective method to develop cultural humility in nursing students. Two final concepts grasped by students that demonstrated cultural humility were: "students saw firsthand that poverty creates health care disparities" and "health promotion teaching projects must consider culture" (Schuessler et al., p. 99).

Applications to Practice

1. Investigate communication strategies used for health education between teachers and students; students and community clients; and health care workers and community members of different cultures.
2. Consider implementing reflective journaling in community clinical experiences over several semesters.
3. Analyze health disparities from the perspective of the client. Teach students to build relationships with community members different from themselves prior to implementing care or health education.

(continued)

EBP 17.1 *(continued)*

4. Cultural humility is an ongoing process. Reflect and analyze on your own experiences as an administrator, educator, nurse, and/or student to continuously build cultural humility.
5. If you were to replicate this study, what would you change in terms of conceptual framework, method, and analysis of findings? Explain.

Source: Schuessler, Wilder, & Byrd (2012).

creativity in illustrating culturally congruent care. It is essential that the faculty develop objectives for the experience, monitor the process, and facilitate debriefing. The debriefing portion at the end of the role play allows analysis of action, recognition of reaction to the role play, and constructive comments (Decker, Gore, & Feken, 2011). Chapter 2 has more discussion about role playing.

Unfolding Scenarios

When using unfolding case scenarios, scenarios are added as students gain in knowledge, skills, and competence throughout the course or courses and the program. This strategy fosters critical thinking and clinical judgment as students build on their learning. Although it is time-consuming to develop unfolding case scenarios, the rewards are worth the effort. In light of the cost in time and money to develop your own scenarios, published case scenarios are available.

APPLICATION OF THE PURNELL MODEL FOR CULTURAL COMPETENCE IN CHN

The *Purnell Model for Cultural Competence* (PMCC) is easy to use and may be applied to all levels of nursing education (Sagar, 2012). Purnell (2008, 2013) views cultural competence as a journey and uses four levels of cultural competence in the model (see Chapter 1).

As an example of the PMCC's applicability in CHN, Phelps and Johnson (2004) used this model to create a website, *Cultural Competency and Haitian Immigrants*, for **public health nursing** personnel in rural Delaware. Delivering electronic staff development resources is a viable alternative to promote cultural competence; this may be used for faculty and students. The PMCC's 12 cultural domains may be used completely or in part when developing or revising a CHN course. Unfolding Case Scenario 17.1 illustrates a PMCC application used in a CHN classroom assignment used in a baccalaureate program.

APPLICATION: UNFOLDING CASE SCENARIO 17.1 USE OF PURNELL MODEL FOR CULTURAL COMPETENCE IN A CLASSROOM ASSIGNMENT

Goal of case scenario: To provide an opportunity for community health nursing students to develop cultural competence in a school setting by utilizing the Purnell Model for Cultural Competence.

Learning Objectives

At the conclusion of this case study, the learner will be able to

1. Apply the **Purnell Model for Cultural Competence** when providing care to an individual and family in a school health setting.
2. Apply the Purnell Model for Cultural Competence to provide care for a school population.
3. Explore the concepts of health disparities, ethnocentrism, participant observation, and acculturation.

Introduction

An urban elementary school has a population of 1,200 diverse students in grades 2 through 5. Students at the school are an evenly distributed blend of many races and ethnicities including Blacks, White Americans, Hispanics/Latinos, and Asian Americans. There is also a wide range in the socioeconomic status of the student population. Approximately 25% of the student population is placed in English as a second language (ESL) classes. Almost 15% of the entire population has special education needs and active Individualized Education Plans (IEPs), as well as 504 plans. Developed by school teams and parents to support the educational goal for students with a disability that "substantially limits one or more of the following life activity: speaking, listening, writing, reading, concentrating, and others" (National Center for Learning Disabilities [NCLD], 2013, Para 2), the 504 plan can be the answer to helping a child succeed in school. The 504 plans are available for K–12 students with a disability; an example of accommodation is extra time on tests or assignments (NCLD, 2013).

Individual and Family Scenario

A 10-year-old Mexican American girl in the fourth grade speaks mainly Spanish and attends the special education program. She has been diagnosed with type 1 diabetes for 3 years. She also has a body mass index (BMI) that falls in the overweight category. The student lives with her mother and 2-year-old brother in a small apartment. The mother works full-time at a local retail market. The student has recently been placed on a diabetic pump.

All doctor's orders are in place for medication administration, pump use, and emergencies. Frequently, the student's glucose level finger stick goes above 400 while in school, which requires either leaving school early or spending extra time in the health office. She usually does not feel well and misses time from

(continued)

class. The nurse is concerned about the frequency of elevated finger sticks and conducts a more detailed assessment. The student reports eating sweetened cereal for breakfast at home; she brings lunch from home that includes chips, a can of soda, a ham sandwich, and fried bananas or a piece of fruit. Her mother calculates carbohydrates each day and also made a comment that "now that she has an insulin pump she can eat whatever she wants because that is what the doctor said."

The nurse determines that nutrition education is critically important to promote optimal health for the student and her family.

1. Do you think culture and language play a role in the student's health, such as the ability to understand doctor's instructions and make good dietary choices? Discuss.
2. What are the possible cultural considerations for the student and the family in the scenario?
3. What additional cultural information needs to be gathered in order to plan for educational interventions? (Refer to the fourth rim of PMCC to explore culture-specific facts from the 12 cultural domains.)
4. Discuss the concepts of **stereotyping** and acculturation in the school health setting.

School Population Scenario

The school nurse has determined there is an increase in childhood obesity based on her observations and screening data gathered from the school health office. The obesity rate is above that of the national levels. The school nurse would like to implement prevention measures to address the obesity issue and improve the overall health of the student population. The nurse begins by establishing a wellness committee.

1. What cultural groups need to be represented and included as members of the wellness committee? Why?
2. What facts need to be gathered during the wellness committee's school assessment in relationship to obesity and health disparities?
3. What cultural considerations need to be addressed in planning for the new obesity prevention measures? (Refer to the fourth rim of PMCC to explore the 12 cultural domains from a population standpoint.)
4. Discuss the concepts of ethnocentrism and participant observation in the school health office and membership on a wellness committee.

Source: Purnell (2013).

CRITICAL THINKING EXERCISES 17.1

Undergraduate Student
1. Has the faculty teaching CHN included content in your current CHN course regarding care for culturally diverse clients? Explain.
2. Do you think there is enough content on cultural diversity and promotion of cultural competence integrated in your CHN class didactic (theory) and in clinical?
3. Have you had opportunities to care for culturally diverse individuals, groups, and families? Did you feel prepared to assist in their care? If not, what preparation in your classes and clinical would have helped? Describe.

Graduate Student
1. Do you have a partnership or collaboration between your SON and a community? If you do, what are the aspects of that collaboration?
2. Has the SON "adopted" the community in this partnership?
3. Does the SON have an outreach program to a local or international community? Is this a mutually beneficial collaboration or partnership?
4. If you are majoring in public health or community health, how is diversity and promotion of culturally and linguistically appropriate services integrated in your curriculum? Describe.

Faculty in Academia
1. How many credits do you have in the CHN course in your nursing program?
2. How do you critically appraise diversity and cultural competence content in the CHN course that you are teaching?
3. Do you have the academic freedom to add TCN concepts into that course? Or does this fall under the duties of the curriculum committee at the division/school of nursing? Explain.
4. Have you been a participant or leader in local or international community partnership? Describe.

Staff Development Educator
1. Do you have CHN students on clinical rotation at your institution or agency? What level are these students?
2. Are the students in CHN required to have components of cultural diversity and promotion of cultural competence as part of orientation?
3. If you are a community agency, what follow-up activities that celebrate diversity do you have for the nurses and ancillary staff? How often are these activities held?
4. How long has it been since you attended a workshop/conference on cultural diversity and promotion of cultural competence among your CHN clients? When are you planning to attend a workshop/conference on this topic?

SUMMARY

Important areas such as health disparities, globalization, and vulnerability have been discussed for inclusion in community health, nursing courses, course planning, or for course revision. The authors reviewed teaching and learning strategies for health promotion of individuals, families, communities, and populations. In addition, the authors illustrated the application of the PMCC in an unfolding case scenario. With the increase in globalization, folk healing and professional care systems go side by side. These systems may clash.

The CCT, more than ever, reveals the vantage point of nursing as the bridge to these two systems in providing culturally and linguistically congruent care.

REFERENCES

Administration on Aging. (2010a). *A statistical profile of Black older Americans aged 65+*. Retrieved July 11, 2013, from www.aoa.gov/AoARoot/Aging_Statistics/minority_aging/Facts-on-Black-Elderly-plain_format.aspx

Administration on Aging. (2010b). *A statistical profile of Hispanic older Americans aged 65+*. Retrieved July 11, 2013, from www.aoa.gov/AoARoot/Aging_Statistics/minority_aging/Facts-on-Hispanic-Elderly.aspx

Administration on Aging. (n.d.a). *A statistical profile of American Indian and Native Alaskan older Americans aged 65+*. Retrieved July 11, 2013, from www.aoa.gov/AoARoot/Aging_Statistics/minority_aging/Facts-on-AINA-Elderly2008-plain_format.aspx

Administration on Aging. (n.d.b). *A statistical profile of Asian older Americans aged 65+*. Retrieved July 11, 2013, from aoa.gov/AoARoot/Aging_Statistics/minority_aging/Facts-on-API-Elderly2008-plain_format.aspx

Agency for Healthcare Research and Quality. (2012). *National healthcare disparities report, 2012*. Retrieved June 1, 2013, from www.ahrq.gov/research/findings/nhqrdr/nhdr12/nhdr12_prov.pdf

Bushy, A., & Napolitano, M. (2010). Rural health and migrant health. In M. Stanhope & J. Lancaster (Eds.), *Foundations of nursing in the community: Community-oriented practice* (3rd ed., pp. 400–418). St. Louis, MO: Elsevier Mosby.

Connor, A., Rainer, L. P., Simcox, J. B., & Thomisee, K. (2007). Increasing the delivery of health care services to migrant farm worker families through a community partnership model. *Public Health Nursing, 24*(4), 355–360.

Connor, A., Layne, L., & Thomisee, K. (2010). Providing care for migrant farm worker families in their unique sociocultural context and environment. *Journal of Transcultural Nursing, 21*(2), 159–166.

Decker, S., Gore, T., & Feken, C. (2011). Simulation. In T. J. Bristol & J. Zerwekh (Eds.), *Essentials for e-learning for nurse educators* (pp. 277–294). Philadelphia, PA: F.A. Davis.

Edberg, M. (2013). *Essentials of health, culture, and diversity: Understanding people, reducing disparities*. Burlington, VT: Jones & Bartlett Learning.

Emerson, R. J. (2007). *Nursing education in the clinical setting*. St. Louis, MO: Elsevier Mosby.

Fadiman, A. (1997). *The spirit catches you and you fall down*. New York, NY: Farrar, Straus and Giroux.

Hawkes, L., May, J. J., Earle-Richardson, G., Paap, K., Santiago, B., & Ginley, B. (2007). Identifying occupational health needs of migrant workers. *Journal of Community Practice, 15*(3), 57–77.

Jenkins, P., Stack, S., May, J. J., & Earle-Richardson, G. (2009). Growth of Spanish-speaking workforce in the northeast dairy industry. *Journal of Agromedicine, 14*(1), 58–65.

Leininger, M. M. (2006). Culture care diversity and universality theory and evolution of the ethnonursing method. In M. M. Leininger & M. R. McFarland (Eds.), *Culture care diversity and universality: A worldwide nursing theory* (2nd ed., pp. 1–41). Sudbury, MA: Jones & Bartlett.

Lesniewski, J., & Martone, J. (2011). Migration, globalization and two intertwined countries: An introduction to the Mexico/U.S case. *Journal of Poverty, 15*(4), 375–381.

Lundy, K. S. (2013). A history of health care and nursing. In K. Masters (Ed.), *Role development in professional nursing practice* (3rd ed., pp. 3–46). Burlington, MA: Jones & Bartlett Learning.

Mills, P., Dodge, J., & Yang, R. (2009). Cancer in migrant and seasonal hired farm workers. *Journal of Agromedicine, 14*(2), 185–191.

Munoz-Laboy, M., Hirsch, J. S., & Quispe-Lazaro, A. (2009). Loneliness as a sexual risk factor for male Mexican migrant workers. *American Journal of Public Health, 99*(5), 802–809.

Nevarez-La Torre, A. (2012). Transiency in urban schools: Challenges and opportunities in educating ESLs with a migrant background. *Education & Urban Society, 44*(1), 3–34.

Onega, L. L., & Barbero, E. D. (2010). Using health education and group process in the community. In M. Stanhope & J. Lancaster (Eds.), *Foundations of nursing in the community: Community-oriented practice* (3rd ed., pp. 188–214). St. Louis, MO: Elsevier Mosby.

Pamies, R. J., & Nsiah-Kumi, P. A. (2009). Addressing health disparities in the 21st century. In S. Kosoko-Lasaki, C. T. Cook, & R. L. O'Brien (Eds.), *Cultural proficiency in addressing health disparities*. Boston, MA: Jones & Bartlett.

Persichino, J., & Ibarra, L. (2012). HIV and Latino migrant workers in the USA. *Ethnic & Racial Studies, 35*(1), 120–134.

Phelps, L. D., & Johnson, K. (2004). Developing local public health capacity in cultural competency: A case study with Haitians in a rural community. *Journal of Community Health Nursing, 21*(4), 203–215.

Purnell, L. (2008). The Purnell Model for Cultural Competence. In L. Purnell & B. Paulanka (Eds.), *Transcultural healthcare: A culturally competent approach* (3rd ed., pp. 19–55). Philadelphia, PA: F.A. Davis.

Purnell, L. D. (2013). The Purnell Model for Cultural Competence. In L. D. Purnell (Ed.), *Transcultural healthcare: A culturally competent approach* (4th ed., pp. 15–44). Philadelphia, PA: F.A. Davis.

Pysklywec, M., McLaughlin, J., Tew, M., & Haines, T. (2011). Doctors without borders: Meeting the health care needs of migrant farm workers in Canada. *Canadian Medical Association Journal, 183*(9), 1039–1042.

Rose, P. R. (2011). *Cultural competency for health administration and public health*. Boston, MA: Jones & Bartlett.

Sagar, P. L. (2012). *Transcultural nursing theory and models: Application in nursing education, practice, and administration*. New York, NY: Springer Publishing.

Schuessler, J. B., Wilder, B., & Byrd, L. W. (2012). Reflective journaling and development of cultural humility in students. *Nursing Education Perspectives, 33*(2), 96–99.

Sebastian, J. G. (2010). Vulnerability and vulnerable populations: An overview. In M. Stanhope & J. Lancaster (Eds.), *Foundations of nursing in the community: Community-oriented practice* (3rd ed., pp. 385–399). St. Louis, MO: Elsevier Mosby.

Shearer, R. G., & Davidhizar, R. (2003). Using role play to develop cultural competence. *Journal of Nursing Education, 42*(6), 273–276.

Stanhope, M., & Lancaster, J. (2010). *Foundations of nursing in the community: Community-oriented practice* (3rd ed.). St. Louis, MO: Elsevier Mosby.

The National Center for Learning Disabilities. (2013). *Is a 504 plan right for my child?* Retrieved September 15, 2013, from www.ncld.org/students-disabilities/iep-504-plan/is-504-plan-right-for-my-child

Young, L. E., & Paterson, B. L. (2007). *Teaching nursing: Developing a student-centered learning environment*. Philadelphia, PA: Lippincott Williams & Wilkins.

United States Department of Health and Human Services, Health Resources Services Administration. (2012). *About healthy people*. Retrieved February 13, 2014 from http://healthypeople.gov/2020/about/default.aspx

United States Department of Health and Human Services, Office of Minority Health. (2010). *National partnership for action to end health disparities*. Retrieved February 2, 2013, from www.healthypeople.gov/2020/about/DisparitiesAbout.aspx

Professional Nursing Transition Course

Priscilla Limbo Sagar

KEY TERMS

Andrews/Boyle Transcultural Nursing
  Assessment for Individuals and Families
Certification
Chagas disease
Coach
Critical care
Medical interpreter
Mentoring
Multistate regulation of nursing

NCLEX-RN®
Nursing licensure compact
Organizational competence
Portfolio
Reciprocity
Resume
Staff competence
Transition
Trypanosoma cruzi

LEARNING OBJECTIVES

At the completion of this chapter, the learner will be able to

1. Apply culturally and linguistically appropriate services (CLAS) standards in the care of clients with complex health problems.
2. Explore assessment tools to evaluate cultural competence of graduating baccalaureate students.
3. Analyze steps in assisting a graduating student in preparation for professional practice.
4. Develop strategies to enhance critical thinking and clinical judgment among graduating students.

OVERVIEW

Professional nursing transition courses in baccalaureate nursing programs are usually the last course prior to graduation. The term **transition** denotes going across, passing over, or passing through (Spross, 2005, p. 193). Senior students are very close to graduation, signaling the end of the quest for a baccalaureate degree. After graduation and licensure, the students become nurse colleagues, adding to the more than 3 million registered professional nurses currently in the United States. Though feeling the promise and exhilaration of a forthcoming professional career, the student is faced with many challenges throughout this transition. Those challenges may include, but are not limited to, pressures and anxiety about passing all courses and graduating on time, passing the National Council Licensing Examination—Registered Nurses (**NCLEX-RN®**), finding a job, and paying student loans. People become vulnerable during transitions (Meleis & Glickman, 2012); in the case of the graduating students, they will lose the familiar environment of being students and guided by faculty. Derived from the Latin *transitus*, this example of life is referred to as "dangerous opportunities" in Chinese culture (Spross, 2005).

As such, there is a huge challenge for faculty to include learning experiences that not only foster higher order critical thinking and clinical judgment but also prepare the student for professional practice. When caring for clients with complex health problems and preparing to transition to professional practice, students need faculty guidance to plan, develop, implement, and evaluate culturally and linguistically appropriate services (CLAS; U.S. Department of Health and Human Services [USDHHS], Office of Minority Health [OMH], 2013). It is essential for faculty and students to be familiar with the document of these enhanced standards as well as the Joint Commission (TJC; The Joint Commission, 2010a, 2010b) accreditation guidelines regarding communication and client and family-centered care. In addition, the student will not only be working with diverse clients, families, and significant others but also with diverse health care workers. Thus, it is vital that students are guided to reflect on their own journey to cultural competence (Hanson & Spross, 2005).

With the huge task of integrating learning from other nursing courses, the senior student needs assistance to plan for and transition to professional practice. Planning for taking the NCLEX-RN® is another important area of preparation. Some of the other vital areas in this planning include refining one's resume, practicing for interviews, preparing a portfolio, and making the most of clinical practice. Most schools offer assistance for preparation of resumes, interviews, portfolios, and image presentation as a professional individual through their career centers.

Integration of TCN Concepts

Schools using theory and models to guide their integration of diversity and cultural competence administer tools to measure the cultural competence of students, usually preprogram, at midpoint, and prior to graduation. Some researchers also suggest testing with a survey tool or tools a year after graduation. During the final semester prior to completion of the program, it is timely to administer the follow-up survey of cultural competence administered at baseline and midprogram. Likewise, a follow-up survey a year or so after graduation is also highly recommended.

Some tools widely used by nursing schools include the tools of Campinha-Bacote (2007) and Jeffreys (2010). Campinha-Bacote developed the *Inventory for Assessing the Process of Cultural Competence Among Healthcare Professionals-Revised* (*IAPCC-R*). The IAPCC-R is a 25-item tool for measuring the level of cultural competence among health care professionals. To assess the cultural competence of student nurses, Campinha-Bacote also created the 20-item *IAPCC-Student Version* (*IAPCC-SV*).

Jeffreys (2010) developed the Transcultural Self-Efficacy Tool (TSET) in 1994, an 83-item tool for measuring and evaluating confidence of students in "performing general transcultural nursing skills among diverse populations" (p. 92). From the TSET, Jeffreys (2010) developed two new tools: *Cultural Competence Clinical Evaluation Tool* (*CCCET*) and *Clinical Setting Assessment Tool-Diversity and Disparity* (*CSAT-DD*). The CCCET contains three subscales that measure dimensions of clinical cultural behavior, namely culturally specific care, cultural assessment, and culturally sensitive and professionally appropriate attitudes, values, or beliefs (Jeffreys, 2010, p. 93). Two of the three CCCET versions are the student version (SV) and teacher version. According to Jeffreys (2010), the CSAT-DD is an easy-to-use tool for data collection regarding the clinical agency, particularly on descriptions of diverse client populations.

Enhancing Critical Thinking and Clinical Judgment

Students in transition courses must have ample opportunities to use critical thinking in class, clinical, or simulation experiences. Course assignments such as reflective journals and unfolding case scenarios can contribute to enhancing critical thinking and clinical judgment. Box 18.1 presents an unfolding case scenario of a migrant worker with **Chagas disease**. This scenario can be used as an assignment for class discussion, clinical conference, or as a makeup assignment for class or clinical absence.

BOX 18.1 A MEXICAN MIGRANT WORKER WITH CHAGAS DISEASE: AN UNFOLDING CASE SCENARIO

Elizabeth Simon, PhD, RN, ANP-BC
Director and Professor, School of Nursing,
Nyack College, Nyack, NY

Goal of Case Scenario

To provide an opportunity for nursing students to develop cultural competence when caring for a migrant worker in critical care by utilizing the Andrews/Boyle Transcultural Nursing Assessment Guide for Individual and Families (*TNAGIF*).

Learning Objectives

At the conclusion of this case study, learners will be able to:

Apply all or components of the Andrews/Boyle TNAGIF to provide care to an individual in a critical care setting.
Explore the concepts of disadvantaged status, ethnocentrism, discrimination, and acculturation.
Develop a culturally and linguistically appropriate plan of care for this client.
Discuss the nursing care of a client with Chagas disease.

Overview of Chagas Disease

Access to health care is a problem for some populations. In migrant populations, health care professionals may deal with common health issues such as occupational hazards related to farm products and pesticides, musculoskeletal injuries, problems of group living, elevated risks for different cancers, and parasite infestations (Mills, Dodge, & Yang, 2009).

One of the common parasitic infestations is Chagas disease. Each year, over 8 million people in America contract the disease. It is caused by the parasite *Trypanosoma cruzi*, transmitted primarily by insects known as "kissing bugs."

Chagas disease represents a serious problem to public health. It affects large rural areas in Latin America and is associated with a high rate of mortality. Individuals are usually affected at the peak of their productive lives (Coura, 2007; Center for Disease Control [CDC], 2013; World Health Organization [WHO], 2013).

(continued)

The acute phase of Chagas disease lasts for 1 to 3 months following an incubation period of 1 to 3 weeks. The clinical manifestations include signs of local invasion by the parasite including the ophthalmoganglionic complex (Romana sign) and inoculation chagoma and general symptoms related to systemic invasion by the parasite, such as fever, hepatosplenomegaly, lymphadenopathy, edema, and signs and symptoms of acute Chagas cardiomyopathy (Hemmige, Tanowitz, & Sethi, 2012).

In the heart, the myocardial fibers are site of parasite reproduction. The severity of myocardial involvement varies widely and it may even be clinically silent. However, it may be so severe as to lead to the patient's death. The cardiovascular signs consist of tachycardia—which is usually greater than can be accounted for by the level of fever—arterial hypotension, and low pulse pressure. Alteration of the heart sounds is encountered, particularly a soft first sound, or equal intensity of sounds, gallop rhythm, and varying degrees of cardiomegaly. Evidence of congestive heart failure may be found if the cardiac involvement has been severe (Bocchi, 2013; Haberland, Munoz Saravia, Wallukat, Ziebig, & Schimke, 2013).

Electrocardiographic disturbances include prolongation of the PR and QT intervals and nonspecific alterations of the T wave and the ST segment. Low-voltage QRS complexes are occasionally encountered. Laboratory findings show leukocytosis, lymphocytosis, and presence of the parasite in the blood. The complement fixation test becomes positive from 15 to 30 days after the onset of infection. The latent phase is the period which follows the cessation of the acute phase and lasts to the beginning of the chronic phase. The complement fixation tests remain positive.

The chronic phase consists of Chagasic cardiomyopathy. This is the most important phase and constitutes the most serious problem, both medically and socially. Clinically, marked cardiomegaly and congestive cardiac failure with mitral and/or tricuspid insufficiency, thromboembolic phenomena, and complex and severe arrhythmias are characteristics of this stage. Patients may develop a stroke or thromboembolism and sudden death. Pacemaker insertion, conservative management, and cardiac transplantation are the current therapies.

The Client

Forty-year-old Romano Rodriguez approached the mobile clinic conducted by Goodwill School of Nursing Community Health and Transcultural Nursing Department in New York. Mr. Rodriguez admitted to only speak "broken English." The nurse practitioner conducted the interview and assessment with the help of a trained **medical interpreter**. The client complains of frequent palpitations and dizzy spells. He passed out once while walking a horse and sustained minor injuries. He recovered from the incident and believed he had pneumonia or a chest cold and would be alright.

(continued)

Following the incident, he was increasingly short of breath during strenuous activities. He was very careful to not fall when he got dizzy. He was worried about his immediate family—his 35-year-old wife and two children aged 8 and 10 years living with him in the "back stretch"—and his extended family in Mexico, who also depended on his income. He had no insurance; according to the client, the children got their "shots" from the department of health.

Upon examination, Mr. Rodriguez appeared as an average built anxious man who was able to communicate using an interpreter. Physical assessment showed BP 100/60; pulse, 62, irregular, weak, and thready; extremities were pale, and cold with poor capillary refill. Apical pulse was displaced to 5th intercostal space (ICS) and anterior axillary line. He had vesicular breathing with bibasilar crackles. Mr. Rodriguez was placed a in mobile clinic stretcher for further focused evaluation. Cardiac examination showed raised jugular vein distention (JVD), S1 softer than S2, with slight hepatosplenomegaly, cardiomegaly, and peripheral edema ++. Upon further review, Mr. Rodriguez admitted to occasionally getting up at night to cough and void. A mobile electrocardiogram (EKG) reading showed low voltage, indicating bradycardia with second degree type 2 block.

Focused history revealed his life in rural Mexico as a farm worker until 2 years ago when he came and started work as a migrant worker in New York. He remembered only one episode of illness 15 years before. At that time, he had fever, swelling, dizzy spells, and a racing heart; he went to a "curandera" and felt better after a week. To stay well, he usually drank chamomile tea and saw the curandera when feeling ill. He admitted to taking over-the-counter antibiotic' in Mexico "when he felt sick." He also added that his family could send him more antibiotics in the mail if that was needed.

Evaluate the utility of the TNAGIF in caring for a client in critical care. What components of the TNAGIF did you use? Why?
What is the disease process that you suspect based on the history and assessment?
How do you establish a connection between a farm worker's occupation and his cardiac symptoms?
What are the possible tests to prove the underlying disease process?
What other therapeutic modalities do you anticipate?
What areas of patient education would you include?
What are socioeconomic and ethical issues surrounding further care? What referrals would you make? Discuss.
Explore other issues surrounding the care of this client.

References for Case Scenario

Bahia, M. T., Andrade, I. M., Martins, T. A. F., Nascimento, Á. F., Diniz, L. F., Caldas, I. S.,...Ribeiro, I. (2012). Fexinidazole: A potential new drug candidate for Chagas disease. *Neglected Tropical Diseases, 6*(11), 1–9.

(continued)

BOX 18.1 A MEXICAN MIGRANT WORKER WITH CHAGAS DISEASE: AN UNFOLDING CASE SCENARIO (continued)

Bocchi, E. A. (2013). Heart failure in South America. Current Cardiology Review, 9(2),147–156.

Center for Disease Control. (2013). *Chagas disease.* Retrieved August 5, 2013 from www.cdc.gov/parasites/chagas/health_professionals/index.html

Coura, J. R. (2007). Chagas disease: What is known and what is needed—A background article (Abstract). Laboratório de Doenças Parasitárias, Instituto Oswaldo Cruz, Fiocruz, Rio de Janeiro, 21045–900, Brasil.

Haberland, A., Munoz Saravia, S. G., Wallukat, G., Ziebig, R., & Schimke, I. (2013). Chronic Chagas disease: From basics to laboratory medicine. *Clinical Chemistry & Laboratory Medicine, 51*(2), 271–294.

Hemmige, V., Tanowitz, H., & Sethi, A. (2012). *Trypanosoma cruzi* infection: A review with emphasis on cutaneous manifestations (Section of Infectious Diseases and Global Health, University of Chicago Medical Center, Chicago). *The International Journal of Dermatology, 51*(5), 501–508.

Mills, P. K., Dodge, J., & Yang, R. (2009). Cancer in migrant and seasonal hired farm workers. *Journal of Agromedicine, 14*(2), 185–191.

Pinto, A. Y., Valente, V. C., Coura, J. R., Valente, S. A., Junqueira, A. C., Santos, L. C.,…& de Macedo, R. C. (2013). Clinical follow-up of responses to treatment with benznidazole in Amazon: A cohort study of acute Chagas disease. *PLoS ONE, 8*(5), 1–9.

World Health Organization. (2013). *Fact sheet: Chagas disease (American trypanosomiasis).* Retrieved August 5, 2013, from www.who.int/mediacentre/factsheets/fs340/en

The Andrews/Boyle Transcultural Nursing Assessment Guide for Individual and Families (Boyle & Andrews, 2012) will be easy to apply when performing assessments of clients with complex health problems. The TNAGIF's 12 areas—*biocultural variations, communication, cultural affiliations, cultural sanctions and restrictions, developmental considerations, economics, educational background, health related beliefs and practices, kinship and social networks, nutrition, religion and spirituality, and values orientation* (Boyle & Andrews, 2012)—may all be used, or may be used selectively to assess, plan, implement, and evaluate culturally congruent client care. Chapter 8 provides detailed strategies for culturally and linguistically appropriate health history and physical assessment.

Assessing Individual Staff and Organizational Competence

Staff at all levels of the organization need to be culturally competent (Ludwig-Beymer, 2012; Marrone, 2013). "Organizational competence" refers to an organization that provides services that are culturally and linguistically responsive to client needs (Ludwig-Beymer, 2012). Organizational competence is essential in reducing racial and ethnic disparities, improving client outcomes and quality of care, and lowering health care costs. A suggested project in this area is the development of a short checklist to assess individual and organizational CLAS compliance using some or all of the 12 domains of Purnell's (2013) Model for Cultural Competence (MCC) or the seven factors from Leininger's Cultural

Care Theory (CCT). It will be interesting to see how an organization fares from the point of view of a graduating student. The student can also be assigned to review application of the MCC (Marrone, 2013) or CCT (Ludwig-Beymer, 2012) as organizing frameworks for organizational cultural competence.

Information regarding basic **certification** in TCN (CTN-A) must be provided for the senior student. To meet the needs of the increasingly diverse population for culturally and linguistically congruent care, certification in TCN will be more in demand in the future (Sagar, in press). In the process of socialization to professional practice, the student must be encouraged to critically appraise available incentives for nurses with specialty certification.

Preparing for the National Council Licensing Examination–Registered Nurses

Students usually have been familiar with NCLEX-type questions since their beginning nursing courses and build more skills, confidence, and success with this type of examination as they get closer to graduation. The student needs to be familiar with the test blueprint and the application process (National Council of State Boards of Nursing [NCSBN], 2013a).

It is helpful for senior students to know that they will need to apply for licensure and registration at the state NCSBN and to schedule to take the NCLEX at the closest Pearson VUE (2013), a large testing company and part of Pearson Publishing. It is essential to become familiar with the licensure guidelines and laws in states where graduates plan to take the NCLEX and practice; these are vital content in this transition course. In addition, **reciprocity** and **multistate regulation of nursing** (MSR) or **nurse licensure compact** (NLC) information needs to be reviewed. To expedite interstate practice and regulation, the NCSBN (2013b, 2013c) created the MSR model in 2000. The NLC is a reciprocal recognition and contract between states to recognize each other's licensees; currently, there are 24 states with NLC (NCSBN, 2013b, 2013c).

Face-to-face or online review for the NCLEX may be a component of Assessment Technologies, Inc. (ATI, 2013) or Health Education Services, Inc. (Elsevier HESI, 2013) programs already being used by the school of nursing (SON). In the event that the SON does not use any of these support programs, the decision to attend a formal review course rests with the senior student.

Transitioning to Professional Practice and Developing Leadership

As the senior students grow in honing their clinical skills, it is important to look ahead at professional practice as registered nurses (RNs). Preceptorship and mentoring are discussed in Chapters 2 and 22. The focus around this time is increasing independence in clinical yet seeking faculty guidance as necessary. The schedule for preceptorship could vary from student to student, depending on each one's areas of interest for future specialization.

Preceptorship. A precepted experience during the last semester in nursing school is beneficial in the transition process from student to professional nurse. In many schools, leadership training is part of the course. In this experience, the student may choose an area in **critical care** or a few areas for the clinical rotation. In addition to enhancing skills in critically ill clients, such a clinical rotation can focus on culturally and linguistically appropriate care.

Preceptorship with the staff development educator is also of great benefit. Table 18.1 shows a planned 8-week leadership rotation practicum within a 6-credit professional nursing transition course; scheduled rotation is necessary to accommodate the large number of students in the graduating class. Some students will start with clinical; others are assigned in the leadership practice. All rotations integrate CLAS standards and institutional

TABLE 18.1   Sample Leadership Rotation Practicum for One Student in a 6-Credit Professional Nursing Transition Course

Weekly Schedule	Area and Preceptor	Practicum Focus
Weeks 1–2	David King, MS, RN Emergency Department Clinical Manager	Managing care in the ED, triage, observation of nonemergency diagnosis seeking ED care
Week 3–4	Cardiothoracic Unit Sally See, MS, CCRN, ANP-C Clinical Manager	Managing care of clients with cardiothoracic problems; Nursing care in compliance with culturally and linguistically appropriate services (CLAS) standards
Weeks 5–6	Telemetry John Kim, MS, ANP-C, CTN-A Clinical Manager	Managing care of clients on telemetry; nursing care in compliance with CLAS standards
Weeks 7–8	Staff Development Victoria Mendoza, EdD, CTN-A Educator	Programs in continuing **staff competence**; organizational CLAS compliance
Weeks 9–15	Preceptorship with staff nurses in the intensive care and coronary care units	Culturally and linguistically appropriate care of a group of patients

compliance (USDHHS, OMH, 2013) and accreditation standards for client-and-family centered communication and linguistic care (TJC, 2010a, 2010b). The leadership practicum is in addition to the regular clinical rotation in the intensive and coronary care units.

Mentoring. An introduction to the vital concept of mentoring may be included in this course. Mentoring is a one-to-one, voluntary relationship; usually between a senior and a junior nurse. The two individuals enter into an agreement where the senior coaches and guides the junior's career choices over a sustained period of time, oftentimes all through a career (Vance 2002, 2011; Vance & Olson, 1998). Chapters 22 and 27 have more discussion on mentoring.

Coaching. The term **coach** is from the word *coche*, a wagon or carriage used as a means of transportation from one place to another (Spross, 2005). Many people are more familiar with coaching in terms of sports. Used in interprofessional education, coaching is aimed at helping people "in transitions or journeys" (Spross, 2005, p. 190).

During the clinical rotation, student nurses are paired with preceptors who are master's prepared. Students observe being coached by preceptors and also observe the preceptor coach patients; Spross (2005) called this "double exposure." Chapter 22 has more discussion on coaching. The preceptor and the faculty need to encourage students and give them opportunities for both reflection-in-action and reflection-on-action (Schon, 1983, 1987).

Getting Ready to Find That First Job

Completing a resume. Although the student may have started a **resume** as a sophomore or a junior, refining that resume at this stage is crucial. The market for RNs has become very competitive—even with the persistent nursing shortage—and the resume may be the first set of information regarding the applicant. An accurate, complete, comprehensive, and well-written resume may be the key to getting selected for a few spots for the interview.

Finding a few solid references from faculty and preceptors is vital at this point. Letters of reference can be compiled in portable document files (PDF), hard copies, or an electronic reference service. When requesting letters of reference, adding the student's potential for graduate school—in addition to classroom, clinical, and ability to work with clients and families—is suggested. The graduate nurse may be starting a master's program sooner than later; seeking letters for references solely for graduate school may be more time consuming.

When listing contact information, an electronic mail (e-mail) address is an important component in addition to the telephone number. Many colleges and universities allow graduates to continue using their student e-mail address. In addition, with the abundance of free e-mail accounts, it is not a problem to get a personal e-mail address. However, addresses that begin with largeassets@...or brownbeauty@...do not sound professional and have no place in a professional resume.

Preparation of a portfolio. A portfolio—the compilation of an individual's professional education, experience, expertise, and accomplishments—can be prepared in the form of a binder holding the documents, stored in a jump drive or cassette disc, or using an electronic portfolio (e-folio) online format. Whether online, electronic, or hard copy, the portfolio must be professional, simple, complete, and attractive. The portfolio should contain samples of the graduating student's project, resume, continuing education (CE) credit certificates, awards, student copy of transcripts, letters of reference, and other proofs of professional accomplishments. Next to the resume, the portfolio may be another key to an invitation for interview.

Proofs of membership and attendance at professional conferences are important to include in the resume and portfolio. For culturally and linguistically congruent programs, the student may be introduced to a local Transcultural Nursing Society (TCNS) chapter or at its annual international conference.

Attending preparation workshops. Colleges and universities have career centers that offer workshops centering on transition to professional practice and for graduate school. These workshops may include topics about dressing for success, mock interviews, and preparation of resumes, among others. While pressed for time due to examinations, presentations, papers, and other course requirements, it is of utmost importance to actively participate in these workshops. The time investment is well worth the effort—considering that these workshops can be instrumental in landing that first job!

Exploring career fairs. Career fairs are usually held at colleges and universities or at central locations from the SON. Attending these fairs and implementing strategies learned about presenting oneself, interviewing, portfolio preparation, and inquiring about available graduate nurse (GN) positions are part of professional growth. It is recommended that the student find out as much about GN positions such as residency or other programs for the nurse while waiting to take the NCLEX. Bridge and residency programs have shown effectiveness in the retention of new nurses.

EBP 18.1

Kardong-Edgren et al. (2010) conducted a descriptive study of 515 senior baccalaureate nursing students enrolled in six geographically dispersed undergraduate baccalaureate nursing programs in the United States. Each program utilized a different curricular and instructional design approach related to teaching cultural competence. These approaches ranged from required cultural coursework inside and outside of the nursing curriculum, integration of cultural concepts across the curriculum, focus

(continued)

EBP 18.1 *(continued)*

on cultural concepts at designated points in the curriculum, clinical experiences with a cultural focus, and cultural immersion experiences out of country.

Each program incorporated selected concepts from Campinha-Bacote's (2003, as cited by Kardong et al.) *Process of Cultural Competence Model*, ranging from an emphasis on two to four of the five constructs of the model, namely: *cultural awareness, cultural knowledge, cultural encounter, cultural skill*, and *cultural desire* (p. 281).

The students completed Campinha-Bacote's *Inventory for Assessing the Process of Cultural Competence Among Healthcare Professionals-R (IAPCC-R)*, which is a 25-item tool used to measure the five constructs of the *Process of Cultural Competence Model*. Along with the IAPCC-R, students also completed a demographic information form inclusive of questions regarding foreign travel, experiences living abroad, past degrees, and course assignments in anthropology as factors that might affect the findings of the study.

Findings indicated that the students from all six programs scored in the culturally aware range, suggesting that no one curricular approach is more effective than another in attaining cultural competence. Moreover, the score differences for each pair of nursing programs was not sufficient to conclude that any one nursing program's score on the IAPCC-R was better than the scores of each of the other nursing programs.

Although not statistically significant, it was noted that one program' which had the oldest students in the sample, 83% of whom had prior degrees utilizing the integrated Culture Care Theory as a framework, received better scores on the IAPCC-R than students in other programs. This potential effect of age and life experience versus prior education on the score was noted in view of the fact that the program with the youngest students in the sample had the lowest scores. Furthermore, it was also observed that this same program had several faculty with certification in transcultural nursing teaching the undergraduate program; this could have been another factor impacting the difference.

In order to validate curricular approaches, Kardong-Edgreen et al. (2010) suggest continued evaluation and critique of this area; measuring cultural awareness instead of competency among graduating students; and cultural validation from vignettes written by representatives from the underserved populations. The researchers also suggest the use of other tools that do not entail self-report by participants.

Applications to Practice

■ Investigate your nursing program's curricular approaches and cultural evaluation tools. If you do not use any of these, which tool are you planning to use? Why?

■ Critically examine your program outcomes related to realistic expectations of student achievement in the area of cultural competence. Do you have cultural awareness rather than cultural competence as a program outcome for graduating nursing students in a baccalaureate program? Explain.

■ If you were to replicate this study, how would you conduct it? What would you change in terms of conceptual framework, sampling, and analysis of findings?

Source: Kardong-Edgreen, Cason, Walsh Brennan, Reifsneider, Hummel, Mancini, & Griffin (2010).

CRITICAL THINKING EXERCISES 18.1

Undergraduate Student

1. You are almost ready to graduate. Do you feel prepared to care for culturally diverse clients when you graduate?
2. Do you think there is enough content of cultural diversity and promotion of cultural competence integrated in your professional nursing transition class (theory) and in clinical?
3. Would you be in favor of including a 3-credit TCN course in your current curriculum? If yes, which course would you be in favor of deleting from your BS in Nursing curriculum? Why?

Faculty in Academia

1. How many credits is your professional nursing transition course for the BS in Nursing program at your school? How many credits are allotted to theory portion? How many credits are for clinical?
2. From student evaluations, are the current practicum hours enough for them to transition to professional practice?
3. Do you have a mentoring program at your SON? Describe.
4. If you were to revise your curriculum, would you make any change in this course? Discuss.

Staff Development Educator

1. Do you require completion of continuing education in cultural diversity and promotion of cultural competence among your critical care nursing staff?
2. When you update your policy and procedure manual, do you include culturally congruent care in each procedure?
3. Do you regularly update your collection of resources on cultural diversity and promotion of cultural competence at your facility? Discuss.
4. Do you have institutional subscription for journals on diversity and cultural competence? How do you give incentives for nurses to read research articles from these journals?

SUMMARY

The senior student in the last semester of graduation is at a crossroad: reluctant to leave the cocoon as a student nurse yet looking ahead at professional nursing practice with anticipation and dread. This chapter discusses important concepts in a professional nursing transition course, usually the last course for a graduating baccalaureate student. As such, this future practitioner needs leadership and management skills, a practicum usually conducted in a critical care setting, and staff development to not only hone and sharpen clinical skills but also to prepare for professional practice. Specifically, the student needs to continue to prepare for taking the NCLEX examination and to embrace resources in preparation for professional practice as an RN.

REFERENCES

Assessment Technologies Incorporated. (2013). *About ATI nursing education.* Retrieved August 22, 2013, from https://www.atitesting.com/About.aspx

Bahia, M. T., Andrade, I. M., Martins, T. A. F., Nascimento, Á. F., Diniz, L. F., Caldas, I. S.,...& Ribeiro, I. (2012). Fexinidazole: A potential new drug candidate for Chagas disease. *Neglected Tropical Diseases, 6*(11), 1–9.

Bocchi, E. A. (2013). Heart failure in South America. *Current Cardiology Review, 9*(2),147–156.

Boyle, J. S., & Andrews, M. M. (2012). Andrews/Boyle transcultural nursing assessment guide for individuals and families. In M. M. Andrews & J. S. Boyle (Eds.), *Transcultural concepts in nursing care* (6th ed., pp. 451–458). Philadelphia, PA: Wolters Kluwer/Lippincott Williams & Wilkins.

Campinha-Bacote, J. (2007). *The process of cultural competence in the delivery of healthcare services: The journey continues.* Cincinnati, OH: Transcultural C.A.R.E. Resources.

Center for Disease Control. (2013). *Chagas disease.* Retrieved August 5, 2013, from www.cdc.gov/parasites/chagas/health_professionals/index.html

Coura, J. R. (2007). Chagas disease: What is known and what is needed—A background article (Abstract; Laboratório de Doenças Parasitárias, Instituto Oswaldo Cruz, Fiocruz, Rio de Janeiro, 21045–900, Brasil). *Memorias do Instituto Oswaldo Cruz, 102*(Suppl 1), 113–122.

Elsevier HESI. (2013). *Elsevier HESI assessment.* Retrieved August 22, 2013, from https://hesifaculty-access.elsevier.com/index.aspx

Haberland, A., Munoz Saravia, S. G., Wallukat, G., Ziebig, R., & Schimke, I. (2013). Chronic Chagas disease: From basics to laboratory medicine. *Clinical Chemistry & Laboratory Medicine, 51*(2), 271–294.

Hanson, C. M., & Spross, J. A. (2005). Clinical and professional leadership. In A. B. Hamric, J. Spross, & C. M. Hanson (Eds.), *Advanced practice nursing: An integrative approach* (pp. 301–339). St. Louis, MO: Elsevier Saunders.

Hemmige, V., Tanowitz, H., & Sethi, A. (2012). *Trypanosoma cruzi* infection: A review with emphasis on cutaneous manifestations (Section of Infectious Diseases and Global Health, University of Chicago Medical Center, Chicago). *The International Journal of Dermatology, 51*(5), 501–508.

Jeffreys, M. R. (2010). Transcultural self-efficacy tool, cultural competence clinical evaluation tool, and clinical setting assessment tool-diversity and disparity. In M. R. Jeffreys (Ed.), *Teaching cultural competence in nursing and health care* (2nd ed., pp. 63–93). New York, NY: Springer Publishing.

Kardong-Edgreen, S., Cason, C. L., Walsh Brennan, A. M., Reifsneider, E., Hummel, F., Mancini, M., & Griffin, C. (2010). Cultural competency of graduating BSN students. *Nursing Education Perspectives, 31*(5), 278–285.

Leininger, M. M. (2006). culture care diversity and universality and evolution of the ethnonursing method. In M. Leininger & M. McFarland (Eds.), *Culture care diversity and universality: A worldwide nursing theory* (pp. 1–41). Sudbury, MA: Jones & Bartlett.

Ludwig-Beymer, P. (2012). Creating culturally competent organizations. In M. M. Andrews & J. S. Boyle (Eds.), *Transcultural concepts in nursing care* (6th ed., pp. 211–242). Philadelphia, PA: Wolters Kluwer/Lippincott Williams & Wilkins.

Marrone, S. R. (2013). Organizational cultural competence. In L. D. Purnell (Ed.), *Transcultural health care: A culturally competent approach* (4th ed., pp. 60–73). Philadelphia, PA: F.A. Davis.

Meleis, A. I., & Glickman, C. G. (2012). Empowering expatriate nurses: Challenges and opportunities—A commentary. *Nursing Outlook, 60,* S24–S26.

Mills, P., Dodge, J., & Yang, R. (2009). Cancer in migrant and seasonal hired farm workers. *Journal of Agromedicine, 14*(2), 185–191.

National Council of State Board of Nursing. (2013a). 2013 NCLEX-RN® detailed test plan candidate version. Retrieved April 5, 2013, from https://www.ncsbn.org/2013_NCLEX_RN_Detailed_Test_Plan_Candidate.pdf

National Council of State Board of Nursing. (2013b). *Nurse licensure compact: The nurse licensure compact (NLC) enables multistate licensure for nurses.* Retrieved August 13, 2013, from https://www.ncsbn.org/nlc.htm

National Council of State Board of Nursing. (2013c). *Five reasons to endorse the nurse licensure compact (NLC).* Retrieved August 13, 2013, from https://www.ncsbn.org/Reasons_to_endorse_the_NLC_(2).pdf

Pearson VUE. (2013). *The NCLEX examination.* Retrieved August 13, 2013, from www.pearsonvue.com/nclex

Pinto, A. Y., Valente, V. C., Coura, J. R., Valente, S. A., Junqueira, A. C., Santos, L. C.,...& de Macedo, R. C. (2013). Clinical follow-up of responses to treatment with benznidazole in Amazon: A cohort study of acute Chagas disease. *PLoS ONE, 8*(5), 1–9.

Purnell, L. D. (2013). The Purnell model for cultural competence. In L. D. Purnell (Ed.), *Transcultural health care: A culturally competent approach* (4th ed., pp. 15–44). Philadelphia, PA: F.A. Davis.

Sagar, P. L. (in press). Transcultural nursing certification: Its role in nursing education, practice, administration, and research. In M. M. McFarland & H. Wehbe-Alamah (Eds.), *Culture care diversity and universality: A worldwide theory of nursing* (3rd ed.). Burlington, MA: Jones & Bartlett.

Schon, D. A. (1983). *The reflective practitioner*. New York, NY: Basic Books.

Schon, D. A. (1987). *Educating the reflective practitioner*. San Francisco, CA: Jossey Bass.

Spross, J. A. (2005). Expert coaching and guidance. In A. B. Hamric, J. A. Spross, & C. M. Hanson (Eds.), *Advanced practice nursing: An integrative approach* (pp. 187–223). St. Louis, MO: Elsevier Saunders.

The Joint Commission. (2010a). *Advancing effective communication, cultural competence, and patient- and family-centered care: A roadmap for hospitals*. Oakbrook Terrace, IL: Author.

United States Department of Health and Human Services, Office of Minority Health. (2013). *Enhanced national CLAS standards*. Retrieved August 16, 2013, from https://www.thinkculturalhealth. hhs.gov/Content/clas.asp

Vance, C. (2002). Leader as mentor. *Nursing Leadership Forum, 7*(2), 83–90.

Vance, C. (2011). *Fast facts for career success in nursing: Making the most of mentoring in a nutshell*. New York, NY: Springer Publishing.

Vance, C., & Olson, R. K. (1998). *The mentor connection in nursing*. New York, NY: Springer Publishing.

World Health Organization. (2013). *Fact sheet: Chagas disease (American trypanosomiasis)*. Retrieved August 5, 2013, from www.who.int/mediacentre/factsheets/fs340/en

TCN Concepts in Simulation

Priscilla Limbo Sagar

KEY TERMS

Cues
Debriefing
Fidelity
Frozen or immediate feedback
Reflection
Reflection-in-action

Reflection-on-action
Roles
Scenario
Simulation
Template
Unfolding simulations

LEARNING OBJECTIVES

At the completion of this chapter, the learner will be able to

1. Analyze his or her own self-efficacy in a specific skill after simulation experience, feedback, and debriefing.
2. Compare and contrast knowledge and skills acquisition between clinical and simulated learning experiences.
3. Analyze the role of reflection in simulation learning.
4. Differentiate between reflection-on-action and reflection-in-action.
5. Explain the use of debriefing in simulation learning.

OVERVIEW

Simulation is an event that is created to reproduce some or almost all of the essential components of a clinical situation to facilitate understanding of the situation and the provide ability to manage it should the situation occur in the client care setting (Morgan, 1995). Realism to an actual setting is the goal of any simulation; this realism classifies it as partial or total immersion (Widemark, 2011). Historically, the use of simulation with a 6-foot wooden figure of an enemy was used for military training in the Roman Empire (Decker, Gore, & Feken, 2011).

The prototype of the high-fidelity (HF) mannequins used in nursing was Mrs. Chase, an adult-sized mannequin used for demonstration of foundation nursing skills at the Hartford Hospital Training School for Nurses (Decker et al., 2011). Resusci Annie, for mouth-to-mouth resuscitation, was introduced in the early 1960s by a plastic toy manufacturer called Laerdal (Cooper & Taqueti, 2004). The rest is history, as the medical simulation industry flourished beyond expectations.

The HF simulation mannequin industry has evolved into a lucrative multibillion dollar industry, estimated by the PR Newswire (2013)—a global provider of news and communications solutions—to be worth 1.9 billion dollars by 2017. The PR Newswire credits advancements in technology for this massive market growth. The increased purchasing power of academic institutions is driving the growth of this market; this increased power results from the (1) expanding focus on training health care professionals, (2) mounting emphasis on client safety, (3) escalating cost of health care, and (4) increasing funding availability. Academics, hospitals, and the military are major users of HF mannequin/patient simulators; academia accounts for the largest market share in 2012 (PR Newswire). The main market for medical simulation products and services is North America, followed by Europe.

Simulation education has gained momentum in academia in the last few decades due to decreasing clinical sites (Caputi, 2011) and access to clients (Jeffries et al., 2011). The American Association of Colleges of Nursing ([AACN], 2008a) emphasizes its support of the complementary nature of clinical and simulation learning as essential to the preparation of a professional nurse. AACN added that simulation experiences give students opportunities for a valuable, safe environment of learning, as well as application of both cognitive and psychomotor skills. Integration of diversity and cultural competence is imperative in academic simulation.

The National League for Nursing (NLN) has been a proponent of simulations in nursing education. With support from Laerdal Medical, NLN (2013) operates the *Simulation Resources Innovation Resource Center (SIRC)*. The SIRC is an electronic learning (e-learning) site where nurse educators not only can learn about development and integration of simulation into their curriculum but also participate in dialogue with experts and peers (NLN, 2013). SIRC offers courses with continuing education credits (CEs) and moderates forums on diverse simulation topics such as faculty and staff training, development of simulation, research, equipment problems, interprofessional education, and enhancing fidelity (NLN, 2013, para 3).

ELEMENTS OF SIMULATION LEARNING

There are six components to a simulation experience: scenario, template, fidelity, roles, cues, and debriefing (Decker et al., 2011). The **scenario** is a case study that portrays "a real life patient care situation" (Decker et al., 2011, p. 285). In the example below, Jose Perez goes to the TB clinic for his checkup.

The **template** is a tool to help faculty plan, develop, and implement a simulation, including the learning objectives as well as the cognitive and psychomotor abilities to successfully complete the simulation (Decker et al., 2011). Other components of the template are:

- "Resources and equipment...to maximize the fidelity;
- Recommended mannequin responses to actions;
- Cues to assist the learner;
- Questions to be proposed during the scenario; and
- Guidelines for feedback" (Decker et al., 2011, p. 280).

Fidelity is the extent that a simulation portrays reality, including use of medical equipment, type of mannequin, and complexity of the simulation (Decker et al., 2011). Tarnow and Butcher (2005) are also strong proponents for a lifelike laboratory experience; they argued that the more lifelike the LRC, the better it is to portray the behaviors anticipated in a nurse–client interaction. The AACN (2008) highlighted the role of reality-based simulation in enhancing student confidence in communication, performance skills, and role development; for example, in Simulation 19.1, in the case of administration of protein derivative (PPD) on a client's arm. Adding these steps lends the portrayal more realism: encircling the bleb with an erasable pen, applying a band-aid, and explaining that the client needs to stay for 30 minutes in the clinic for assessment of untoward effects.

Cues include "assessment data, diagnostics or hints provided to direct or redirect the simulation" (Decker et al., 2011, p. 281). These may be employed as a reminder to participants in the action to be pursued.

The characters assumed by participants in a simulation are called **roles**, which can be passive (such as a participant) or active (such as the roles of a nurse, physician, or other members of the health team). Participants may give cues to guide other members of the simulation (Decker et al., 2011).

Debriefing. Debriefing is the planned, facilitated session whereby participants examine their actions, address emotional reactions to the simulation, and receive constructive feedback (Decker et al., 2011). The aim of the feedback session is to guide the student to consistently engage in reflection, the ability to explore approaches to resolving issues at hand. There are many definitions of **reflection**; one that describes the concept of reflection succinctly is by Dewey (1933) as cited by Cohen (2005): the "active, persistent, and careful consideration of any belief or supposed form of knowledge in the light of the grounds that support it…" (p. 316). Shellenbarger, Palmer, Labant, and Kuzneski (2005) warned that if faculty were to efficiently integrate reflection in education, the faculty themselves must regularly engage in reflection. In so doing, faculty may not only better understand student perspectives and reflective activities but may achieve their own personal growth in the process (Shellenbarger et al., 2005).

Schon (1987) exhorted the type of education that prepares professionals to manage the constantly changing problems of real world practice. Schon (1987) used the example of "ivory tower" where rigor and theory reside; theories sometimes do not solve the actual problems in the "lowly swamp" of practice. Schon argued that continual problem solving prepares a student for effective practice. To prepare reflective practitioners, Schon (1983, 1987) illustrated the utilization of two types of reflective thinking: reflection-in-action and reflection-on-action.

Reflection-in-action, reflection while in the middle of an action, whereby the individual engages in critical thinking, asks the meaning of the action, gathers information about how the intervention is making a difference, and appraises the client's response (Tarnow & Butcher, 2005). For example, a nurse performing a lung sound assessment notices adventitious sounds in a patient with congestive heart failure, recalls a similar incident as a nursing student when she observed a client so quickly go into fluid overload, promptly obtains an order for intravenous (IV) diuretic, and closely assesses the client thereafter.

Reflection-on-action occurs after the incident, giving the individual time to look back on the experience, examine the comprehension of the experience, and analyze what else can be used to approach such an experience (Schon, 1983, 1987; Tarnow & Butcher, 2005). For example, a nurse used the language access services (LAS) and asked for a Pakistani interpreter for a client from Pakistan who was of Punjabi descent. After the incident, the interpreter commented that, in the future, due to dialects and regional differences, the client might have benefited more from an interpreter who spoke Punjabi rather than an Urdu interpreter like him. This nurse in forthcoming situations will be more discerning of this aspect of culturally and linguistically appropriate care.

The faculty needs to review the objectives of the experience and provide ground rules for the simulation; this faculty should initiate the debriefing. If appropriate feedback is not given, the learner could have a distorted perception of the experience and may repeat mistakes and fixations (Decker et al., 2011). Feedback can be given during or at the end of a simulation session. **Frozen** or **immediate feedback** is given at the bedside "to emphasize a teaching point, defuse a deteriorating situation, or limit potential embarrassment" (Decker et al., 2011, p. 289).

Integration of TCN Concepts

Nurse educators are entrusted to prepare practitioners so they are ready to care for the increasingly diverse U.S. population. The more realistic the simulation, the more learning is expected to occur (AACN, 2008; Tarnow & Butcher, 2005). Incorporating diversity in the simulation laboratory or LRC—to reelect the burgeoning diversity of the population—is imperative and must be integrated in planning, implementation, and evaluation of simulation programs. Compliance with culturally and linguistically appropriate services (CLAS) standards (United States Department of Health and Human Services [USDHHS], Office of Minority Health [OMH], 2013) must be incorporated, not just in the classroom, but in all learning situations at the LRC. Faculty and staff can use available guides and tools from the AACN (2008b, 2011) and the NLN (2009, 2010).

Reflecting Diversity in the LRC

When planning the purchase of mannequins for the LRC, dolls must be ethnically diverse. Faculty need to explore options and give feedback to mannequin manufacturers such as Laerdal (Norway), CAE (formerly Canadian Aviation Electronics), Simulaids (United States), & Kyoto Kagako (Japan) for specifications of mannequins reflecting ethnic diversity such as those found in actual clients in clinical settings.

Nursing is an art and a science. Works of arts that reflect caring, such as painting or sculpture, may be placed in the LRC; this may increase the development of aesthetics knowledge among nursing students (Tarnow & Butcher, 2005). These works of arts must be representative of diverse cultures, ethnicities, gender, and gender and sexual orientation. Through interactions with mannequins during simulations, students grow to be more comfortable with clients in health care settings (Tarnow & Butcher, 2005). An example would be placing the IV training arm that does not allow for IV infusion alongside a full mannequin, thus encouraging and promoting more student interaction during a simulated IV skill training.

The integration of CLAS standards (USDHHS, OMH, 2013) needs to be assessed in terms of the mannequin population of the LRC. Mannequin names and signage in the LRC must mirror the diversity of ethnicity, gender, and sex reflective of actual client care settings in the locality. A copy of the enhanced CLAS standards must be in the LRC; these standards must be integrated in all learning experiences in the LRC.

Personalization of mannequins can be illustrated in their specific names, hard copies of their charts or electronic medical record (EMR), medication boxes, or special clothing or bed covers. To elaborate, if a community has a Native American population, the bed cover for a mannequin can be reflective of Native American heritage. Signage examples include offering the Bill of Patient Rights in languages of ethnocultural groups predominant in the community. Signs indicating the availability of interpreters and translators must be visible. A double phone for interpretation and translation, or a likeness of one used in institutions or agencies, must also be in the LRC. Table 19.1 can be used by faculty to evaluate the diversity of their LRC. The maximum possible score is 20 points; this score suggests an LRC that resembles actual client settings. It is suggested that faculty adapt this proposed evaluation tool to the ethnocultural groups prevalent in a particular community.

Using Professional Standards, Mandates, and Guidelines in Simulations

The use of **unfolding simulations** can show evidence of effective integration of Quality and Safety Education for Nurses (QSEN) in unfolding simulation-centered care of older adults (Forneris et al., 2012). AACN essentials, NLN competencies, and QSEN concepts may similarly be integrated with TCN concepts in designing simulation learning. The *Inner City*, a virtual diverse community (Table 19.2), illustrates this integration.

TABLE 19.1   Proposed Evaluation Tool. Diversity in the LRC

Criteria	Score	Comments

1. Mannequins reflect ethnic and racial diversity (0-5 points)
  a. White
  b. African American
  c. Hispanic
  d. Asian
  e. Native American		

2. Mannequin names show ethnic and racial diversity (0-5 points)
  a. White
  b. African American
  c. Hispanic
  d. Asian
  e. Native American		

3. Furniture, paintings, and other artifacts reflect ethnic and racial diversity (0–3 points)		
4. Signage reflects ethnocultural population in the community (0–2 points)		
5. Availability of interpreters and translators at no extra cost to the patient (0–2 points)		

6. Bill of Rights displayed prominently (0–3 points)
  a. In English
  b. In language common in the community		

Total Score (A maximum possible score of 20. The closer the score is to 20, the more indicative it is of a LRC that resembles actual client settings.)		

TABLE 19.2 Integration of QSEN Competencies and Standards of TCN in Unfolding Simulations

The Inner City Community Unfolding Simulations	Quality and Safety Education for Nurses (QSEN) Competencies	Transcultural Nursing Standards (TCN)	American Association of Colleges of Nursing (AACN) Essentials; End of Program Competencies for Baccalaureate Graduates	National League for Nursing (NLN) Competencies
Simulation 19.1. Jose Perez Visits TB Clinic (Filipino)	**Patient-centered care:** sensitive care; respect for diversity; recognize personal attitudes about clients from different ethnic, cultural, and social backgrounds; own level of communication; empowering clients **Evidence-based practice:** use of this in culturally and linguistically congruent care **Safety:** cultural safety	**Critical reflection:** reflective thinking; culturally congruent care **Knowledge of cultures:** assessments; policies and procedures Client advocacy and empowerment **Cross-cultural communication:** effective listening; perception of time and space; values of modesty	Information management and patient care technology Interprofessional collaboration and communication to improve patient outcomes **Cultural competencies** **1–5:** apply knowledge; use relevant data sources; safe and quality outcomes for diverse populations; advocacy for social justice; and continuous cultural competence development	**Core values:** diversity, caring **Professional identity:** advocacy; safe, quality care for diverse clients, families, and communities
Simulation 19.2. Kim An visits Mental Health Clinic (Korean)	**Patient-centered care:** sensitive care; respect for diversity; recognize personal attitudes about clients from different ethnic, cultural, and social backgrounds; own level of communication; empowering clients **Evidence-based practice:** use of this in culturally and linguistically congruent care **Safety:** cultural safety	**Critical reflection:** reflective thinking; culturally congruent care **Knowledge of cultures:** assessments; policies and procedures	Information management and patient care technology Interprofessional collaboration and communication to improve patient outcomes **Cultural competencies** **1–5:** apply knowledge; use relevant data sources; safe and quality outcomes for diverse populations; advocacy for social justice; and continuous cultural competence development	**Core values:** diversity, caring **Professional identity:** advocacy; safe, quality care for diverse clients, families, and communities

(continued)

TABLE 19.2 Integration of QSEN Competencies and Standards of TCN in Unfolding Simulations *(continued)*

The Inner City Community Unfolding Simulations	Quality and Safety Education for Nurses (QSEN) Competencies	Transcultural Nursing Standards (TCN)	American Association of Colleges of Nursing (AACN) Essentials; End of Program Competencies for Baccalaureate Graduates	National League for Nursing (NLN) Competencies
Simulation 19.3._ Dietary Education for Ada Myers (African American)				
Simulation 19.4. Caring for Mahmoud Mustafa (Afghan)				

Sources: American Association of Colleges of Nursing (2008a); American Association of Colleges of Nursing (2008b); National League for Nursing (2010); Quality and Safety Education for Nurses (2013); TCNS Expert Panel on Global Nursing & Health (2010).

SIMULATION 19.1   JOSE PEREZ VISITS A TB CLINIC AT INNER CITY

At the completion of this simulated scenario, the learner will:

1. Outline the nursing care for a patient with tuberculosis (TB).
2. Demonstrate the appropriate steps to administer a PPD.
3. Rate the importance of patient education to prevent multiple drug resistant (MDR) TB.

Jose Perez, a 50-year-old immigrant from the Philippines, presents at the Inner City tuberculosis clinic. He has been having night sweats and fever and has been "feeling weak for two months." Jose, a graduate of a 4-year business program in the Philippines, immigrated to the United States 2 years ago and has been working as a housekeeper in a nursing home. He lives with his sister Jinky in the basement of her and her husband's two-bedroom house.

Jinky is 47 years old and works as a nurse at the Newbury Medical Center, the only hospital in Inner City. Jinky is married to Arthur Garrido, a 55-year-old carpenter from Puerto Rico. Jinky and Arthur have two children: Annabeth, 13, and Cristina, 11.

Jose is 5'9 and weighs 200 lbs. Vital signs: 190/100, 70, RR = 22. He is not taking any medications.

Clinic Nurse: How long have you noticed these symptoms of night sweats, fever, weakness? Do you have any cough? Any sputum? Color, consistency, amount? Did you notice any blood in your sputum?

Jose: About 2 months. I thought I had the flu.

To the clinic nurse:

1. What else would you assess?
2. How would you administer the PPD on Jose's forearm?
3. Describe the protocol for reporting TB cases in your county?
4. Who else would need to be notified?

To the students on observation:

1. Describe how you would do the history and physical assessment differently. Why?
2. What would you include in your client education?
3. Analyze the treatment regimen for TB. Have you heard of some clients who stopped taking their medications before the course of treatment was completed?

Debriefing

1. How did you feel as you were placing the PPD on Jose's forearm?
2. If you were to repeat the PPD procedure, what would you change? Why?
3. How important is patient education for a patient with tuberculosis?
4. What strategies for self-care would you implement when caring for a client with TB?

SIMULATION 19.2 KIM AN VISITS THE MENTAL HEALTH CLINIC

At the completion of this simulated scenario, the learner will:

1. Outline the nursing care for a depressed client.
2. Demonstrate the appropriate therapeutic communication strategies for this client.
3. Apply Choi's Theory of Cultural Marginality in the care of Kim An.

Kim An, a 16-year-old Korean girl, is a junior at a local high school. Kim's parents, Kim Kuan (50 years old) and Sue (47 years old), migrated from Korea when Kim was about 3 years old. Kim has two siblings: Britney, 13 years old, and David, 10 years old, both born in the United States. Kim Kuan

(continued)

SIMULATION 19.2   KIM AN VISITS THE MENTAL HEALTH CLINIC   (continued)

and Sue help each other run a market at Inner City. Kim Kuan expects the children to help out with the market on weekends. Kim Kuan does not care whether the children have homework or that they need to be out with their friends; Sue thinks that the children could be more 'Americanized' with peers for easier adjustment.

At home, Kim, Britney, and David speak only Korean with their parents; at school, they only speak English—even to each other when they are alone. The three children have heard people making fun of their parents' accent. The children eat only Korean food at home. However, at school the children eat only American food such as hamburgers, fries, and pizza and drink soda all the time even though the selection has some "Oriental foods."

Kim has been increasingly depressed the last couple of months. She has been feeling like she is astride between two cultures: the Korean and the American cultures.

Kim Kuan and Sue, quite proud of their children because they are doing extremely well at school, are saving a quarter of their income for the children's college fund. The couple dreams of the three children finishing college. Kim has already looked at colleges with her parents. Secretly, Kim has been dreading going away to a faraway college. However, she is also concerned about going to a community college nearby. She feels this is going to be too close to home and she will not be independent. However, she knows she will be missing her mother's cooking as well as the close Korean community. Kim has visited Korea three times and in her heart she is proud to be a Korean. When she is in Korea, however, she does not feel at home. She always feels the desire to go back to the United States where things are more familiar. When she is in the United States, she feels she wants to go to Korea, the country of her birth.

Kim dreads going away to college and becoming independent of her parents. At the same time, she is increasingly getting tired of helping at the grocery store and not being able to go out with her friends. Kim's parents forbid her from going out and dating. Kim likes the company of her peers and is particularly fond of a boy at school, 16-year-old Nathan, who is third generation Irish American.

Britney, on the other hand, already plans to go to Harvard University to become a doctor. The parents compare Kim and Britney all the time; they tend to favor Britney for her motivation and clear goals ahead. David has no plans of going to college at all; he plans to be in business and own a large chain of supermarkets and become a millionaire by the time he is 30 years old. He does not dare mention this dream to his parents. He knows they will be disappointed; going to college is expected of him.

Kim came to the clinic today to see the psychiatrist. Her mother, Sue, came with her. Sue speaks heavily accented Korean and has limited English proficiency (LEP). Kim did not want Sue to be with her. Kim is not embarrassed being with her mother, but she feels self-conscious because her mother can only speak "broken" English.

Debriefing

1. How would you apply the Theory of Cultural Marginality (Choi, 2008, 2013) in this simulation scenario: for Kim An, her parents, and her siblings?
2. What is your plan of care for Kim An?
3. Analyze the stigma of mental illness in various cultures. Why is it easier to report somatic problems than mental problems?

EBP 19.1

The study by Reising, Carr, Shea, and King (2011) aimed to determine the differences between simulation technologies and traditional or round table discussion in communications and problem solving skills involving nursing and medical students. In their study, Reising et al. (2011) used the Jeffries simulation model in which both students and educators bring distinct qualities to a learning experience that influence the situation and need to be considered in determining the results. The study employed simulation technology and traditional interaction methods using sample groups consisting of medical students and baccalaureate nursing students.

The convenience sample included 20 second-year medical students and 48 senior nursing students. The students were divided into teams typically made up of two medical students and three or four nursing students that were assigned to either a round table discussion group or a simulation group. The simulation groups used a mannequin in a hospital-type bed and cardiac monitoring equipment.

Each of the groups were provided with a scenario that involved a cardiac arrest, a situation that both groups were expected to function in as a team (Reising et al., 2011). At the conclusion of the scenario the groups of students completed a survey providing quantitave as well as qualitative data in areas such as perception of role on the clinical team; changes in perception of role on the team; stress of the situation; and professionalism in communication between team members and in group interaction (Reising et al., 2011).

Reising et al. (2011) reported the major quantitative differences were findings that indicate students who were exposed to the simulation technology reported experiencing higher levels of stress than the round table group. Additionally, the qualitative data suggested differences in the simulation group, particularly for nursing students in roles perception. Also reported among the simulation group was an enhanced sense of time, providing for greater realism in the encounter. In reference to the Jeffries model used, the impact of student qualities was equal to the educational design on the outcomes (Reising et al., 2011).

Reising et al. (2011) acknowledged these limitations: small sample of 60 participants; self-reports as means of all data collected; and tools used were inadequate to capture concepts of interprofessional communication. Further studies are recommended to explore interprofessional learning.

Applications to Practice

■ As the nursing profession continues to expand beyond traditional roles and settings, the interface between nursing and medicine is continually changing. It is essential that these two disciplines learn to communicate effectively and collaborate efficiently. What other strategy can be used to provide these opportunities? Explain.

■ In which other situations might simulation technologies be used in intercollaboration training between allied health students? Discuss.

(continued)

EBP 19.1 *(continued)*

■ If you were to replicate this study, what would you do differently in terms of conceptual framework, sampling, and analysis of findings?

_____

Source: Reising, Carr, Shea, & King (2011).

CRITICAL THINKING EXERCISE 19.1

Undergraduate Student
1. You often hear faculty at your school say that the more the situation approximates reality, the more effective learning should be. Do you feel that the simulation portion of your learning is reality-based? Explain.
2. Do you think there is enough content of cultural diversity and promotion of cultural competence integrated in the simulation portion of your curriculum?
3. Would you be in favor of increasing the hours for simulation learning in your course? If yes, would you be in favor of deleting some hours from your clinical time? Why?

Graduate Student
1. Are simulated experiences used in your graduate program? If they are used, are they for replacement of a face-to-face class or classes? Explain.
2. How are your simulated learning experiences similar or different than the examples in this book? Compare and contrast.
3. Are you in favor of the simulated portion of your curriculum? Explain.
4. Do you take interprofessional courses in your curriculum? Describe.

Faculty in Academia
1. How many hours do you allocate for simulated learning experiences in the BS in Nursing program at your school?
2. Do you develop your simulated scenarios or do you purchase a program or programs?
3. Are TCN concepts built into your simulations or in those programs that you are using? Discuss.
4. How much diversity is reflected in your LRC?

Staff Development Educator
1. Do you have a simulation laboratory for staff orientation and continuing competence? Describe.
2. Is your simulation laboratory part of a grant? Describe.
3. Are TCN concepts integrated in your simulated learning? If not, how do you plan to incorporate diversity and promotion of cultural competence in staff orientation and continuing competence training?
4. When are you planning to attend a workshop/conference on this topic?

When designing a simulation scenario, it is best to incorporate all domains of learning—cognitive, affective, and psychomotor—for more effective learning (Decker et al., 2011). Simulations 1 and 2 are more advanced in terms of development. Faculty can add to these scenarios and develop more to populate the very diverse community of Inner City.

SUMMARY

This chapter outlined the history of simulation, its use in nursing, and its evolution into a multibillion dollar industry. The Institute of Medicine advocated for interprofessional education. Reflection in developing critical thinking and clinical judgment is illustrated. The knowledge, skills, and attitudes of QSEN; AACN essentials for baccalaureate education and the cultural competency toolkit; NLN baccalaureate competencies; and transcultural standards were reviewed for applicability in some simulation scenarios.

Adherence to the CLAS standards is an imperative when planning, implementing, and evaluating simulation learning. Reality-based simulation is emphasized as an effective way to teach cognitive, psychomotor, and affective concepts. It is time, then, that simulation must carefully integrate culturally and linguistically congruent care for clients, families, and communities. Nurse educators are, after all, preparing graduates to care for the nation's increasingly diverse population. The simulations at LRCs are complementing what we teach in the classroom and clinical settings.

REFERENCES

American Association of Colleges of Nursing. (2008a). *The essentials of baccalaureate education for professional nursing practice.* Washington, DC: Author.
American Association of Colleges of Nursing. (2008b). *Cultural competency in baccalaureate nursing education.* Washington, DC: Author.
American Association of Colleges of Nursing. (2011). *Toolkit for cultural competence in master's and doctoral nursing education.* Washington, DC: Author.
Caputi, L. (2011). Program approval and accreditation. In T. J. Bristol & J. Zerwekh (Eds.), *Essentials for e-learning for nurse educators* (pp. 295–306). Philadelphia, PA: F.A. Davis.
Choi, H. (2008). Theory of cultural marginality. In M. J. Smith & P. R. Liehr (Eds.), *Middle range theory for nursing* (3rd ed., pp. 243–259). New York, NY: Springer Publishing.
Choi, H. (2013). Theory of cultural marginality. In M. J. Smith & P. R. Liehr (Eds.), *Middle range theory for nursing* (3rd ed., pp. 289–307). New York, NY: Springer Publishing.
Cohen, J. A. (2005). The mirror as metaphor for the reflective practitioner. In M. H. Oermann (Ed.) & K. T. Heinrich (Associate Ed.), *Annual review of nursing education: Strategies for teaching, assessment, and program planning* (pp. 313–330). New York, NY: Springer Publishing.
Cooper, J. B., & Taqueti, V. R. (2004). A brief history of the development of mannequin simulators for clinical education and training. *Quality and Safety in Health Care, 13*(Suppl1), i11–i18. doi: 10.1136/qshc.2004.009886. Retrieved May 20, 2013, from www.ncbi.nlm.nih.gov/pmc/articles/PMC1765785/pdf/v013p00i11.pdf
Decker, S., Gore, T., & Feken, C. (2011). Simulation. In T. J. Bristol & J. Zerwekh (Eds.), *Essentials for e-learning for nurse educators* (pp. 277–294). Philadelphia, PA: F.A. Davis.
Forneris, S. G., Crownover, J. G., Dorsey, L., Leahy, N., Maas, N. A., Wong, L....Zavertnik, J. E. (2012). Integrating QSEN and ACES: An NLN simulation leader project. *Nursing Education Perspectives, 33*(3),184–187.
Jeffries, P. R., Beach, M., Decker, S. I., Dlugasch, L., Groom, J., Settles, J., & O'Donnell, J. M. (2011). Multi-center development and testing of simulation-based cardiovascular assessment curriculum for advanced practice nurses. *Nursing Education Perspectives, 32*(5), 316–322.

Morgan, P. G. (1995). Creating a laboratory that simulates the critical care environment. *Critical Care Nurse, 16*(6), 76–81.

National League for Nursing. (2009). *Diversity toolkit.* Retrieved August 22, 2013, from NLN website: www.nln.org/facultyprograms/Diversity_Toolkit/index.htm

National League for Nursing. (2010). *Competencies for baccalaureate graduates.* Retrieved February 3, 2013, from www.nln.org/facultyprograms/competencies/comp_bacc.htm

National League for Nursing. (2013). *Simulation innovation resource center: FAQs.* Retrieved August, 26, 2013, from sirc.nln.org/mod/resource/view.php?id=258

PR Newswire. (2013, June 11). *Healthcare/medical simulation market worth $1.9 billion by 2017.* Retrieved August 26, 2013, from www.prnewswire.com/news-releases/healthcaremedical-simulation-market-worth-19-billion-by-2017–210968801.html

Quality and Safety Education for Nurses. (QSEN). (2013). *Pre-licensure KSAs.* Retrieved July 28, 2013, from http://qsen.org/competencies/pre-licensure-ksas/

Reising, D. L, Carr, D. E., Shea. R. A., & King, J. M. (2011). Comparison of communication outcomes in traditional versus simulation strategies in nursing and medical students. *Nursing Education Perspectives, 32*(5), 322–327.

Schon, D. A. (1983). *The reflective practitioner.* New York, NY: Basic Books.

Schon, D. A. (1987). *Educating the reflective practitioner.* San Francisco, CA: Jossey Bass.

Shellenbarger, T., Palmer, E. A., Labant, A. L., & Kuzneski, J. L. (2005). Use of faculty reflection to improve teaching. In M. H. Oermann (Ed.) & K. T. Heinrich (Associate Ed.), *Annual review of nursing education: Strategies for teaching, assessment, and program planning* (pp. 343–357). New York, NY: Springer Publishing.

Tarnow, K. G., & Butcher, H. K. (2005). Teaching the art of professional nursing in the learning laboratory. In M. H. Oermann (Ed.) & K. T. Heinrich (Associate Ed.), *Annual review of nursing education: Strategies for teaching, assessment, and program planning* (pp. 375–392). New York, NY: Springer Publishing.

TCNS Expert Panel on Global Nursing & Health. (2010). *Standards of practice for culturally competent nursing care.* Retrieved February 3, 2013, from www.tcns.org/TCNStandardsofPractice.html

United States Department of Health and Human Services, Office of Minority Health. (2013). *Enhanced national CLAS standards.* Retrieved August 16, 2013, from https://www.thinkculturalhealth.hhs.gov/Content/clas.asp

Widemark, E. (2011). Web-based environments. In T. J. Bristol & J. Zerwekh (Eds.), *Essentials for e-learning for nurse educators* (pp. 133–164). Philadelphia, PA: F.A. Davis.

CHAPTER

TCN Concepts in Undergraduate Nursing Programs

20

Priscilla Limbo Sagar and Julie Coon

KEY TERMS

Associate
Baccalaureate
Curricular design
Diploma
Instructional approaches
Licensed practical nurse

National Council Licensure Examination for
  Licensed Practical Nurses or NCLEX-PN®
National Council Licensure Examination for
  Registered Nurses or NCLEX-RN®
Registered Nurse to Bachelor of Science
  (RN–BS) in Nursing

LEARNING OBJECTIVES

At the completion of this chapter, the learner will be able to

1. Discuss the integration of transcultural concepts in licensed practical nursing, diploma, associate degree, baccalaureate, and baccalaureate completion programs.

2. Analyze methods of an interprofessional transcultural health care courses offered for nursing and allied health students.

3. Collaborate with an interprofessional team in the promotion and acquisition of awareness, knowledge, and skills in cultural diversity and cultural competence.

4. Examine the current evidence-based practices regarding integration of transcultural nursing concepts in undergraduate nursing programs.

OVERVIEW

It is imperative to integrate transcultural nursing in all programs that prepare nurses. The increasing body of knowledge related to transcultural nursing coupled with the growing emphasis on the need for the profession to embrace diversity as both a practice and professional value has clearly impacted nursing education curricula at the undergraduate level.

The American Association of Colleges of Nursing ([AACN], 2008a, 2008b) and National League for Nursing ([NLN], 2005, 2009a, 2009b), as the national organizations that guide nursing education, have both issued position statements, guidelines, and toolkits designed to provide support for nursing programs as they strive to integrate transcultural nursing standards into curricula at the undergraduate level. In **baccalaureate** programs specifically, the AACN and the NLN, as well as their respective accrediting bodies, the Commission on Collegiate Nursing Education ([CCNE], 2013) and Accreditation Commission for Education in Nursing ([ACEN], 2013), formerly the National League for Nursing Accreditation Commission (NLNAC), expect programmatic integration of transcultural nursing (TCN) concepts.

Integration of TCN Concepts

Transcultural nursing education experts have provided a plethora of teaching strategies that can be utilized to increase cultural competence as a fundamental component of nursing practice (Andrews, 2012; Davidhizar & Giger, 2001; Davidhizar & Shearer, 2005; Eshelman & Davidhizar, 2006; Hughes & Hood, 2007; Jeffreys, 2010a, 2010b; McFarland, & Leininger, 2002; Purnell, 2007; Sagar, 2012). The number of diverse instructional applications clearly reflects the extensive research that has been conducted by the most notable scholars in TCN and serves to provide excellent models for nurse educators who recognize the need for intentional approaches to the inclusion of transcultural content into respective undergraduate nursing programs.

Empirical evidence to support **curricular design** and instruction in the area of transcultural nursing is an emerging field as nurse educators endeavor to demonstrate relationships between **instructional approaches** based on established transcultural nursing theories or models and student learning outcomes. McFarland and Leininger (2002) proposed three approaches for effectively integrating TCN within the academic setting at the undergraduate level: (1) integration of transcultural concepts, skills and principles within an existing curriculum; (2) incorporation of selected culture care modules within a curriculum; and (3) offering a series of coordinated, substantive transcultural nursing courses with field experiences. Although there are limited examples in the literature of the second and third approaches, it is noted that the majority of applications and research-based studies reflect the first approach. Jeffreys (2010a) suggests that the first approach has received the most emphasis based on the perception that it has the broadest and most immediate application across academic settings and degree programs. Jeffreys (2010a) also notes that "an integrated approach has the potential to positively affect the greatest number of 'future' students" (p. 117). In addition, Pacquiao (2007) highlighted the impact of cultural competence education and the desired outcome to increase diversity in the nursing workforce.

A review of the current literature reveals that there are studies at both the associate degree and baccalaureate levels of nursing education, but to date, no published research has been conducted among licensed practical nursing students with an emphasis on TCN concepts. The primary research emphasis has been on baccalaureate nursing education at the undergraduate level. Most studies conducted within baccalaureate and associate degree nursing programs focused on the measurement of student knowledge, attitudes, behaviors, and competencies as a result of cultural competence instructional techniques (DeRuyter, 2008; Hughes & Hood, 2007; Lipson & Desantis, 2007; Talley, 2002; Thompson, Boore, & Deeny, 2000; Wittig, 2004). Other studies (Kardong-Edgren & Campinha-Bacote, 2008; Kardong-Edgreen et al., 2010; Lipson & Desantis, 2007) examined multiple curricular designs in regard to the outcomes related to cultural competency. Successful use of the

Culture Care Theory (Leninger, 2006) was used to recruit, engage, and retain minority and financially disadvantaged students (McFarland, Mixer, Lewis, & Easley, 2006). Finally, it is significant to note that ongoing research devoted to the refinement of instruments to measure the acquisition of cultural competence specifically in nursing students is being conducted with notable outcomes in the areas of reliability and validity (Jeffreys, 1999, 2010a, 2010b; Jeffreys & Smodlaka, 1998). A synopsis of Kardong-Edgreen' s (2007) current research related to cultural competence of undergraduate nursing faculty is presented in **EBP 20.1**.

EBP 20.1

Kardong-Edgreen (2007) conducted a randomized, stratified, descriptive, cross-sectional survey of 170 baccalaureate nursing faculty selected from schools on the National League for Nursing Accrediting Commission (NLNAC) 2000 Directory of Accredited Nursing Programs. For every school selected, the researcher randomly chose six undergraduate faculty from the school's website.

This study used Campinha-Bacote's model (2007) and its five constructs of cultural desire, cultural awareness, cultural knowledge, cultural skill, and cultural encounters as framework. In addition, Kardong-Edgreen used Campinha-Bacote's (2003) Inventory for Assessing the Process of Cultural Competence Among Healthcare Professionals-Revised (IAPCC-R, 2003). The mailed survey asked for (1) comfort level when caring for individuals from other cultures; (2) cultural content in one's own academic preparation; and (3) cultural content in current program employment. The study likewise compared cultural competence of faculty teaching in the states with the most immigrants to the cultural competence of faculty teaching in the states with the least immigrants.

Kardong-Edgreen used the Center for Immigration Studies by Camarotta and McArdle (2003, as cited in Kardong-Edgreen, 2007), to stratify the sample into faculty from the states with the most immigrants (n = 87) and from the states with the least immigrants (n = 83). Identified as states with the most immigrants were California, New York, Florida, Texas, New Jersey, Massachussetts, Arizona, Michigan, Washington, Colorado, and Pennsylvania. States with the least immigrants included Louisiana, Iowa, Oklahoma, New Mexico, Tennessee, Kentucky, Arkansas, Delaware, Maine, Montana, New Hampshire, North Dakota, South Carolina, Nebraska, and Mississippi.

The participants' ages ranged from 25 to 69 years old. Immersion and working with peoples from diverse cultures frequently accounted for increasing comfort level in teaching and working with diverse clients. Specific reasons cited included travel, working within and with people of other cultures, and interactions with students.

Findings indicate that 16% of the respondents reported no cultural content in their own academic preparation. Despite this lack of preparation, 88% of the respondents currently integrate cultural content into the program. Some faculty evidence cultural desire and actively seek educational experiences to prepare them to teach cultural content (Kardong-Edgreen, 2007). The researchers acknowledged self report as a limitation of this study. Among the participants, 80% would like further education in meeting patients' cultural needs.

(continued)

EBP 20.1 *(continued)*

Applications to Practice

■ Recall your "informal" preparation in TCN. Describe. Does this help you in integrating TCN concepts in your current job as faculty/nursing professional development (NPD) specialist?

■ Do you have "formal" preparation in TCN---that is, taking courses regarding TCN, diversity, cultural competence—in the undergraduate and graduate levels of your nursing education? How many courses or continuing education (CE) credits did you take?

■ Is there a conceptual theory or model you use in integrating cultural concepts? If there is none, how are cultural concepts integrated?

■ If you were to replicate this study, how would you conduct it? What would you change in terms of conceptual framework, sampling, and analysis of findings?

Source: Kardong-Edgreen (2007).

SELECTED RESEARCH STUDIES

Cultural Competence Among Nursing Students

Wittig (2004) conducted an open-ended survey to determine the knowledge, skills, and attitudes among associate degree nursing students believed to be essential when providing culturally competent health care for Native American clients. Conceptual analysis revealed interrelated and connected themes: knowledge (4), skills (2), and attitudes (2). These findings actually supported the assertion that the current nursing curriculum at this institution fostered the development of cultural competence among nursing students who are future practitioners in multicultural settings.

DeRuyter's (2002) ethnonursing study examined the cultural care education and experiences of African American students in eight predominantly European American associate degree nursing programs. Leininger's Culture Care Theory (2006) was used as a guide to describe the worldview, beliefs, values, and meanings of the ways of life of the nine key and 19 general informants. The eight patterns identified were further refined into three themes that were found to reflect specific situational and belief factors related to the educational outcomes of African American students.

Talley (2002) conducted a cross-sectional, nonexperimental, survey design study to test theorized sources of self-efficacy by examining factors that might explain the variance in a proposed model of perceived cultural self-efficacy in nursing students. The sample included 351 nursing students enrolled in eight associate degree and baccalaureate degree programs. Stepwise multiple regressions were used to measure relationships among cross-cultural experience, performance feedback in cultural diversity education, model competence, and perceived cultural self-efficacy as measured by the Bernal and Froman Cultural Self-efficacy Scale (CSES, 1988), as cited in Talley (2002). Performance feedback of cultural diversity education was measured with the Performance Feedback Scale (PFS) and model competence was measured by the Model Evaluation Scale (MES). Findings suggested that three factors positively influence a nursing student's cultural self-efficacy: (1) cross-cultural experiences; (2) cultural diversity education in their nursing programs that includes positive performance feedback from nursing faculty; and (3) role modeling by culturally competent nurses (Talley, 2002).

Studies Outside of the United States

Lim, Downie, and Nathan (2004) conducted a study using the Transcultural Self-Efficacy Tool (TSET) designed by Jeffreys (1999) with a sample of 196 Australian first-and fourth-year students in a nursing program. Findings indicated that fourth-year students with increased didactic information and clinical backgrounds had a more positive perception of their self-efficacy in providing transcultural care than the first-year students. In addition, Lim et al. (2004) found that demographic variables such as age, gender, country of birth, languages spoken at home, and past work experience did not affect nursing students' perception of self-efficacy in providing transcultural care. This research indicates that formal educational preparation and structured clinical experience are essential in giving nursing students the opportunity to develop self-efficacy in providing culturally congruent care to diverse client populations.

In a descriptive study of 622 nursing students from three different university-based nursing schools in Turkey, Ayaz, Bilgili, and Akin (2010) explored the cultural diversity that students encountered while providing care to patients. Ayaz et al. (2010) also investigated the students' knowledge of transcultural nursing. Cultural differences have been prevalent in Turkey, and some problems arise in patient care, resulting in a greater focus on the promotion of cultural competence in providing health care to patients. The researchers used a survey method for data collection and percentages and chi-square for data analysis. The data revealed that most students (85.5%) had encountered cultural differences while providing patient care; of these, 73.8% of the students did not know the definition of cultural differences. According to the students, the highest degree of cultural differences experienced were in dialect and pronunciation, language, traditions and customs, and the religious belief of the sect. Ayaz et al. (2010) also found that the grade of the students had a significant effect on the experience of cultural diversity. The researchers recommended that educational programs could minimize the negative effects of cultural diversity by including a separate course for students to address this serious issue in their country.

Thompson, Boore, and Deeny (2000) conducted a survey study among 74 undergraduate nursing students from Northern Ireland to measure the impact of a 3-month international experience in another country as an option to teach TCN. Thompson et al. (2000) found that the international experience not only exerted a significant impact on students' global perspective and career development but also enhanced their understanding of cultural and political issues within Northern Ireland.

STRATEGIES FOR DIFFERENT EDUCATIONAL PROGRAMS

LPN Programs

Licensed practical nurse (LPN) programs, whether offered in technical schools, community colleges, high schools, or hospital-based schools, are approximately 1 year in length. **Licensed practical nurses** (LPNs) and licensed vocational nurses (LVNs), depending on the state in which they work, provide basic medical care under the supervision of registered nurses and physicians (Bureau of Labor Statistics, 2012).

The curricula consisting of nursing, biology, pharmacology, and related content, plus supervised clinical experience, are already packed with content; integrating TCN concepts will not only require faculty commitment but their utmost creativity. Sagar (2012) proposed a virtual field trip to Ellis Island. For programs in closer proximity to Liberty and Ellis Islands, a physical visit is possible (Table 20.1). Reflective journals as a course assignment may assist students in exploring their thinking, awareness, and feelings about the challenges of immigration and starting over in a new country.

Graduates of practical nursing programs must take and successfully pass the **National Council Licensure Examination for Practical Nurses or NCLEX-PN®** for licensure and work as LPNs or LVNs. Graduates of associate and baccalaureate programs take the **National Council Licensure Examination for Registered Nurses or NCLEX-RN®**. There is a varying degree of cultural diversity and competence content in the NCLEX-PN and NCLEX-RN. Chapter 5 contains more discussion about the NCLEX.

Associate Degree/Diploma Programs

Generally, associate degree nursing (ADN) and **diploma** programs require 65 to 68 credits for graduation. In such a tight curriculum, the integration of TCN content poses a huge challenge for nurse educators. However, if instructors are passionate enough for TCN, integration is possible. Seamless articulation, as illustrated in Box 20.1, could be vital in integration of TCN concepts at the ADN or diploma levels of nursing education. This integration will give students background knowledge, awareness, and continuity when they transition to the RN–Bachelor of Science (BS) in Nursing program. Faculty-to-faculty collaborations are likewise illustrated in Box 20.1 in an unfolding case scenario about Eagle Community County College and in Chapter 4 and Appendix 10.

Baccalaureate Programs

Baccalaureate programs require a minimum of 120 credits for graduation. Although there is more potential for TCN integration in the longer curricula of baccalaureate education, many schools still do not have a separate TCN course. The usual reason cited is overcrowded

TABLE 20.1 Sample Assignment Guide for a Reflective Journal in an LPN Program

Assignment: Reflective Journal #1
Complete a tour of Liberty and Ellis Islands through a physical or a virtual visit. Answer the following guide questions. Allow yourself to think deep and explore your feelings.
Name:
How did you complete your visit? Physical tour? Virtual tour?
How does Ellis Island function as a reminder of the roots for many immigrants and their descendants?
Do you have any ancestors who came to this country through Ellis Island? If not, how did they migrate?
Select a set of artifacts at Ellis Island such as luggage samples or health care materials and tools. What feelings did those objects and artifacts evoke in you?
While Ellis Island has been closed since 1954 as a gateway for immigrants, do you think it is still a powerful reminder of immigrant struggles? How is coming through Kennedy International Airport different from undergoing entrance through Ellis Island? Discuss.

Source: Statue of Liberty–Ellis Island Foundation (2013).

> **BOX 20.1 APPLICATION OF THE GIGER AND DAVIDHIZAR TRANSCULTURAL ASSESSMENT MODEL IN AN UNFOLDING CASE SCENARIO FOR AN ASSOCIATE DEGREE PROGRAM AT EAGLE COUNTY COMMUNITY COLLEGE**
>
> The Department of Nursing at Eagle County Community College (ECCC) offers an associate in nursing degree with 68 credits. ECCC has an articulation agreement with Fidelity College Sunrise School of Nursing's RN-BS fully online completion program. Faculty at ECCC are aware that FCSSN may be offering a 3-credit elective transcultural health care course in a semester or two—a proposal was approved at the FCSSN faculty divisional committee and is pending college-wide curriculum and faculty senate approvals.
>
> The ECCC faculty has recently voted to undergo curriculum revision and has adopted Giger and Davidhizar's Transcultural Assessment Model (2008, 2013) for its simplicity and applicability to their associate degree curriculum. The faculty plans to integrate the TAM's six cultural phenomena of biological variations, environmental control, time, social orientation, space, and communication (Giger & Davidhizar, 2008, 2013).
>
> For teaching strategies, ECCC faculty plan to use role plays, case studies, and games to teach TCN content in all their NUR courses. Their templates for role plays include scenario, reflection, and debriefing to facilitate critical thinking. The six phenomena of the TAM lend themselves well, in their totality or by selecting specific areas, to role plays as a teaching and learning strategy (Sagar, 2012). A sample role play is provided in Box 20.2.
>
> _____
>
> *Sources*: Giger & Davidhizar (2008); and Sagar (2012).

curricula (McFarland & Leininger, 2002). The most common method is integration of TCN concepts in existing nursing courses (Jeffreys, 2010a). The development of a 3-credit transcultural health care course for nursing and allied health students is reviewed in Chapter 4.

Offering courses where there is opportunity for interprofessional education is endorsed by the Institute of Medicine in its *Future of Nursing* report (2010). Interprofessional education provides opportunities for collaboration and teamwork in solving real-life problems in practice; this teamwork and collaborative work enhance future partnerships in improving client outcomes.

Allied Health Programs

In allied health, cultural diversity and promotion of cultural competence content have been gaining momentum (Andrews & Friesen, 2011). Muñoz, DoBroka, and Mohammad (2009) planned, developed, and implemented a 3-credit course on cultural competence for nursing, education, and social work students at a university in the midwestern United States. Muñoz et al. (2009) suggested seeking support from administrators and advisers, especially in the course's initial offering when there is a problem with small enrollment. The synopsis of this research is in EBP 4.1, Chapter 4.

When developing an interprofessional transcultural health care course, the content should be reflective of an interprofessional focus. Academic policies in regards to grading and preparation of assignments must be flexible; use nursing department policy for student nurses but specify a clause that other students will adhere to their own departmental grading and other policies. An actual separate 3-credit course is in Appendix 17 for baccalaureate programs for nursing, physical therapy, premedicine, and other allied professions.

APPLICATION: GIGER AND DAVIDHIZAR TRANSCULTURAL ASSESSMENT MODEL

The sample role play below uses Giger and Davidhizar's Transcultural Assessment Model ([TAM], 2008, 2013) in Box 20.1. This role play is appropriate for use with diploma, associate, and baccalaureate nursing and allied health students or in staff development settings.

BOX 20.2 SAMPLE ROLE PLAY

Student A is dressed as a 60-year-old Muslim man from Bangladesh. He was admitted the day before for acute myocardial infarction and is currently on bed rest. The male student nurse, assigned to assist in his care as per the client's request, was about to remove the basin with warm water that the client just used. The client planned to use a rug when he prays after his ablutions. He was also planning to request that his bed face Mecca for prayers. Answers are designated by number; for example, "answer 1" is designated as A1, and so forth. Questions are assigned a number consecutively in a similar manner.

Student A, A1: "I have displeased the evil spirits."

Student A, A2: "I need to see the folk healer to exorcise the evil spirits."

Student A, A3: "It is proper to both use folk healer and come to the hospital for treatment."

Student A, Q1: "Is it possible to change the position for my bed so I can face Mecca to pray?"

Student B is dressed as a male student. He is wearing scrubs and has a stethoscope around his neck. In his haste, he forgot to knock on the client's door prior to entering the room. In addition, the student kicked the prayer rug on the floor to get it out of his way. The student began asking the client about assessment questions; he needs answers for his first assessment paper.

Student B, Q1: "What do you think caused your illness?"

Student B, Q2: "You just mentioned evil spirits and displeasing them. What are your beliefs in appeasing those spirits?"

Student B, Q3: "Is it appropriate to use western healing with your folk healing?"

Student B, A1: "I will need to check with my instructor and my nurse. I will let you know as soon as possible."

(continued)

BOX 20.2 SAMPLE ROLE PLAY (continued)

Reflection

Student C is wearing a laboratory coat and will ask as the facilitator to moderate the discussion following the role play. She has prepared the following guide questions and discussed them with the faculty:

1. How is *communication* as a cultural phenomenon involved in this scenario? Describe.
2. How is *environmental control* as a cultural phenomenon involved in this scenario? Discuss.
3. How are *social organizations* as cultural phenomenon involved in this scenario? Discuss.
4. How is *space* as a cultural phenomenon involved in this scenario? Discuss.
5. Reenact the scenario.

Faculty Debriefing

1. Reflect on this role play. Describe your feelings.
2. Analyze what you learned. What other learning needs do you have?
3. Discuss the clinical application of this role play.
4. Examine the changes needed in your knowledge, skills, and attitudes in order to integrate culturally congruent care in all your client interactions.

Source: Statue of Liberty–Ellis Island Foundation (2013).

CRITICAL THINKING EXERCISES 20.1

Undergraduate Student
1. Have you had opportunities in clinical to care for culturally diverse patients? Do you feel prepared to care for these patients?
2. Do you have course assignments in transcultural nursing? If you do, how much toward the course grade do those assignments count?
3. Are transcultural concepts included in your course exams?
4. Would you feel prepared to answer TCN questions in the NCLEX-RN/NCLEX-PN? Why?

Faculty in Academia
1. How many credits do you have in your associate degree program?
2. If you were to select a theory or model when applying TCN concepts in your curriculum, whose theory or model would you use? Why?
3. What teaching strategies will you use to develop awareness, knowledge, and skills about cultural diversity and promotion of cultural competence among your students? Discuss your rationales for use of these strategies.

(continued)

CRITICAL THINKING EXERCISES 20.1 (continued)

Staff Development Educator
1. Do you have LPN/associate/diploma students on clinical rotation at your hospital or agency? Do these students have opportunities to care for diverse clients?
2. Are you having problems accepting clinical rotations from any level of nursing programs such as for LPN, AD, diploma, and baccalaureate? Why? Describe.
3. Do you have any required portion of hospital orientation devoted to activities that celebrate diversity? How often are these activities required for students and faculty?

SUMMARY

The U.S. population is one of the most diverse globally and will increasingly be so in the next 50 years. It is a tremendous challenge to educate nurses and other health care professionals to provide culturally and linguistically congruent care to these populations. This chapter explored integration of TCN concepts in LPN, diploma, associate, and baccalaureate nursing programs, drawing from available research and TCN experts. The authors included research regarding integration of TCN concepts as well as studies attempting to measure cultural competence among undergraduate nursing students. In addition, integration of TCN concepts is discussed for students in allied health.

REFERENCES

Accreditation Commission for Education in Nursing. (2013). *ACEN standards and criteria: Baccalaureate.* Retrieved August 22, 2013, from www.acenursing.net/manuals/SC2013_BACCALAUREATE.pdf

American Association of Colleges of Nursing. (2008a). *The essentials of baccalaureate education for professional nursing practice.* Washington, DC: Author.

American Association of Colleges of Nursing. (2008b). *Cultural competency in baccalaureate nursing education.* Washington, DC: Author.

Andrews, M. M. (2012). Cultural competence in the health history and physical examination. In M. M. Andrews & J. S. Boyle (Eds.), *Transcultural concepts in nursing care* (6th ed., pp. 38–72). Philadelphia, PA: Wolters Kluwer/Lippincott Williams & Wilkins.

Andrews, M. M., & Friesen, L. (2011). Finding electronically available information on cultural competence in health care. *Online Journal of Cultural Competence in Nursing and Health Care, 1*(4), 27–43. Retrieved January 27, 2013, from www.ojccnh.org/1/4/27–43.pdf

Ayaz, S., Bilgili, N., & Akin, B. (2010). The transcultural nursing concept: A study of nursing students in Turkey. *International Nursing Review, 57*(4), 449–453.

Bureau of Labor Statistics, United States Department of Labor. (2012). *Occupational outlook handbook, 2012–13 edition* (Licensed Practical and Licensed Vocational Nurses). Retrieved December 12, 2012, from www.bls.gov/ooh/healthcare/licensed-practical-and-licensed-vocational-nurses.htm

Commission on Collegiate Nursing Education. (2013). *Standards for accreditation of baccalaureate and graduate nursing programs.* Retrieved September 20, 2013, from www.aacn.nche.edu/ccne-accreditation/Standards-Amended-2013.pdf

Davidhizar, R. E., & Giger, J. N. (2001). Teaching culture within the nursing curriculum using the Giger-Davidhizar model of transcultural nursing assessment. *Journal of Nursing Education, 40*(6), 282–284.

Davidhizar, R. E., & Shearer, R. (2005). When your nursing student is culturally diverse. *Health Care Manager, 240*(4), 356–363.

deRuyter, L. M. (2008). *Cultural care education and experiences of African American students in predominantly Euro American associate degree nursing programs* (Doctoral dissertation). Duquesne University, Pittsburgh, PA.

Eshelman, J., & Davidhizar R. E. (2006). Strategies for developing cultural competency in an RN-BS program. *Journal of Transcultural Nursing, 17*(2), 179–183.

Giger, J. N., & Davidhizar, R. E. (2008). *Transcultural nursing: Assessment and intervention* (5th ed.). St. Louis, MO: Mosby Elsevier.

Giger, J. N., & Davidhizar, R. E. (2013). *Transcultural nursing: Assessment and intervention* (6th ed.). St. Louis, MO: Mosby Elsevier.

Hughes, K. H., & Hood, L. J. (2007). Teaching methods and an outcome tool for measuring cultural sensitivity in undergraduate nursing students. *Journal of Transcultural Nursing,18*(1), 57–62.

Institute of Medicine. (2010, October 5). *The future of nursing: Leading change, advancing health.* Washington, DC: National Academies Press.

Jeffreys, M. R. (1999). Construct validation of the transcultural self-efficacy tool. *Journal of Nursing Education, 38*(5), 222–227.

Jeffreys, M. R. (2010a). *Teaching cultural competence in nursing and health care* (2nd ed., pp. 45–59). New York, NY: Springer Publishing.

Jeffreys, M. R. (2010b). Factor analysis of the transcultural self-efficacy tool (TSET). *Journal of Nursing Measurement, 18*(2), 120–139.

Jeffreys, M. R., & Smodlaka, L. (1998). Exploring the factorial composition of the trancultural self-efficacy tool. *International Journal of Nursing Studies, 35*(4), 217–225.

Kardong-Edgreen, S. (2007). Cultural competence of baccalaureate nursing faculty. *Journal of Nursing Education, 46*(8), 360–366.

Kardong-Edgreen, S., & Campina-Bacote, J. (2008). Cultural competency of graduating U.S. Bachelor of Science nursing students. *Contemporary Nurse, 28*, 37–44.

Kardong-Edgreen, S., Cason, C. L., Walsh Brennan, A. M., Reifsneider, E., Hummel, F., Mancini, M., & Griffin, C. (2010). Cultural competency of graduating BSN students. *Nursing Education Perspectives, 31*(5), 278–285.

Leininger, M. M. (2006). Culture care diversity and universality and evolution of the ethnonursing method. In M. Leininger & M. McFarland (Eds.), *Culture care diversity and universality: A worldwide nursing theory* (pp. 1–41). Sudbury, MA: Jones & Bartlett.

Lim, J., Downie, J., & Nathan, P. (2004). Nursing students' self-efficacy in providing transcultural care. *Nurse Education Today, 24*(6), 428–434.

Lipson, J. G., & Desantis, L. A. (2007). Current approaches to integrating elements of cultural competence in nursing education. *Journal of Transcultural Nursing, 18*(1), 10S–20S.

McFarland, M. R., & Leininger, M. M. (2002). Transcultural nursing: Curricular concepts, principles and teaching and learning activities for the 21st century. In M. Leininger & M. McFarland (Eds.), *Transcultural nursing: Concepts, theories, research, and practice* (3rd ed., pp. 527–561). New York, NY: McGraw-Hill.

McFarland, M., Mixer, S., Lewis, A. E., & Easley, C. (2006). Use of the culture care theory as a framework for the recruitment, engagement, and retention of culturally diverse nursing students in a traditionally European American baccalaureate nursing program. In M. Leininger & M. McFarland (Eds.), *Culture care diversity and universality: A worldwide nursing theory* (pp. 239–254). Boston, MA: Jones & Bartlett.

Muñoz, C. C., DoBroka, C. C., & Mohammad, S. (2009). Development of a multidisciplinary course in cultural competence for nursing and human service professions. *Journal of Nursing Education, 48*(9), 495–503.

National League for Nursing. (2005). Core competencies of nurse educators with task statements. New York, NY: Author. Retrieved January 26, 2011, from www.nln.org/aboutnln/core_competencies/cce_dial3.htm

National League for Nursing. (2009a). *A commitment to diversity in nursing and nursing education.* Retrieved August 22, 2013, from www.nln.org/aboutnln/reflection_dialogue/rfl _dial3.htm

National League for Nursing. (2009b). *Diversity toolkit.* Retrieved August 22, 2013, from www.nln. org/facultyprograms/Diversity_Toolkit/index.htm

National League for Nursing. (2009b). *Diversity toolkit.* Retrieved January 26, 2011, from www.nln. org/aboutnln/reflection_dialogue/rfl_dial3.htm

Pacquaio, D. (2007). The relationship between cultural competence education and increasing diversity in nursing schools and practice settings. *Journal of Transcultural Nursing, 18*(1), 28S–370S.

Purnell, L. D. (2007). Commentary on "Current approaches to integrating elements of cultural competence in nursing education." *Journal of Transcultural Nursing, 18*(1), 23S–24S.

Sagar, P. L. (2012). *Transcultural nursing theory and models: Application in nursing education, practice, and administration.* New York, NY: Springer Publishing.

Statue of Liberty–Ellis Island Foundation. (2013). *Ellis Island-history.* Retrieved January 3, 2013, from www.statueofliberty.org/Ellis_History.html

Talley, L. K. (2002). *Cross-cultural experience, performance feedback, model competence, and cultural self-efficacy: Analysis of a model* (Doctoral dissertation). Texas Woman's University, Denton, TX.

Thompson, K., Boore, J., & Deeny, P. (2000). A comparison of an international experience for nursing students in developed and developing countries. *International Journal of Nursing Studies, 37*(6), 481–492.

Wittig, D. (2004). Knowledge, skills, and attitudes of nursing students regarding culturally congruent care of Native Americans. *Journal of Transcultural Nursing, 15*(1), 54–61.

TCN Concepts in Graduate Nursing Programs

Priscilla Limbo Sagar

Advanced practice nurses (APNs)
Clinical specialist
Consultation
Family nurse practitioner (FNP)
Midwife

Nurse anesthetist
Nurse practitioner (NP)
Nursing centers (NCs)
Primary health care
Translation

LEARNING OBJECTIVES

At the completion of this chapter, the learner will be able to

1. Trace the history of the global development of advanced practice nursing.
2. Integrate biological variations and safety in specific ethnocultural groups in client's therapeutic regimen.
3. Assess use of generic folk remedies and how this impacts prescribed medications and diet.
4. Collaborate with an interprofessional team in managing client health problems.
5. Devise culturally sensitive strategies in the recruitment and retention of minority participants in research.
6. Develop strategies to ensure the performance of the proper steps of translation and back translation of a given instrument.

OVERVIEW

To examine graduate education in nursing, it is imperative that we glimpse at the beginning of the professionalism of nursing in the United States. It has been a long time since the establishment of the first university level school of nursing in the United States at the University of Minnesota in 1909. In the last two decades, there was a marked expansion of both master's and doctoral programs; doctoral programs increased from 220 to 518 institutions and master's programs increased from 180 to 417 (American Association of Colleges of Nursing [AACN], 2006). Globally, there are approximately 6,000 schools of nursing (World Health Organization [WHO], 2006).

Graduate students in the master's and doctoral programs will be—if they are not already—our future practitioners, educators, administrators, and researchers. A nurse prepared at the graduate level is expected to not only be able to serve as a proficient clinician but also as a faculty member in academia, as a role model for novice nurses, as a nurse administrator managing nursing practice, or as a researcher enhancing the knowledge base for the profession (Radzyminski, 2005).

Advanced practice nursing is emerging globally to answer health care needs in terms of lower cost, easier access, service for the underserved, and health maintenance (Sheer & Wong, 2008). In the United States, an approximate 56,000 **nurse practitioners (NP)** practiced in primary care in 2010 compared to only 29,000 physicians (Yee, Boukus, Cross, & Samuel, 2013). The demand for NPs is increasing; care by NPs not only compares favorably with physicians' but also with a proven addition of spending more time with the clients and developing closer relationships (Kiplinger Washington Editors, 2002). The AACN and later the Institute of Medicine (IOM, 2010), called for redirecting Medicare funds from diploma nursing education to the education of NPs at the graduate level and from acute inpatient care to outpatient clinics where many NP students rotate for clinical practice (AACN, n.d.).

This makes it imperative to ensure that graduate curricula contain structured course content in providing culturally and linguistically appropriate services (International Council of Nurses [ICN], 2007; U.S. Department of Health and Human Services, Office of Minority Health, 2013). Germain (2004), applying Leininger's (2006) Culture Care Theory, exhorted the APN's responsibilities as a healer and caregiver in bridging the challenges of caring for diverse populations. Furthermore, the graduate curricula must also develop an improved understanding of relationships between systems, policies, and populations and how these could be used for better health outcomes (Radzyminski, 2005).

Integration of TCN Concepts

The National League for Nursing ([NLN], 2009a, 2009b) provides guidelines and faculty toolkits for the inclusion of diversity and cultural competence in baccalaureate, master's, and doctoral education. The AACN (2009, 2011) has a specific graduate toolkit for master's and doctoral education. **Primary health care** affords an effective framework to maintain health in minority populations (McMurray, 2008). According to the American Academy of Nurse Practitioners (AANP), 89% of NPs in the United States are educated in primary care; of these, more than 75% are actually practicing in primary care settings (Yee et al., 2013).

In master's level programs, transcultural nursing (TCN) concepts need to be integrated in whatever programs are used in preparing **advanced practice nurses (APN)** anesthetists, **clinical specialists,** midwives, NP educators, or combination programs. In addition to threading TCN concepts in vertical and horizontal formats, the offering of separate TCN courses is imperative. Graduate curricula also need to include *Healthy People 2020's* (USDHHS, 2012) mission, goals, and priority health indicators.

Concepts that can be threaded into curricula include lack of diversity among nurses and other health professionals; worsening faculty shortage; disparities in access and quality of care; development of advanced practice nursing globally; complementary and alternative modalities; areas for inclusion research in multicultural populations; care of diverse populations such as lesbian, gay, bisexual, and transgender (LGBT) clients; and efforts to integrate TCN in graduate curricula. The degree of integration depends on the mission and goals of the college or university and that of the school of nursing (SON).

Lack of Diversity Among Nurses

Despite the expansion of graduate education in nursing, there is not much headway about increasing diversity among nursing students. The Sullivan Commission (2004) emphasizes the lack of diversity among nurses and other health care professionals. Notably, this commission report cites that this very lack of diversity and "mirroring" of the clients caused the disparity in access and quality among minority populations. Table 21.1 shows the race/ethnicity of students enrolled in AACN schools offering baccalaureate, master's, and doctoral (research focused) programs in nursing during the years 2002, 2007, and 2011.

Worsening Faculty Shortage

There is an acute shortage of nurse educators; this shortage is predicted to worsen in the next few years. Therefore, it is very important to encourage graduate students to consider a career in academia. There has been graying of the nurse faculty—60% of the existing nursing faculty are 50 years old or older Faculty shortages will increase in the near future (American Nurses Association [ANA], 2011; USDHHS, HRSA, 2010) and are liable to impact the dwindling supply of nurses. A review of Chapter 22, especially Table 22.1, evidencing the "graying of U.S. faculty," will give exigency to this persistent shortage as one of the most difficult and challenging periods in nursing.

The shortage of nurses, however, is not unique to the United States. The WHO (2006) estimates that there are 57 countries with critical shortages of health professionals; these shortages are equivalent to a worldwide deficit of 2.4 million doctors, nurses, and midwives (p. 6). WHO (2006) specifically calls for a decade-long plan of action from 2006 to 2015 from all stakeholders in the areas of preparation of workforce; enhancing productivity; and managing attrition and migration.

Disparities in Quality and Access of Care

Globally, there are 59.2 million full-time paid health workers (WHO, 2006). However, there are glaring inequities in the distribution of human resources for health. The WHO indicates that while the United States and Canada only have 10% of the global burden of disease (GBD), they have 52% of the world's financial resources and 37% of global health workers. In comparison, Asia has 29 GBD, 1% financial resources, and 12% of the health workforce; Africa has 24 GBD with 3% of health service (WHO, 2006). The continuing exodus of health care professionals, mainly nurses, from developing nations to developed countries—termed as nurse drain—is one of the causes of this uneven distribution (Ea, Griffin, L'ePlattenier, & Fitzpatrick, 2008; Tiwari, Sharma, & Zodpey, 2013). Chapter 27 reflects foreign-educated nurses (FENs) and their ongoing migration.

Nursing centers (NCs) across the nation are primary care facilities run by nursing schools and managed by NP faculty. NCs obtain vital seed money from the Nurse

TABLE 21.1 Race/Ethnicity of Students Enrolled in Baccalaureate, Master's, and Doctoral (Research Focused) Programs in Nursing During the Years 2002, 2007, and 2011

	Generic Baccalaureate	Master's	Doctoral
White			
2011	111,417 (72%)	56,075 (73.4%)	3,020 (75.3%)
2007	97,796 (74%)	41,795 (76.5%)	2,773 (79%)
2002	60,911 (52.3%)	25,546 (61.3%)	2,269 (71.6%)
Black/African American			
2011	15,860 (10.3%)	9,661 (12.6%)	478 (11.9%)
2007	15,574 (11.8%)	6,436 (11.8%)	357 (10.2%)
2002	9,338 (8%)	2,903 (7%)	215 (6.8%)
Hispanic or Latino			
2011	10,774 (7.0%)	3917 (5.1%)	189 (4.7%)
2007	7,747 (5.9%)	2,659 (4.9%)	126 (3.6%)
2002	4,649 (4.0%)	1,349 (3.2%)	64 (2.0%)
Asian/Native Hawaiian/ Pacific Islander			
2011	13,576 (8.8%)	5,361 (7%)	236 (5.9%)
2007	10,099 (7.6%)	3,379 (6.2%)	217 (6.2%)
2002	4,409 (3.8%)	1,552 (3.7%)	115 (3.6%)
American Indian or Alaska Native			
2011	835 (0.5%)	509 (0.7%)	55 (1.4%)
2007	894 (0.7%)	353 (0.6%)	35 (1.0%)
2002	460 (0.4%)	197 (0.5%)	16 (0.5%)

Source: Prepared from the American Association of Colleges of Nursing (2012).

Education Act (NEA), the single largest source of federal funding for nursing education (AACN, n.d.). NCs are not only essential clinical training sites for NP students but also the source of basic health services to their proximate communities, including high-risk, vulnerable, and underserved populations (AACN, n.d.). APNs can promote health and alleviate the basic health care needs of people in these places. Nurses have a long history as trailblazers and pioneers, including advocacy for the underserved and vulnerable.

Lillian Wald and Mary Brewster epitomized the care for the underserved and vulnerable population with the establishment of the Henry Street Settlement in 1893. Wald was an indefatigable activist for legislative reforms for equity in access and distribution of available resources (Lundy, 2013). What is less publicized is Wald's commitment to diversity in hiring African Americans, initially Elizabeth Tyler, and later Edith Carter in 1906, to work with

African American families at the settlement (Lundy, 2013). In succeeding years, Wald hired 25 other African American nurses and gave them equal pay as the other nurses (Lundy, 2013). The Henry Street Settlement later evolved into the Visiting Nurse Service of New York (VNSNY). Today, the VNSNY is the largest, not-for-profit home care agency in the United States, providing skilled nursing care, rehabilitation therapy, and home health aide services (VNSNY, 2013).

Development of Advanced Practice Nursing Globally

Worldwide, APN education is developing, a proof that across nations there is increasing recognition of the value of nursing in improving health outcomes, NPs and APNs alleviate deficiency in human resources and health care among developed and developing countries (Pulcini, Jelic, Gul, & Loke, 2009). It is very interesting and enlightening to see the global development of APN. Table 21.2 shows the development of APN in selected countries and continents.

To explore international trends in the developing role of the NP-APN, including types of education and regulation, among others, Pulcini et al. (2009) conducted a cross-sectional descriptive survey among active members of the International NP-APN Network of the ICN. Fifty percent of the 91 respondents from 32 countries identified the master's degree as the most common level of preparation; 48% had licensure maintenance or renewal, whereas most require continuing education (CE) or clinical practice (Pulcini et al., 2009).

Research in Multicultural Populations

Doctoral students in research-focused programs are expected to add to the body of knowledge in professional nursing. Research in particular is much needed to shed more light into the persistent disparities in health care and access among African Americans, Hispanics, Native Americans, and Asians (Agency for Health Care Policy and Research, 2012). Furthermore, there is a huge need for nurse researchers prepared to conduct research with multicultural populations (Leipre, Van Horn, Hu, & Upadhyaya, 2008). Fortier and Bishop (2003) outlined three main categories in their report on the AHRQ research agenda: (1) culturally sensitive interventions, (2) language assistance, and (3) organizational supports for cultural competence. Category 1 includes "competence education and training; racial, ethnic and linguistic concordance; and community health workers and culturally competent health promotion" (Fortier & Bishop, pp. 11–12). Included in category 2 of this report are the impact of trained versus untrained interpreters; cost of language assistance; **translation** of prescription and medication errors, and others (pp. 12–13). Some of the research topics suggested under category 3 are institutionalization of cultural competence activities; surveys and instruments to measure satisfaction or quality of services; and cultural competence self-assessment (Fortier & Bishop, p. 13).

Dialogue regarding cultural issues and the conduct of research is vital. After its formation, a four-member Race and Gender Committee (RGC) at the University of North Carolina at Greensboro organized three seminars and workshops to promote a dialogue of cultural issues pertaining to teaching and research: (1) innovative teaching strategies, (2) recruitment and retention of minority populations in research, (3) instrumentation, (4) language barriers, and (5) grant requirements (Leipre et al., 2008). Among the 70 attendees were faculty, undergraduate, and graduate students. The RGC committee endorsed a systematic approach consisting of needs assessment, planning, implementation, and evaluation of activities. Leipre et al. (2008) also suggested utilization of all existing resources across the institution.

TABLE 21.2 Development of APN in Selected Countries and Continents

Location	Initial Development	Role Titles	Regulation	Level of Education
Africa	2000	NP	Not reported	Master level
America				
Canada	1970s	CNS, NP, APN	Provincial, territorial state	Master level
United States	1940s	CNS, NP, nurse anesthetist, nurse midwife, nurse case manager		Master level, DNP
Asia				
China	1990s in Hong Kong and Taiwan	CNS, NP, APN	Professional certification (HK) National legislation in Taiwan	Master level
Japan	2000	CNS	Professional certification	Master level
Korea	1950	APN	National regulation	Master level
Australia	1990	CNS, NP, APN	State/territory	Master level
Europe				
Belgium	1980s	APN, NP		Master level
Netherlands	1997	APN, NP		Master level
United Kingdom	1991	CNS, NP, ANP	National	Master level

Sources: Adapted from Sheer & Wong (2008); Keeling & Bigbee (2005).

Culturally valid tools are important in obtaining accurate information. To ensure that none of the content is lost during the translation process, the translation of an instrument from one language to another requires back translation to the original. The process of back translation is usually performed by a bilingual individual (Laranjeira, 2012). See EBP 25.1 for more details regarding this research.

Complementary and Alternative Medicine

APNs need to be knowledgeable about complementary and alternative medicine (CAMs) when managing care of clients. There is increasing evidence that clients use CAM along-side western medicine. The interactions and side effects of herbal medications are areas needing inclusion (Campinha-Bacote, 2007). Chapter 14 has additional information about CAMs.

Although the literature suggests that many clients use traditional healing modalities, community health workers (CHWs), research studies exploring the impact of CHWs, and traditional healers are almost nonexistent (Fortier & Bishop, 2003). Specifically, the AHRQ recommends studies that examine the impact of CHW and culturally competent health promotion (CCHPP) programs that improve the access, quality, and use of services (Fortier & Bishop, 2003). These topics are of utmost importance to both master's, and doctoral students. For master's students in the education track, these are important curricular threads in all levels of nursing education. NPs and NP students must include these in their plans for managing client and family care. For doctoral students, these are crucial research areas to add to the body of knowledge in outcome-based, culturally sensitive interventions.

Health Care for Lesbian, Gay, Bisexual, and Transgender Clients

As primary health care providers, APNs will be managing care of lesbian, gay, bisexual, and transgender, (LGBT) clients and their families. The care of LGBT families is generally missing in undergraduate and graduate curricula. The Gay, Lesbian, Straight Education Network (GLSEN, 2011) conducted a survey of 8,584 students of LGBT identity between the ages of 13 and 20 years old from grades 6 to 12 in 50 states as well as the District of Columbia. Sadly, this GLSEN study revealed the continuing evidence of discrimination, harassment, and bullying of LGBT individuals among students. When reading this and similar studies, the importance of exploring the quality of care received by LGBT families cannot be ignored. See Chapter 8, EBP 8.1, for a synopsis of the GLSEN study and for more discussion of LGBT.

Efforts to Integrate TCN in Graduate Curricula

This book contains some examinations of research studies that examine curricular integration of TCN. Campbell-Heider et al. (2006) described the development, implementation, and evaluation of a new family nurse practitioner (FNP) curriculum at the State University of New York at Buffalo. This university implemented a program that built theory and clinical cultural competence utilizing an eclectic approach. Twelve students completed surveys in the form of *cultural quiz, Xenophilia Scale* (Kosmitzki & Pratto, 1994, as cited in Campbell-Heider et al. [2006]), and *Cross Cultural Worldmindedness (CCWM;* Der-karabetian, 1992, as cited in Campbell-Heider et al. [2006]) in the beginning, at the middle, and after completion of the curriculum of the program. Campbell-Heider et al. (2006) illustrated their quest to improve an FNP curriculum seeking to continually foster cultural competence among its graduates. This is a prime example of measuring cultural competence among graduate students.

Sumpter and Carthon (2011) conducted focus groups of undergraduate and graduate students to evaluate student perspectives and recommendations regarding curricular integration of cultural competence (EBP 21.1). Little research has been completed to explore student perceptions of cultural competence in the nursing curricula. The efforts to integrate cultural competence in curricula are geared to prepare graduates to care for diverse populations.

EBP 21.1

Sumpter and Carthon (2011) conducted a qualitative descriptive study as part of the University of Pennsylvania School of Nursing (UPSON) school-wide strategic plan from 2003–2008 to integrate cultural competence in its agenda for research, practice, and education. To fully develop an appreciation of this study and understand its context, it is necessary to review the background of this study.

Background. In line with this goal, UPSON hired a director of diversity affairs and provided an intensive faculty development program of workshops, seminar series, and training sessions. In addition, the school invested in financial resources to support faculty attendance at diversity conferences; to obtain **consultations** with national and international experts; and to engage in diversity recruitment efforts. Furthermore, in 2002, the UPSON formed a Master Teachers Taskforce on Cultural Diversity (MTTCD). The MTTCD's goal was to assess the school curriculum and to offer recommendations for approaches in integrating cultural competence. Important stakeholders comprised the MTTCD: faculty, course directors, program directors, and students. The taskforce, in a period of 5 years, ventured on collecting data about the status of cultural competence in the UPSON curricula. The taskforce culminated with a *Blueprint for Integration of Cultural Competence in the Curriculum (BICC)*. The results of the Sumpter and Carthon (2011) study was used in the development of the BICC.

Inclusion criteria for participants required that they had completed at least one semester of courses at UPSON. The recruitment of participants was done electronically via listservs and flyers at the UPSON. There were five doctoral focus group participants: one male, four females; three White, and two Hispanics; two first-year and three second-year students. The five undergraduate focus group participants did not state their race or ethnicity and were all females; two were second degree and three were traditional baccalaureate students. The UP Institutional Review Board approved the study.

Each focus group lasted between 1.5 to 2 hours and audio-taped and recorded for field notes. Both interview guides were made up of five questions. The baccalaureate guides centered on clinical practice whereas the doctoral guides

(continued)

focused on research. Two moderators conducted the focus groups, one facilitating the discussion and the other acting as recorder. Participants were requested to evaluate the presentation of curricular cultural content in their nursing courses. Students were asked for their concrete recommendations at the end of the focus groups.

Three themes emerged from the focus groups: (1) broadening definition of cultural competence, (2) integrating cultural competence, and (3) missed opportunities (Sumpter & Carthon, 2011, pp. 45–46). The students in the focus groups verbalized concerns about the depth of meaning of cultural competence. Doctoral students voiced concerns about effective recruitment and retention of participants from diverse ethnic groups. Among missed opportunities, students pointed to the need for faculty training in advanced cultural competence and for faculty sharing of personal experiences with diverse populations.

The researchers acknowledged the small number of focus groups as a limitation of this study (Sumpter & Carthon, 2011). To minimize this limitation, the researchers included BSN and doctoral students and used a structured interview guide.

Applications to Practice

■ Investigate your nursing program in terms of integration of diversity and cultural competence.

■ Have you ever conducted a focus group or survey regarding student feedback about curricular integration of cultural concepts? Discuss.

■ If you were to replicate this study, how would you conduct it? What would you change in terms of conceptual framework, sampling, and analysis of findings?

Source: Sumpter & Brooks Carthon (2011).

CRITICAL THINKING EXERCISES 21.1

Graduate Student

1. You often hear that minority health professionals go back and practice in their own community. Describe the advantages of this.
2. What may arise when a practitioner comes back to one's own community to initiate change? Explain.
3. Do you think there is enough content of cultural diversity and promotion of cultural competence integrated in your graduate classes (theory) and in clinical practice?
4. Would you be in favor of integrating TCN concepts in all courses in your current graduate curriculum? If yes, which course would you be in favor of integrating and in which courses do you feel that TCN concepts are not needed? Explain your position.

(continued)

CRITICAL THINKING EXERCISES 21.1 (continued)

Faculty in Academia

1. How many credits do you have in the MS in Nursing program at your school? Is there a separate TCN course or courses? Are TCN concepts threaded throughout the curriculum?
2. How many credits do you have in the Doctoral in Nursing program? Is there a separate TCN course or courses? Are TCN concepts threaded throughout the curriculum?
3. If you do not have a separate TCN course in your graduate program or programs, are you planning to add a 3-credit TCN course? Which current course would you delete? Why?
4. How do you critically appraise diversity and promotion of cultural competence in your graduate curricula? Is student feedback integrated in curricular revision? Describe.

Staff Development Educator

1. Do you have a preceptorship program for master's and/or doctoral students? Describe the criteria for preceptor assignment. Are preceptors remunerated?
2. How do you reinforce and encourage specialty certification in nursing? Are there financial and other rewards for being certified? How are certified nurses recognized?
3. Are you certified in transcultural nursing? If you are certified in TCN, do you plan to renew your certification? Why or why not?

SUMMARY

This chapter examines the huge responsibilities of graduate students as they prepare for their roles as APNs, educators, administrators, and researchers—all change agents in the nursing profession. As change agents, nurses need to be proactive in the implementation of culturally and linguistically appropriate care to all clients. To prepare for this role, graduate students, curricula must include formal, structured courses in diversity and cultural competence.

Graduate students must be proponents of research for minority and vulnerable populations and for ensuring that participants in these research areas are ethically and morally recruited and protected throughout and after the research studies. Further research priorities are suggested in these three main areas: culturally sensitive interventions, language assistance for clients, and organizational support for cultural competence.

REFERENCES

Agency for Healthcare Research and Quality. (2012). *National healthcare disparities report, 2012.* Retrieved June 1, 2013, from www.ahrq.gov/research/findings/nhqrdr/nhdr12/nhdr12_prov.pdf

American Association of Colleges of Nursing. (2006). *The essentials of doctoral education for advanced nursing practice.* Washington, DC: Author. Retrieved July 24, 2013, from www.aacn.nche.edu/publications/position/DNPEssentials.pdf

American Association of Colleges of Nursing. (2009). *Tool kit for cultural competence in masters and doctoral nursing education.* Washington, DC: Author.

American Association of Colleges of Nursing. (2011). *Tool kit for cultural competence in masters and doctoral nursing education.* Washington, DC: Author.

American Association of Colleges of Nursing. (2012). *Race and ethnicity of students*. Washington, DC: Author. Retrieved September 5, 2013, p. 258, table source from www.aacn.nche.edu/research-data/EthnicityTbl.pdf

American Association of Colleges of Nursing. (n.d.). *Fact sheet: Nurse practitioners: The growing solution in health care delivery*. Retrieved September 30, 2013, from www.aacn.nche.edu/media-relations/fact-sheets/nurse-practitioners

American Nurses Association. (2011). *Fact sheet: Registered nurses in the US: Nurses by the numbers*. Retrieved August 2, 2013, from http://nursingworld.org/NursingbytheNumbersFactSheet.aspx

Campbell-Heider, N., Reman, K. P., Austin-Kech, T., Sackett, K., Feeley, T. H., & Wilk, N. C. (2006). Measuring cultural competence in a family nurse practitioner program. *Journal of Multicultural Nursing & Health, 12*(3), 24–34.

Ea, E. E., Griffin, M., L'Eplattenier, N., & Fitzpatrick, J. J. (2008). Job satisfaction and acculturation among Filipino registered nurses. *Journal of Nursing Scholarship, 40*(1), 46–51

Fortier, J. P., & Bishop, D. (2003). *Setting the agenda for research on cultural competence in health care: Final report* (Edited by C. Brach). Rockville, MD: USDHHS, OMH, Agency for Healthcare Research and Quality. Retrieved July 5, 2013, from www.ahrq.gov/research/findings/factsheets/literacy/cultural/cultural.pdf

Gay, Lesbian, & Straight Education Network. (2011). *The 2011 national school climate survey: Key findings on the experiences of lesbian, gay, bisexual, and transgender youth in our nation's school*. Retrieved May 15, 2013, from http://www.glsen.org/binary-data/GLSEN_ATTACHMENTS/file/000/002/2106-1.pdf

Germain, M. (2004). A cultural variable in practice. In L. A. Joel (Ed.), *Advanced practice nursing: Essentials for role development* (pp. 430–454). Philadelphia, PA: F.A. Davis.

International Council of Nurses. (2007). *Position statement: Cultural and linguistic competence*. Retrieved September 6, 2013, from www.icn.ch/images/stories/documents/publications/position_statements/B03_Cultural_Linguistic_Competence.pdf

Keeling, A. W., & Bigbee, J. L. (2005). The history of advanced practice nursing in the United States. In A. B. Hamric, J. A. Spross, & C. M. Hanson (Eds.), *Advanced practice nursing: An integrative approach* (pp. 3–45). St. Louis, MO: Elsevier Saunders.

Kiplinger Washington Editors. (2002). *Nurse practitioners for routine health care*. Retrieved July 13, 2013, from www.npcentral.net/press/kiplinger.shtml

Laranjeira, C. A. (2012). Translation and adaptation of the fatigue severity scale for use in Portugal. *Applied Nursing Research, 25*, 212–217.

Leininger, M. M. (2006). Ethnonursing: A research method to study the theory of culture care. In M. M. Leininger & M. R. McFarland (Eds.), *Culture care diversity and universality: A worldwide nursing theory* (2nd ed., pp. 43–81). Sudbury, MA: Jones & Bartlett.

Leipre, J., Van Horn, E. R., Hu, J., & Upadhyaya, R. C. (2008). Promoting cultural awareness and knowledge among faculty and doctoral students. *Nursing Education Perspectives, 29*(3), 161–164.

Lundy, K. S. (2013). A history of health care and nursing. In K. M. Masters (Ed.), *Role development in professional nursing practice* (3rd ed., pp. 3–46). Burlington, MA: Jones & Bartlett Learning.

McMurray, A. (2008). Culture-specific care for indigenous people: A primary health care perspective. *Contemporary Nurse, 28*, 165–172.

National League for Nursing. (2009a). *A commitment to diversity in nursing and nursing education*. Retrieved August 22, 2013, from www.nln.org/aboutnln/reflection_dialogue/rfl _dial3.htm

National League for Nursing. (2009b). *Diversity toolkit*. Retrieved August 22, 2013, from www.nln.org/facultyprograms/Diversity_Toolkit/index.htm

Pulcini, J., Jelic, M., Gul, R., & Loke, A. Y. (2009). An international survey on advanced practice nursing education, practice, and regulation. *Journal of Nursing Scholarship, 42*(1), 31–39.

Radzyminski, S. (2005). Advances in graduate nursing education: Beyond the advanced practice nurse. *Journal of Nursing Scholarship, 21*(2), 119–125.

Sheer, B., & Wong, F. K. Y. (2008). The development of advanced nursing practice globally. *Journal of Nursing Scholarship, 40*(3), 204–211.

Sullivan Commission. (2004). *Missing persons: Minorities in the health professions: A report of the Sullivan Commission on diversity in the healthcare workforce*. Retrieved January 6, 2013, from www.jointcenter.org/healthpolicy/docs/Sullivan.pdf

Sumpter, D. C., & Brooks Carthon, J. M. (2011). Lost in translation: Student perceptions of cultural competence in undergraduate and graduate nursing curricula. *Journal of Professional Nursing,* 27(1), 43–49. doi: 10.10.16/j.profnurs.201009.005

Tiwari, R. R., Sharma, K., & Zodpey, S. P. (2013). Situational analysis of nursing education and work force in India. *Nursing Outlook,* 129–136. Retrieved May 19, 2013, from http://download.journals.elsevierhealth.com/pdfs/journals/0029–6554/PIIS0029655412001753.pdf

U.S. Department of Health and Human Services, Health Resources Services Administration. (2010). *The registered nurse population: Initial findings from the 2008 National Sample Survey of registered nurses.* Retrieved July 27, 2013, from http://bhpr.hrsa.gov/healthworkforce/rnsurveys/rnsurveyfinal

U.S. Department of Health and Human Services, Health Resources Services Administration. (2012). *About Healthy People 2010.* Retrieved July 27, 2013, from www.healthypeople.gov/2020/Consortium/HP2020Framework.pdf

U.S. Department of Health and Human Services, Office of Minority Health. (2013). *Enhanced national CLAS standards.* Retrieved August 16, 2013, from https://www.thinkculturalhealth.hhs.gov/Content/clas.asp

Visiting Nurse Service of New York. (2013). *Providing non-stop care to a city in need.* Retrieved September 1, 2013, from www.vnsny.org/why-vnsny/vnsny-difference/vnsny-providing-nonstop-care-to-a-city-in-need/.pdf

World Health Organization. (2006). *Working together for health: The world health report 2006.* Retrieved June 1, 2013, from www.who.int/whr/2006/06_overview_en.pdf

Yee, T., Boukus, D., Cross, I., & Samuel, D. (2013). *Primary care workforce shortages: Nurse practitioner scope-of-practice laws and payment policies* (National Institutes for Health Care Reform). Retrieved September 30, 2013, from www.nihcr.org/PCP-Workforce-NPs

TCN Concepts in Faculty Orientation and Mentoring

22

Priscilla Limbo Sagar

Apprentice
Faculty of color
Faculty data form
Faculty orientation
Mentee
Mentoring
Portfolio
Preceptorship
Promotion

Scholarship
Scholarship of application
Scholarship of discovery
Scholarship of integration
Scholarship of teaching
Service
Teaching effectiveness
Tenure

At the completion of this chapter, the learner will be able to

1. Analyze the faculty's role in promoting transcultural nursing (TCN) knowledge among students and colleagues.
2. Evaluate materials for faculty orientation and mentoring.
3. Appraise the role of mentoring in faculty retention.
4. Discuss the three spheres of responsibilities in academia, namely teaching, scholarship, and service, and ways to effectively meet criteria for promotion and tenure for each sphere.
5. Develop documentation for annual evaluations and reappointments.
6. Organize portfolio materials ahead of time for promotion and tenure.

OVERVIEW

In 2011, more than 75,587 qualified applicants were unable to begin nursing school due to faculty shortage; lack of clinical sites, classroom space, and clinical preceptors; and budgetary restrictions (American Association of Colleges of Nursing [AACN], 2012). The AACN further elaborated that of these qualified applicants prevented from starting school, 58,327 were for baccalaureate, 2,906 for registered nurse–baccalaureate in nursing (RN-BS), 13,198 for master's, and 1,156 for doctoral education. This presents a huge problem since one million nurses will be needed in 2014 to fill U.S. health care needs. Nationwide, 60% of the current nursing faculty are 50 years old or older and faculty shortage will intensify in the near future (American Nurses Association [ANA], 2011; U.S. Department of Health and Human Services [USDHHS], Health Resources Services Administration [HRSA], 2010b). The nurse faculty vacancy rate was 6.9 in 2010 (ANA, 2011); a similar but more specific statistic put the vacancy rate at 7.9% in baccalaureate and 5.6% in associate degree programs (National League for Nursing [NLN], 2010). When surveyed regarding the primary obstacle to program expansion, deans and directors for undergraduate programs cited the shortage of clinical sites; deans and directors for graduate programs alluded to faculty shortage (NLN, 2012).

The average ages of nurse faculty have been progressively increasing. For doctorally prepared faculty and respective ranks, the current averages are 60.5 years for professors, 57.1 years for associate professors, and 51.5 years for assistant professors; for master's degree-prepared nurse faculty, the average ages are a few years lower at 57.7 for professors, 56.4 for associate professors, and 50.9 for assistant professors (AACN, 2013). Similarly, in a study by the NLN (2009b), a majority of faculty were in the 46 to 60 and 60 plus age brackets. Table 22.1 outlines the age of nurse educators by rank according to the NLN (2009b) survey. By comparison, the average age of nurses in the practice arena is 45.5 years (ANA, 2011). Overall, nurses in the 55-year-old and older category plan to leave the nursing profession within 3 years; an additional 54,539 anticipate quitting their jobs and are unsure if they will stay in nursing thereafter (USDHHS, HRSA, 2010a).

Lower salary is one of the reasons nurses cite for not choosing the academic setting. Although the average salary of registered nurses is $66,973 (USDHHS, HRSA, 2010a, 2010b), the average salary of nurse educators at the rank of assistant professor of nursing is $55,499 (NLN, 2009c). Faculty with master's preparation receive 33% less than nurse anesthetists, 17% less than head nurses and nurse midwives, and about 12% less than nurse practitioners (NLN, 2009c).

The nurse faculty shortage has reached critical proportions. To attract and retain nurse academicians, it is imperative for nurses to encourage and nurture colleagues and future nurses for academic careers. The continuing faculty shortage is causing nurses in the practice arena to enter academia (Duphily, 2011). Many of these nurses with master's degrees do not have preparation in nursing education. Beres (2006), as cited in Duphily

TABLE 22.1 Age of Nurse Educators by Rank, NLN Survey

Rank	Under Age 30	Age 30–45	Age 46–60	Age 60 and Older
Professor	0.1%	10%	67%	22%
Associate professor	1%	27%	61%	12%
Assistant professor	2.4%	34%	55%	9%
Instructor	1.8%	25%	60%	13%

Source: Developed from National League for Nursing (2009a).

(2011), suggested tapping on the resource of staff development educators (SDEs) who may be considering academia as their next career. In addition to expert clinical knowledge, SDEs already have the experience and skills in planning, implementing, and evaluating educational programs and staff competencies.

In addition to the faculty shortage, there is a huge concern about the lack of minority faculty not just in nursing but in allied health. *Missing Persons* is how the Sullivan Commission (2004) eloquently referred to the marked lack of African Americans, Hispanics, and Native Americans among professional providers in our health care system. The disparities in health care access and quality among these very groups are attributed to the lack of their mirror images among health care professionals. While one-third (34%) of the U.S. population belongs to a racial or ethnic minority (U.S. Census Bureau, 2012), minorities among health professionals show only 9.4% of nurses, 6.1% of physicians, 6.9% of psychologists, and 5% of dentists (Sullivan Commission, 2004; U.S. Commission on Civil Rights, 2010). Parallel disparities are revealed among faculty members in the health professions: less than 10% of baccalaureate and graduate nursing faculties, 8.6% of dental faculties, and 4.2% of medical school faculties (Sullivan Commission, 2004). Although there are some increases among minority enrollments in baccalaureate, master's, and doctoral programs, these are not enough to keep pace with the increasing diversity of the U.S. population. If these trends were to persist, health professionals of the future will bear even less resemblance with population served than it currently does (Sullivan Commission, 2004).

INTEGRATING TRANSCULTURAL CONCEPTS IN FACULTY ORIENTATION AND MENTORING

Faculty orientation to the teaching role and to the division, department, or school of nursing has generated importance with the revolutions in higher education, health care, and information technologies; these create new paradigms in teaching and in the faculty role (Finke, 2005). Many colleges and universities have general orientation programs along with structured division or department-specific orientation activities. The importance attached to diversity and inclusivity may be apparent in the college or university mission and goals and in the school philosophy, mission, goals, and program outcomes.

Orientation: Beginnings in Academia

Orientation is essential whether embarking as a novice faculty or beginning a new job as a seasoned faculty. Finke (2005) analyzed the faculty role and concluded that orientation programs are essential to (1) help new faculty attain teaching competencies, (2) promote socialization to the teaching role, and (3) provide for faculty participation as contributing members of the academic community. Orientation programs that are sustained and last over time tend to be more effective.

During orientation, a look ahead in preparing for **promotion** and **tenure** at the particular college or university needs to be discussed thoroughly; the progress in meeting the institution's expectations can be mapped out as a guide. A timeline is likewise suggested so the new faculty can start developing a plan to meet those guidelines. For example, a plan for promotion in 3 years, for promotion and tenure in the sixth year, and for promotion on the 11th year (Table 22.2). Copies of guidelines for promotion and tenure, institutional peer review process, faculty annual report, and faculty handbook need to be provided and

TABLE 22.2 Length of Service and Projected Application for Promotion and/or Tenure

Length of Service	Rank
3 years	Assistant professor
6 years	Associate professor and tenure
11 years	Professor

reviewed with the new faculty. Many or all of these documents are available on the college or university portal. The faculty needs to be advised to compile documentation of teaching effectiveness; scholarship activities; and service to the profession and the community. In addition to integrating these into the faculty data form—or annual faculty report for contract renewal—these are components to include in the portfolio (a collection of the faculty work evidencing performance and progress) required for promotion and tenure. Materials in the faculty portfolio center on meeting standards and guidelines for teaching, scholarship, and service. The portfolio format depends on the college or university: electronic, compact disk (CD), or hard copy of materials in a binder. The expectations of a division or department should be consistent with the larger institution to avoid conflict (Sauter & Applegate, 2005).

During orientation, it is suggested that the three triads of teaching, scholarship, and service in academia be thoroughly integrated in the systematic **mentoring** plan for the new faculty. In the midst of the faculty shortage, measures are indeed imperative to recruit, nurture, and retain faculty. A faculty member who experienced nurturing and mentoring is more likely to nurture and mentor students or faculty colleagues.

Mentoring: "Nurses Do Not Eat Their Young"

On the shadow side, nurses have seen some colleagues "eat" young and novice nurses. On the sunny side, mentoring is alive and well in nursing. Mentoring has proven its effectiveness not only in nursing academia but also in nursing practice, administration, and research. In some schools of nursing, mentoring is a formal program; in other schools, mentoring relationships are conducted in an informal manner.

Mentoring is not new in nursing; many successful nurses can count at least a mentor or two who has helped them get to where they are as staff nurses, nurse educators, administrators, or researchers. **Mentoring** occurs in a one-to-one relationship; this can be exemplified by a senior and a junior faculty freely entering into an agreement where the senior instructs and guides the junior's career choices over a sustained period of time, oftentimes throughout a career (Vance, 2002, 2011; Vance & Olson, 1998). The person being mentored is called a **mentee.** Mentoring is different from preceptorship. While also on a one-to-one relationship, **precepting** is usually for a school semester or for a year. **Preceptorships,** with definite goals and objectives, are usually contractual or informally arranged; the person who is precepted is often called an **apprentice** (Barnum, 2006).

Mentoring is a necessity in education, practice, administration, and research. In nursing education, the mentoring of new faculty is essential because nurses are not generally prepared in graduate programs for a role in academe (Finke, 2005). Faculty development is vital and should begin with the orientation of new faculty. Mentoring is imperative as the new faculty begin to juggle the three aspects of the academic role: teaching, scholarship, and service.

Duphily (2011) posed the questions of reduction of workload, salary for mentoring position, assignment of mentors, and duration of mentorship. Although mentoring is considered a vital aspect in nurturing the next generation of faculty, it is a consuming responsibility in an already bulging schedule of teaching, advising students, and performing committee work, in addition to being expected to provide service not only to the college or university but to the profession and the community at large.

In TCN, mentoring had been modeled by none other than its foundress, D. Madeleine Leininger. During her decades of TCN leadership up until her passing, Dr. Leininger mentored so many nurses who later themselves mentored others, further contributing to the vast body of TCN knowledge. Before her passing in 2012, Dr. Leininger had entrusted Dr. Marilyn McFarland and Dr. Hiba Wehbe-Alamah with the next editions of *Transcultural Nursing: Concepts, Theories, Research, and Practice* and *Culture Care Diversity and Universality: A Worldwide Nursing Theory* (Andrews, 2012).

Balancing Acts: Teaching, Scholarship, and Service

The challenge of balancing faculty roles in the three triads of teaching, scholarship, and service is daunting; this is doubly daunting for a novice faculty. What counts as scholarship? This may differ in colleges and universities; sometimes it may even vary among departments or divisions in the same institution. Ernest Boyer's definition of scholarship is used in many colleges and universities to give new meaning to scholarship. To define **scholarship**, Ernest Boyer has expanded the vision of scholarship from the traditional teaching and research used in many colleges and universities. Boyer (1997) proposed four separate yet overlapping aspects of scholarship, namely: **scholarship of discovery, scholarship of integration, scholarship of application,** and **scholarship of teaching.** Moreover, Boyer (1997) strongly advocated for collaborative and creative interprofessional education that required a team approach, and in which the

> ...discovery of knowledge, the integration of knowledge, the application of knowledge, and great teaching would be fully honored, powerfully reinforcing one another...a new vision of scholarship is required, one dedicated not only to the renewal of the academy,...but to the renewal of society. (p. 81)

The Institute of Medicine (IOM, 2010) emphasized the importance of interprofessional education in its *Future of Nursing* report. In Table 22.3, examples of faculty activities are listed to illustrate Boyer's (1997) vision of scholarship under the four intersecting aspects of discovery, application, integration, and teaching.

Juggling: Meeting Expectations for Teaching Effectiveness

In most smaller colleges, teaching rather than research is the focus of the faculty role. **Teaching effectiveness** is measured in terms of student evaluations of classroom, laboratory, or clinical teaching; grade distribution; and pedagogical approaches to teaching.

The AACN (2008, 2011) and the NLN (2009a, 2009b) have compiled faculty toolkits for integrating diversity and cultural competence in nursing curricula. These will be very helpful when planning for existing course revisions as well as developing new courses. The pedagogical approaches to teaching and learning are vital areas for new faculty to learn, such as engaging the learners and serving as facilitators of learning.

TABLE 22.3 Sample Documentation of Scholarship TCN Utilizing Boyer's Teaching as a Scholarly Endeavor

Aspects of Scholarship	Documentation of Accomplishment
Discovery Research and generation of new knowledge	Dissertation: The Lived Experience of Vietnamese Nurses: A Case Study Research: Transcultural Content in Baccalaureate Curricula Throughout the United States Research: History of Nursing in the Philippines and Viet Nam
Integration Interprofessional collaboration and synthesis of knowledge; interprofessional education	Development of advanced certification exam in transcultural nursing including reliability and validity study. Sabbatical project: Creation of a Multicultural Center HLT 3000: course for nursing, premedicine, physical therapy, and other allied health students
Application Service to profession of nursing at the local, regional, national, and international levels; publications; leadership in professional organizations, community, national panels and boards	Workshop: Cultural Competence: A Journey Workshop: Cultural Competence: Continuing the Journey Publication (book): *Transcultural Nursing Theory and Models: Application in Nursing Education, Practice, and Administration* Publication (book): *Transcultural Nursing Strategies* President: TCNS Northeast Chapter Standard setting panel: American Nurses Credentialing Center adult health exam Site evaluator: Commission on Collegiate Nursing Education
Teaching Evidence of effective teaching and dissemination of knowledge; sharing with colleagues, presentation, publication; outcomes of working with students; increasing use of technology in education	Publication of a senior baccalaureate student's reflective journals in *Transcultural Nursing Strategies* Publication of a senior RN-BS student's Module on Post-Traumatic Stress Disorder (PTSD) in *Transcultural Nursing Strategies* Book chapters with other faculty in intro to nursing, nursing skills, childbearing, child-rearing, undergraduate, and mental health in *Transcultural Nursing Strategies* Presentation with three other faculty: Bringing Water to the Villages of the World: Applying Leininger's Cultural Care Theory and Models in Nursing Education New courses developed: NUR 5400-Transcultural Nursing, HLT3000-Transcultural Healthcare Developing blended and totally online courses: Bridge to Foundations Nursing Practice; Community Health; Adult Health Seminar; NUR 5040.

Sources: Adapted from: Boyer (1997); Finke (2005).

Brown and Doane (2007) pointed out that a way for educators to engage the learners is for them to approach and live knowledge, exemplifying a quote from Yeats (as cited in Brown & Doane, 2007): "Education is not the filling of a pail, but the lighting of a fire." This entails inciting passion for learning as a journey and not as an end point, always keeping that flame aglow. This applies to education in general and TCN in particular.

To elaborate, what Brown and Doane are emphasizing is the value of knowledge for its practical contribution, for making individuals more effective. In this type of learning, educators need to consistently foster among students that knowledge is not to be obtained but something to be fostered. Educators need to place students at the center of learning and actively engage them as participants in the learning process.

Brown and Doane (2007) likewise place emphasis on the purposeful alignment of education and nursing practice as "nursing education...flowing out of nursing practice" (p. 99). This concept of deliberate alignment of education and practice is vital in academia; both mentor and mentee need to reflect on this partnership. For the mentor, this is a reminder of the continuing commitment in this alignment; for the mentee, this is an initial commitment or a renewal of the need to partner with colleagues in practice in order to enrich the academe. This alignment informs educators of skills critically needed at the bedside; the collaboration enlightens staff development of new trends and resources in education. Recent practice of joint faculty appointments in the university and the hospital bridges this partnership. Another way to achieve such partnership is soliciting school advisory board members from affiliating agencies, all potential employers of SON graduates. It is enlightening to listen to dialogues from both sides at advisory board meetings.

Juggling: Meeting Scholarship Expectations

A proof of being ahead of his time, Boyer (1997) voiced concerns about the lack of minority faculty; he predicted then that tomorrow's faculty will have even more challenges in diverse classrooms. Boyer's concern, echoing in the 1990s, is consistent with what the Sullivan Commission (2004) had eloquently painted as "missing persons" among health care professionals. The ethnocultural diversity in nursing and allied health—its faculty, its workforce, its student enrollments—do not mirror their recipients of care. This lack of mirroring is believed to be one of the causes for the persistent disparities in health care access and quality (Sullivan Commission, 2004).

Currently, evidence suggests that the intellectual and cultural sensitivity of students is deepened when they have opportunities to learn in educational settings with ethnic and racial diversity (U.S. Commission on Civil Rights, 2010). Conversely, it is encouraging for students to see faculty that mirror their diversity; the success of someone from the same background—ethnic or cultural or gender or gender orientation—could inspire and motivate an individual to succeed. Workforce diversity will allow clients to see practitioners sharing the same diversity (Warner, 2005); many believe that this will lessen the disparity in health care access and quality among minority populations. These predominantly Euro American educational settings may prompt many people to ask about experiences of both faculty and students of color. The critical grounded theory study by Hassouneh and Lutz (2013) gives glimpses of how it is to be a **faculty of color** in these schools (EBP 22.1).

Juggling: Meeting Service Expectations

Service to the college or university and to the community at large forms the third corner in the faculty triad. The new faculty may explore service at the school, division, or department; college or university; local, national, or global community; or regional, national, or international organizations of interest. The local chapter or an at-large-chapter of Sigma Theta Tau International Honor Society of Nursing (STTI) is another venue for service. At STTI chapters, the position of faculty counselor may be available as a starting position.

As a rule of thumb, during the first couple of years of a faculty appointment, involvement in service is influenced by other factors in the faculty's life. These first 2 years are characterized by intense learning opportunities and periods of adjustment; however, the faculty must remember to not "spread herself so thin" in the three triads of faculty role, thus preventing early burnout as a nurse academician. Fortunately, at this time, being members of STTI and the Transcultural Nursing Society (TCNS) may be enough for service, especially if the faculty is engaged in other service areas, such as being advisor to a student organization at the school, and a local community involvement, such as facilitating the farmer's market once a week into an inner city.

Joining the TCNS affords access to educational resources including a subscription to the *Journal of Transcultural Nursing*, a discount to TCNS conferences, and a chance to get involved in service as an officer both at the chapter and international organizations. TCNS has 10 chapters and 3 regional liaisons within the United States and an alliance in Australia (TCNS, 2013). For future international and chapter conferences and to contact various chapters, consult the TCNS website at www.tcns.org. Many chapters are involved with mentoring programs that increase awareness of cultural competence and of available resources for culturally and linguistically appropriate services. There is informal mentoring in the Northeast Chapter of TCNS.

EBP 22.1

Hassouneh and Lutz (2013) conducted a study to explore the experiences of faculty of color (FOC) in mostly EuroAmerican schools of nursing in the United States. Using a combination of critical and ground theory approaches, their study sought to explore social processes in the background of social and historical injustices and was aimed at lessening domination and oppression (Hassouneh & Lutz, 2013). The study received Institutional Review Board (IRB) approval.

The 23 participants consisted of 15 African Americans, four Asian Americans, one Native American, and three Latina faculty from nine states and all regions of the United States. The three men and 20 women participants ranged in age from 33 to 65 years old. The academic ranks of the participants were listed as full professors (3), associate professors (5), assistant professors (9), and instructors (6) working at public colleges and universities (private, research intensive, and teaching focused) and community colleges. Recruitment of participants was done through personal contacts, professional organizations, and snowball sampling.

(continued)

In-depth interviews of eight participants were done via face-to-face meetings and by phone for 15 participants. Interviews, lasting from 60 to 90 minutes with an average of 90 minutes, were audio-taped and transcribed verbatim. Topics used for interview guides were "experiences of FOC over time; relationships with others; respect and value; decision making and change; job satisfaction; and recruitment and retention of faculty and students of color." (Hassouneh & Lutz, 2013, p. 155). Data were collected throughout a 22-month period.

The grounded theory of *Surviving and Resisting Controlling Influences: Experiences of FOC in Predominantly Euro-American Schools of Nursing* illucidates the processes that FOC experience in their struggle to survive and fight racism in their schools. Three main processes emerged: *Patterns of Exclusion and Control, Balancing Survival and Resistance,* and *Having Influence* (p. 156). Under Patterns of Exclusion, participants cited "Good Old Girls" challenged by the FOC and maintaining the status quo. FOC experience exclusionary and controlling actions. In Balancing Survival and Resistance, FOC employ awareness of the rules of the game, engaging and disengaging, and managing outcomes. In Having Influence, the FOC (1) influence survival and success of students and FOC and (2) affect practices in SONs and influence health in communities (Hassouneh & Lutz, p. 156). Findings further indicated that FOC work is often "underappreciated, unrewarded, and hidden" (Hassouneh & Lutz, p. 156).

Limitations include intersectionality between individual factors such as race, ethnicity, gender, and class; others were not investigated in terms of possible effects to the FOC. In addition, second interviews were not done with all participants, and many of the participants were African Americans and were juniors in ranking. All these factors need to be analyzed when evaluating the generalizability and transferability of findings.

Applications to Practice

■ Observe some practices at your division/department/school of nursing. Could you relate some of those practices to the findings of this study? Explain.

■ Analyze the composition of your college/university faculty. How many among the full-time faculty are FOC or immigrants? How many among the adjunct or part-time faculty are FOC?

■ Analyze the composition of your division/department/school of nursing faculty. How many among the full-time faculty are FOC or immigrants? How many among the adjunct or part-time faculty are FOC?

■ If you were to replicate this study, how would you conduct it? What would you change in terms of conceptual framework, sampling, and analysis of findings?

Source: Hassouneh & Lutz (2013, June).

CRITICAL THINKING EXERCISES 22.1

Undergraduate Student
1. Compare and contrast the similarities and differences between mentors and preceptors.
2. Do you think preceptors should be paid for their services? Why or why not?
3. Would you be in favor of becoming a preceptor after a year of working as a staff nurse? If yes, what are some of the strategies and rationales you will implement? Why?
4. Do you plan to pursue a master's degree in nursing?

Graduate Student
1. Do you plan to work as a faculty in academia upon graduation? If yes, explain. If not, why?
2. If you do plan to work as an advanced practice nurse, will you consider working part-time in academia? If yes, why? If no, why not?
3. What type of incentives should be in place before you consider a career in academia? Discuss.

Faculty in Academia
1. Have you had mentors throughout your baccalaureate, master's, and doctoral nursing education? Describe your experiences as a mentee.
2. Have you mentored anyone? Describe your experiences as a mentor.
3. Do you suggest mentoring as a component of a faculty orientation program?
4. How long have you been employed in the academic setting? Do you plan to remain in academia?

Staff Development Educator
1. Have you had mentors throughout your baccalaureate, master's, and doctoral nursing education? Describe your experiences as a mentee.
2. Have you mentored anyone? Describe your experiences as a mentor.
3. Do you employ preceptors in your institution? Describe your arrangement with educational institutions in terms of preceptor remuneration, incentives, and recognition.

SUMMARY

There is a nurse faculty shortage of critical proportion. The shortage is predicted to get worse in the near future as faculty reach retirement age. The triad of the faculty role in teaching, scholarship, and service is explained in this chapter, including strategies on how to plan to meet criteria under each triad for promotion and tenure. Using Boyer's (1990) four expanded notions of scholarship—discovery, integration, application, and teaching—a guide was developed and presented to keep track of meeting the college or university expectations for promotion and tenure. The chapter also explores the role of faculty orientation and mentoring to assist in recruitment, retention, and transition to productive faculty roles.

REFERENCES

American Nurses Association. (2011). *Fact sheet: Registered nurses in the US: Nurses by the numbers.* Retrieved August 2, 2013, from http://nursingworld.org/NursingbytheNumbersFactSheet.aspx

American Association of Colleges of Nursing. (2008). *Cultural competency in baccalaureate nursing education.* Washington, DC: Author.

American Association of Colleges of Nursing. (2011). *Toolkit for cultural competence in master's and doctoral nursing education.* Washington, DC: Author.

American Association of Colleges of Nursing. (2012). *Nursing faculty shortage fact sheet.* Retrieved April 19, 2013, from www.aacn.nche.edu/media-relations/FacultyShortageFS.pdf

American Association of Colleges of Nursing. (2013). *Salaries of instructional and administrative nursing faculty in baccalaureate and graduate programs in nursing.* Retrieved July 27, 2013, from www.aacn.nche.edu/research-data/standard-data-reports

Andrews, M. M. (2012). Editorial- Madeleine. *Online Journal of Cultural Competence in Nursing and Healthcare, 2*(4), 1–2. doi:10.9730/. Retrieved March 19, 2013 from http://www.ojccnh.org/2/4/v2n4e1.pdf

Barnum, B. S. (2006). Precepting, not mentoring or teaching: Vive la difference. In J. P. Flynn & M. C. Stack (Eds.), *The role of the preceptor: A guide for nurse educators and clinician* (pp. 1–14). New York, NY: Springer Publishing.

Boyer, E. (1997). *Scholarship reconsidered: Priorities of the professorate.* Princeton, NJ: Carnegie Foundation for the Advancement of Teaching.

Brown, H., & Doane, G. H. (2007). From filling a bucket to lighting a fire: Aligning nursing education and nursing practice. In L. E. Young & B. L. Paterson (Eds.), *Teaching nursing: Developing a student-centered learning environment* (pp. 97–118). Philadelphia, PA: Lippincott Williams & Wilkins.

Duphily, N. (2011). From clinician to academic: The impact of culture on faculty retention in nursing education. *Online Journal of Cultural Competence in Nursing and Healthcare, 1* (3), 13–21. Retrieved March 19, 2013, from www.ojccnh.org/1/3/index.shtml

Finke, L. M. (2005). Teaching in nursing: The faculty role. In D. M. Billings & J. A. Halstead (Eds.), *Teaching in nursing: A guide for faculty* (2nd ed. pp. 3–20). St. Louis, MO: Elsevier Saunders.

Hassouneh, D., & Lutz, K. F. (2013, June). Having influence: Faculty of color having influence in schools of nursing. *Nursing Outlook, 61*(3), 153–163. Retrieved July 29, 2013, from http://dx.doi.org/10.1016.j.outlook.2012.10.002

Institute of Medicine. (2010). *The future of nursing: Focus on education.* Washington, DC: National Academy of Sciences.

National League for Nursing. (2009a). *Age of full-time nurse educators by rank, 2009.* Retrieved July 28, 2013, from www.nln.org/researchgrants/slides/pdf/FC0809_F07.pdf

National League for Nursing. (2009b). *Race-ethnicity of minority full-time nurse educators by rank, 2009.* Retrieved July 28, 2013, from www.nln.org/researchgrants/slides/pdf/FC0809_F09.pdf

National League for Nursing. (2009c). *Executive summary: Findings from the 2009 faculty census.* Retrieved July 28, 2013, from www.nln.org/researchgrants/slides/fc_exec_summary_0809.pdf

National League for Nursing. (2010). *2010 NLN nurse educator shortage fact sheet.* Retrieved July 28, 2013, from www.nln.org/governmentaffairs/pdf/NurseFacultyShortage.pdf

National League for Nursing. (2012). *Executive summary: Findings from the annual survey of schools of nursing academic year 2011–2012.* Retrieved July 28, 2013, from www.nln.org/researchgrants/slides/execsummary2012.pdf

Sauter, M. K., & Applegate, M. H. (2005). Educational program evaluation. In D. M. Billings & J. A. Halstead (Eds.), *Teaching in nursing: A guide for faculty* (2nd ed., pp. 543–599). St. Louis, MO: Elsevier Saunders.

Sullivan Commission. (2004). *Missing persons: Minorities in the health professions: A report of the Sullivan Commission on diversity in the health care workforce.* Retrieved July 26, 2013, from http://health-equity.pitt.edu/40/1/Sullivan_Final_Report_000.pdf

Transcultural Nursing Society. (2013). *TCNS area contacts.* Retrieved August 3, 2013, from www.tcns.org/AreaContacts.html

U.S. Census Bureau. (2012). *U.S. Census Bureau projections show a slower growing, older, more diverse nation a half century from now.* Retrieved August 3, 2013, from www.census.gov/newsroom/releases/archives/population/cb12–243.html

U.S. Commission on Civil Rights. (2010). *Healthcare disparities: A briefing before the United States Commission on Civil Rights.* Retrieved July 26, 2013, from www.usccr.gov/pubs/Healthcare-Disparities.pdf

U.S. Department of Health and Human Services, Health Resources Services Administration. (2010a). *The Registered Nurse population: Initial findings from the 2008 National Sample Survey of registered nurses.* Retrieved July 27, 2013, from http://bhpr.hrsa.gov/healthworkforce/rnsurveys/rnsurveyfinal.pdf

U.S. Department of Health and Human Services, Health Resources Services Administration. (2010b). *HRSA study finds nursing workforce is growing.* Retrieved July 27, 2013, from www.hrsa.gov/about/news/pressreleases/2010/100922nursingworkforce.html

Vance, C. (2002). Leader as mentor. *Nursing Leadership Forum, 7*(2), 83–90.

Vance, C. (2011). *Fast facts for career success in nursing: Making the most of mentoring in a nutshell.* New York, NY: Springer Publishing.

Vance, C., & Olson, R. K. (1998). *The mentor connection in nursing.* New York, NY: Springer Publishing.

Warner, J. R. (2005). Forces and issues influencing curriculum development. In D. M. Billings & J. A. Halstead (Eds.), *Teaching in nursing: A guide for faculty* (2nd ed., pp. 109–124). St. Louis, MO: Elsevier Saunders.

CHAPTER

Staff Orientation and Professional Development

23

Priscilla Limbo Sagar

KEY TERMS

Blended
Employee orientation program (EOP)
Evidence-based practice (EBP)
Fully online
Intranet
Mentor
Mentoring
Nurse residency program (NRP)

Nursing professional development (NPD)
Preceptor
Preceptorship
Staff development
Staff orientation
Transcultural nursing society (TCNS) scholar
Transcultural self-efficacy

LEARNING OBJECTIVES

At the completion of this chapter, the learner will be able to

1. Analyze transcultural nursing (TCN) concepts for inclusion in staff orientation.
2. Discuss the roles of preceptor and preceptee during the orientation phase.
3. Collaborate with an interprofessional team in integrating cultural competence at individual and organizational levels.
4. Differentiate between preceptors and mentors.
5. Critique strategies and modalities of delivering continuing education offerings for staff development.

OVERVIEW

The American Nurses Association (ANA) and the National Nursing Staff Development Organization ([NNSDO], ANA & NNSDO, 2010) describes **nursing professional development (NPD)** as a specialty nursing practice that promotes the "professional development of nurses...in lifelong learning activities to enhance their professional competence and role performance" (p. 3). NPD's core is **evidenced-based practice (EBP)**, the assembling of the best research evidence; expertise in education and practice; and client values to facilitate decision making (ANA & NNSDO, 2010; DiCenso, Ciliska, & Guyatt, 2005; Sackett, Straus, Richardson, Rosenberg, & Haynes, 2000). The end goal of NPD is to safeguard public safety and to enhance quality of care (ANA & NNSDO, 2010). Figure 1.6 in Chapter 1 illustrates the model of NPD specialist practice.

Staff orientation as an area of professional development requires much planning, creativity, and expenditures of resources. Nursing staff education supports and enhances client care and is vital to the development of quality clinical experience for affiliating students (Pugnaire-Gros & Young, 2007). Since the orientation of new employees is expensive, one strategy that is being implemented to enhance nurse retention is nurse residency programs.

Nurse residency programs. The University Health System Consortium (UHC) and the American Association of Colleges of Nursing (AACN) Residency Program was developed out of chief nursing officers' passion for a better educated workforce (AACN, 2013; UHCS/AACN, 2008). This collaboration between AACN and UHCS aims to 1) "expand capacity in baccalaureate programs and 2) develop a residency program to take the novice learner from new graduate to more competent provider" (AACN, 2013, para 1). Presently, there are 92 sites in 30 states that offer the one year residency; to date, more than 26,000 nurses have completed the **nurse residency program (NRP)**. An evidence-based, formal curriculum serves as the framework for the residency. The NRP has an impressive retention of new nurses at 94.3% for the first year of employment at 28 participating organizations (UHCS/AACN, 2008; AACN, 2011), while the general retention rate for new graduate nurses is 30% (AACN, 2013). According to the UHCS and AACN, the NRPs, long-range goal is to alleviate the nursing shortage. NRPs are sometimes referred to as transition-to-practice programs or bridge programs.

In support of AACN's longtime advocacy for NRPs, the Institute of Medicine (IOM, 2010) suggested that the Secretary of Health and Human Services divert money from diploma education to support the implementation of NRPs in rural and underserved areas. Furthermore, the IOM exhorted health care organizations, the Health Resources Service Administration (HRSA) Center for Medicare and Medicaid Services, and philanthropic organizations to fund the development of NRPs in all settings of health care. The effectiveness of these NRPs needs to be monitored in the areas of "improving nurse retention, expanding competencies, and improving patient outcomes" (IOM, 2010, recommendation 3, p. 3).

Staff Orientation

The ANA and NNSDO (2010) define **staff orientation** as the "educational process of introducing individuals who are new to the organization or department to the philosophy, goals, policies, procedures, role expectations, and other factors needed to function in a specific work setting" (p. 45). Staff orientation is the best time to teach the mission and goals of an institution regarding diversity and promotion of cultural competence in both the individual and organizational levels. Orientation programs may involve (1) newly licensed graduate nurses, (2) expert nurses transferring to other units or new institutions, or (3) nurses returning to practice. These groups will have varying needs in terms of orientation. Orientation programs generally have a didactic portion—this may consist of face-to-face classroom learning, self-learning modules, or a blend of the two—and a clinical segment (Mackin & Schmidt, 2006). The clinical portion usually employs preceptors. In some instances, a mentor may also be assigned.

A **preceptor** is a specialist in a profession who provides practical training to a student or novice (Nichols, Davis, & Richardson, 2009) in a one-to-one, time-limited relationship or an assigned duty in a facility as part of orientation to a job or a different role (Barnum, 2006). This contractual relationship involves clear professional objectives. Preceptor programs may vary in structure and process among institutions. Mackin and Schmidt (2006) proposed a **preceptorship** program that is truly integrated with the mission and goals of the facility as well as the philosophy and conceptual framework of the nursing department. In such a program, role modeling by example from staff educators for new staff members is paramount. For example, if the nursing department embraces diversity, examples of how this is done in practice must be manifested for clients, colleagues, and other employees. Criteria for preceptor selection must be in place inclusive of educational preparation, experience, desire, and willingness to help another nurse's professional growth, transition to practice, and readiness to care for clients. Preceptor selection in a facility with a highly competent pool of staff will be less of a problem (Mackin & Schmidt) than in another facility with a smaller pool of competent nurses.

Mentoring, on the other hand, is not an outcome of an assignment, but may result from a preceptorship; a senior person and a junior individual enter in a voluntary one-on-one relationship whereby the mentor coaches and "guides the protégé's career over a sustained period of time" (Barnum, 2006, p. 2). Vance (2002)—a longtime author and leader in mentoring—succinctly stated that the leader mentor engages a vital "development role in the professional socialization and personal career development..." (p. 84) of the protégé. Mentorship promotes safe, quality, evidence-based practice while adding to the scientific body of nursing knowledge. Currently, mentoring relationships are common in nursing academia, practice, administration, and research. These mentoring relationships can occur formally and informally between novice and expert, between peers, and among experts (Vance, 2011).

Mentoring is very much alive in nursing; we need to mentor students and colleagues and ensure that culturally and linguistically appropriate care is part of the equation. This author had experienced the encouragement and support of mentors along the way and firmly believes in giving back as she herself mentors students and professional colleagues. The beauty of mentorship is in the giving and giving back as we ourselves nurture the profession of nursing. More discussions about mentoring can be found in Chapter 22.

There is a shortage of certified transcultural nurses (CTNs) with basic and advanced certification to act as preceptors or mentors in TCN since there are only about 59 nurses with advanced certification (CTN-A) and 22 with basic (CTN-B) certification (Transcultural Nursing Society [TCNS], 2013a). Out of these 81 CTNs, only four nurses practice outside of the United States: one each in Australia, Canada, Israel, and Saudi Arabia (TCNS, 2013a). Eighty-one CTNs are too few—since there are 3,163,133 total registered nurses in the United States alone (USDHHS, HRSA, 2010)—to be able to function as preceptor or mentor for other nurses (Sagar, in press).

The availability of CTN certification is vital information to share among nurses. Administrators, nursing and otherwise, must ensure that incentives for specialty certification must be in place to encourage nurses to pursue this as part of continuing competence and lifelong learning. Among employers of foreign-educated nurses (FENs), preceptorship was cited as having the most impact in successful transition to U.S. practice (Commission on Graduates of Foreign Nursing Schools [CGFNS, 2005], as cited in Davis & Richardson, 2009).

Integration of TCN Concepts

The integration of TCN content in orientation programs will take much creativity on the part of staff educators. Structured orientation programs need to include diversity and promotion of cultural competence. According to Jeffreys and Karczewski (2010), there are five important steps in integrating cultural competence in an **employee orientation program** (EOP):

■ "Assess present employees and clients;
■ Assess existing EOP;
■ Identify trends;
■ Review literature; and
■ Revise EOP" (pp. 287–290).

Employee characteristics (such as age, ethnicity, gender, socioeconomic status, religion, primary language, educational background, and previous work experience) and affective factors (including values and beliefs, **transcultural self-efficacy [TSE]** need to be assessed (Jeffreys & Karczewski, 2010). TSE refers to the individual's perceived confidence in his or her own skills to provide culturally congruent care for diverse populations (Jeffreys, 2010).When designing an EOP, examples that are reflective of client populations, such as their clinical and cultural problems and issues, will be more beneficial. Continuing competence will be discussed more in Chapter 24.

Generally, EOPs are guided by accreditation and agency mandates. The existing cultural competence components should be evaluated for timeliness, relevance, and to ensure they are evidence-based. The teaching and learning strategies must be examined, taking into consideration employee characteristics, learner centeredness, and reflective techniques of relevance to the adult learner (Jeffreys & Karczewski, 2010). The NNSDO standards 1 through 6 can be used to assess, plan, implement, and evaluate compliance with the culturally and linguistically appropriate services (CLAS) standards (USDHHS, OMH, 2013)—as part of orientation and continuing professional **staff development** (Table 23.1).

TABLE 23.1 Standards of Practice for Nursing Professional Development and Suggested Activities for TCN Competence

NNSDO Standard	Suggested Activities for TCN Competence
Assessment. Collects data and information related to educational needs and other pertinent situations.	Local, regional, national, global diversity trends
Identification of issues and trends. Analyzes issues, trends, and data to determine the needs of Individuals Groups Communities	Enhanced CLAS standards facility compliance Language access services (LAS) Organizational compliance
Outcome identification. From 7/15/13-1/15/14	Development of tool to survey multidisciplinary use of the LAS
Planning	Drafts 1, 2, 3: Development of tool to survey multidisciplinary use of the LAS
Implementation	Use of LAS by physicians, nurses, pharmacists, social workers for 2 months
Evaluation	Survey: actual use of LAS by physicians, nurses, pharmacists, social workers

Source: Adapted from American Nurses Association, American Nurses' Association, and National Nursing Staff Development Organization (2010).

Collaboration and Sharing of Resources

Collaboration and sharing of resources in health care has become the rule rather than the exception. This type of collaboration and sharing has infinite possibilities in TCN. Minority nursing and nursing professional organizations, for example, may be available for preceptorship and mentoring programs for new graduates or for newly recruited FENs. In a case study, Sagar (2012) illustrated collaborations between state and minority nursing organizations in easing the transition of newly recruited FENs to U.S. nursing practice (Appendices 19 and 20).

The Transcultural Nursing Society (TCNS, 2013b) has 10 chapters and three regional liaisons throughout the United States, as well as a cooperative alliance in Australia. Some chapters have pooled resources to sponsor workshops. Other chapters have sponsored the annual TCNS conference. Individual or institutional memberships in TCNS include subscription to the *Journal of Transcultural Nursing;* this quarterly journal publishes original TCN research and other articles on diversity and culture. The TCNS website at www.tcns.org offers vast resources inclusive of information for membership, certification, conferences, workshops, and publications. Mentorship is available, including for those who are planning to seek basic (CTN-B) or advanced (CTN-A) certification in transcultural nursing.

When investigating and planning for professional TCN workshops, TCNS has a listing of transcultural nurse scholars with diverse expertise in nursing education, practice, administration, and research. The designation as a **TCNS scholar** recognizes an individual who demonstrates excellence in leadership to advance transcultural nursing and health care research, education, practice, and/or administration on national or global levels. Established in 2004 by TCNS, the TCN scholars' goal is "to promote the advancement of a body of knowledge; initiate and disseminate research, teaching and learning; and the clinical applications of transcultural nursing and health care globally" (TCNS, 2013c, para 2).

Adoption of Delivery Method: Face-to-Face, Blended, Fully Online

For orientation, online and face-to-face modules for diversity and development of cultural competence may be offered (see Module 3.1 Culturally and Linguistically Appropriate Services (CLAS) Standards and Module 3.2 Generic Folk Practices: Theory of Hot and Cold in Chapter 3). TCN content may also be delivered using traditional practices such as face-to-face lectures, simulation, role plays, and case studies. Resorting to **blended** (half face-to-face, half online) or **fully online** delivery is another staff development option, using available technology such as the **intranet**—a computer network within an organization—or the web. Each modality has strengths and limitations; the NPD specialist has to be mindful of the learner's skill sets and type of learning preferred. Some institutions use a combination of the modalities as well as commercially prepared professional development materials.

Free CE may also be accessed through various sites, such as the cultural competence project, *Online Journal of Cultural Competence in Nursing and Health care,* and the U.S. Department of Health and Human Services, as well as other credible sites. Table 24.1 in Chapter 24 contains a listing of free online resources. Membership in state (New York State Nurses Association), national (American Nurses Association), and international (Sigma Theta Tau International Honor Society of Nursing, Transcultural Nursing Society) professional organizations usually includes subscription to journals and online access of databases where nurses can obtain original research articles on diversity and promotion of cultural competence.

Complying With Standards and Guidelines

CLAS. Compliance with culturally and linguistically appropriate services (CLAS) standards needs to be integrated in staff orientation and in all staff development. A copy of the enhanced CLAS (USDHHS, OMH, 2013) must be attached as an appendix to the institutional policy for CLAS. There must be signage posted in strategic places—in languages commonly used in the community—for interpreter and translator availability; this service is provided at no extra cost to the client. The goal of CLAS is to promote equity in health care. Compliance with CLAS includes individual as well as organizational cultural competence.

Annual requirements or "mandatories" refer to life and safety issues designated by the Joint Commission (TJC, 2010a, 2010b, 2013) and the Occupational Safety and Health Administration (U.S. Department of Labor, OSHA, n.d.; O'Shea & Smith, 2002). Included in the mandatory list are fire and safety, back injury prevention, control of infection, electrical safety, and radiation and magnet safety. Other clinical issues include fall prevention and medication error prevention (O'Shea & Smith, 2002). Cultural diversity has become one of the most vital areas of staff development. CE is calculated by dividing the total number of minutes by 50 (Bulmer, 2002). As a general guideline, CE offerings must be evaluated for relevance with the institution's thrust for excellence, prevailing accreditation standards (Bulmer, 2002), and evidence-based practice. In addition, the IOM (2010) emphasized the responsibilities of health care and other organizations to offer programs that are adaptable, flexible, accessible, and impact clinical outcomes. Partnership between academic institutions and health care organizations should foster interprofessional competency programs (IOM, 2010).

All educational services, including continuing education courses, need to be evaluated to determine the level of achievement of learner's objectives. Evaluation is valuable in appraising the quality of education (Wilson, Crockett, & Curtis, 2002), including employee orientation programs. Narayanasamy's (2003) research (EBP Box 23.1) provided a glimpse into nurses' feelings and perceptions about the cultural aspect of client care as well as the inclusion of cultural competence training in the orientation and continuing competence training among nurses.

EBP 23.1

Narayanasamy (2003) conducted a study of 126 registered nurses (RNs) in England in four settings of nursing practice: adults (90), mental health (15), children (15), and learning disabilities (6). The RNs responded to a 4-item cultural care questionnaire that dealt with nurses' feelings about cultural considerations in patient assessments; perception in length of time since recognition of cultural needs; degree of meeting cultural needs; and desire for further education in meeting patient cultural needs.

Findings indicate that 80% of the participants considered cultural needs when performing patient assessments. However, the RNs varied in their last recognition of cultural needs: past week (29%), past month (37%), and past 6 months (22%). Up to 1% of the nurses never recognized cultural needs; other nurses who had not taken consideration of patients' cultural needs cited "several years" (6%) and "past year" (4%). There is a wide range in the degree of feelings pertaining

(continued)

to meeting patients, needs, ranging from not met at all (2%) to poorly met (31%), adequately met (44%), well met (15%), or completely met (5%). Among the participants, 80% desired further education in meeting patients' cultural needs.

Religious needs (28%) ranked highest among the five nursing situations wherein participants responded to patients' cultural needs. The rest of the situations were dietary (26%), culture specific (15%), dying (14%), and communication problems (13%). Because 29 of the participants left this incomplete, the rankings are inconclusive. Narayanasamy (2003) attributed this to poor recall or lack of transcultural care practice.

The small percentage attributed to communication problems needs further investigation since language is essential to navigating the health care system. The Joint Commission (2010b) conducted a study of Florida hospitals; results indicate that despite the availability of interpretation services, health care providers used family members as interpreters. Follow-up research regarding TCN practices among nurses and other health care professionals needs to be a priority for the future.

Applications to Practice

■ Investigate the ability of interpretation and translation services in your practice setting.
■ Analyze your own assessment tool when admitting a new patient. What areas are included in terms of cultural assessment? Do these areas differ from the areas in this study?
■ If you were to revise your assessment tool, what other areas from a TCN theory or model would you include? Explain.

Source: Narayanasamy (2003).

CRITICAL THINKING EXERCISES 23.1

Undergraduate Student
1. You are required to attend orientation sessions every semester and whenever you are assigned in a new affiliating agency.
2. Are these orientation sessions inclusive of preparation to care for culturally diverse clients? Elaborate.
3. Do you think there is enough content of cultural diversity and promotion of cultural competence integrated in the orientation and follow-up programs in your clinical rotations? What other components are lacking? Discuss.

(continued)

CRITICAL THINKING EXERCISES 23.1 *(continued)*

Graduate Student
1. If you were to design an orientation program, what other components would you include in addition to those mentioned here? Why?
2. From the standpoint of a master's prepared nurse—or from someone in the master's program—what are the pressing problems in terms of integrating TCN in education, practice, administration, and research? Describe.
3. From the standpoint of a doctorally prepared nurse—or from someone in the doctoral program—how would you address the problems in question number 2? Explain.

Faculty in Academia
1. How much input do you have in orientation programs with affiliating agencies? Discuss.
2. Have you sought student feedback regarding orientation programs of affiliating agencies on a regular basis? How?
3. Is student feedback integrated in planning future orientation? Discuss.
4. How do you critically appraise orientation programs and their alignment with your program objectives?

Staff Development Educator
1. When planning student orientation, how much input do you allow from affiliating agencies? Discuss.
2. What follow-up activities do you have for students on orientation to ensure that they are comfortable in their learning activities at your facility?
3. How long is your orientation program for new graduates? For new staff transferring from other units or from other facilities?
4. Do you have a bridge program for new graduates? Do you offer this bridge program to newly recruited FENs? Discuss.
5. Do your preceptor and mentoring programs include integration of CLAS standards? Describe.

SUMMARY

Orientation programs are guided by agency and accreditation mandates. This chapter outlines strategies in planning, implementation, and evaluation of orientation programs as part of nursing professional development. There is a focus on ensuring that orientation programs contain TCN concepts to prepare nurses to meet culturally and linguistically appropriate care for increasingly diverse clients in health care. Both preceptorship and mentoring are briefly explored as possibilities to ease the transition to practice for new graduates, for those in new positions, or for newly recruited FENs.

REFERENCES

American Association of Colleges of Nursing. (2011). *UHC/AACN nurse residency program update.* Retrieved October 5, 2013, from www.aacn.nche.edu/leading-initiatives/education-resources/NurseResidencyProgramUpdate.pdf

American Association of Colleges of Nursing. (2013). *Nurse residency program*. Retrieved October 5, 2013, from www.aacn.nche.edu/education-resources/nurse-residency-program

American Nurses Association & National Nursing Staff Development Organization. (2010). *Nursing professional development: Scope & standards of practice*. Silver Spring, MD: Nursesbooks.org.

Barnum, B. S. (2006). Precepting, not mentoring or teaching: Vive le difference. In J. P. Flynn & M. C. Stack (Eds.), *The role of the preceptor: A guide to nurse educators, clinicians, and managers* (2nd ed., pp. 1–14). New York, NY: Springer Publishing.

Bulmer, J. M. (2002). Credentialing. In K. L. O'Shea (Ed.), *Staff development nursing secrets* (pp. 95–99). Philadelphia, PA: Hanley & Belfus.

Davis, C. R., & Richardson, D. R. (2009). Preparing to leave your home country. In B. L. Nichols & C. R. Davis (Eds.), *What you need to know about nursing and health care in the United States* (pp. 1–19). New York, NY: Springer.

DiCenso, A., Guyatt, G., & Ciliska, D. (2005). *Evidence-based nursing: A guide to clinical practice*. St. Louis: MO: Elsevier Mosby.

Institute of Medicine. (2010). *The future of nursing: Leading change, advancing health*. Retrieved October 20, 2012, from www.nap.edu/catalog.php?record_id=12956

Jeffreys, M. R. (Ed.). (2010). *Teaching cultural competence in nursing and health care* (2nd ed.). New York, NY: Springer Publishing.

Jeffreys, M. R., & Karczewski, C. (2010). Case exemplar: Linking strategies-spotlight on employee orientation programs to enhance cultural competence. In M. R. Jeffreys (Ed.), *Teaching cultural competence in nursing and health care* (pp. 285–302). New York, NY: Springer.

Mackin, J., & Schmidt, C. D. (2006). Precepting in acute care. In J. P. Flynn & M. C. Starck (Eds.), *The role of the preceptor: A guide to nurse educators, clinicians, and managers* (2nd ed., pp. 54–110). New York, NY: Springer Publishing.

Narayanasamy, A. (2003). Transcultural nursing: How do nurses respond to cultural needs? *British Journal of Nursing, 12*(3), 185–194.

Nichols, B. L., Davis, C. R., & Richardson, D. R. (2009). Foreign educated nurses in the health care system. In B. L. Nichols & C. R. Davis (Eds.), *What you need to know about nursing and health care in the United States* (pp. 1–19). New York, NY: Springer Publishing.

O'Shea, K. L., & Smith, L. (2002). The mandatories. In K. L. O'Shea (Ed.), *Staff development nursing secrets* (pp. 185–195). Philadelphia, PA: Hanley & Belfus.

Pugnaire-Gros, C., & Young, L. E. (2007). Teaching the McGill Model of Nursing and Client Centered Care: Collaborative strategies for staff education and development. In L. E. Young & B. L. Paterson (Ed.), *Teaching nursing: Developing a student-centered learning environment* (pp. 97–118). Philadelphia, PA: Lippincott Williams & Wilkins.

Sackett, D. L, Straus, S. E., Richardson, W. S., Rosenberg, W., & Haynes, R. B. (2000). *Evidence-based medicine: How to practice and teach EBM*. Edinburgh, Scotland: Churchill Livingstone.

Sagar, P. L. (2012). *Transcultural nursing theory and models: Application in nursing education, practice, and administration*. New York, NY: Springer Publishing.

Sagar, P. L. (in press). Transcultural nursing certification: Its role in nursing education, practice, and administration. In M. M. McFarland & H. Wehbe-Alamah (Eds.), *Culture care diversity and universality: A worldwide theory of nursing* (3rd ed., pp. xx-xx). Sudbury, MA: Jones & Bartlett.

The Joint Commission. (2010a). *Advancing effective communication, cultural competence, and patient-and family-centered care: A roadmap for hospitals*. Oakbrook Terrace, IL: Author.

The Joint Commission. (2010b). *Cultural and linguistic care in area hospitals*. Oakbrook Terrace, IL: Author.

Transcultural Nursing Society. (2013a). *Certification in transcultural nursing*. Retrieved August 29, 2013, from www.tcns.org/Certification.html

Transcultural Nursing Society. (2013b). *Area organizations*. Retrieved August 29, 2013, from http://tcns.org/AreaOrganizations.html

Transcultural Nursing Society. (2013c). *TCNS scholars*. Retrieved August 29, 2013, from http://tcns.org/files/TCNS_Scholars_Directory_for_web.pdf

U.S. Department of Health and Human Services, Health Resources Services Administration. (2010). The registered nurse population: Initial findings from the 2008 National Sample Survey of registered nurses. Retrieved July 27, 2013, from http://bhpr.hrsa.gov/healthworkforce/rnsurveys/rnsurveyfinal.pdf

U.S. Department of Health and Human Services, Office of Minority Health. (2013). *Enhanced national CLAS standards*. Retrieved August 16, 2013, from https://www.thinkculturalhealth.hhs.gov/Content/clas.asp

U.S. Department of Labor, Occupational Health and Safety Administration. (n.d.). *OSHA laws and regulations*. Retrieved August 31, 2013, from https://www.osha.gov/law-regs.html

University Health System Consortium/American Association of Colleges of Nursing. (2008). *Nurse residency program: Executive summary*. Retrieved October 5, 2013, from www.aacn.nche.edu/leading-initiatives/education-resources/NurseResidencyProgramExecSumm.pdf

Vance, C. (2002). Leader as mentor. *Nursing Leadership Forum, 7*(2), 83–90.

Vance, C. (2011). *Fast facts for career in nursing: Making the most of mentoring in a nutshell.* New York, NY: Springer Publishing.

Wilson, R., Crockett, C., & Curtis, B. (2002). Evaluation. In K. L. O'Shea (Ed.), *Staff development nursing secrets* (pp. 149–159). Philadelphia, PA: Hanley & Belfus.

Continuing Competence for Nursing

Priscilla Limbo Sagar

KEY TERMS

Competence
Competency
Continuing competence
Continuing education
Lifelong learning

Mandatories
Professional portfolio
Specialty certification
Staff development specialist
Workplace learning

LEARNING OBJECTIVES

At the completion of this chapter, the learner will be able to

1. Describe the benefits of staff continuing competence education in improving client outcomes.
2. Discuss the benefits of specialty certification, including the basic and advanced certification in transcultural nursing (TCN).
3. Compare mandatory programs for continuing licensure for allied health practitioners, such as physicians, physical therapists, and chiropractors, to those of nursing.
4. Review his or her own staff development policy for continuing staff competence.
5. Discuss evidence-based practice utilized by the institutions to comply with accrediting bodies.
6. Compile learning resources for staff development continuing competence.

OVERVIEW

In 2012, the Board of Directors of the American Board of Nursing Specialties (ABNS, 2012) not only endorsed the *Statement of Continuing Competence for Nursing: A Call to Action* but also encouraged its member organizations to utilize this as the initial point in evaluating and enhancing their assessment and recertification programs. The

Continuing Competence Task Force (CCTF) of the National Board for Certification of Hospice and Palliative Nurses (NBCHPN, 2011) developed the statement. **Continuing competence**, as defined by the CCTF, is "the ongoing commitment of a registered nurse to integrate and apply the knowledge, skills, and judgment with the attitudes, values, and beliefs required to practice safely, effectively, and ethically in a designated role and setting" (NBCHPN, 2011, para 6). To differentiate competence from competency, **competence** is the potential ability to effectively function, whereas **competency** pertains to actual functioning in a specific situation; hence, competence is a prerequisite to competency (Schroeder, as cited by NBCHPN, 2011). Continuing competence is aligned with **lifelong learning**, a concept threaded throughout the curricula instilled early and throughout nursing schools, and highly encouraged by the Institute of Medicine (IOM, 2010) in its *Future of Nursing Report*.

The National Council of State Boards of Nursing (NCSBN, 2005) has acknowledged continued competence as a crucial issue for boards of nursing (BONs) and has been examining this topic since 1985. Although medicine did not pursue the issue of continuing competence until 1998 (NCSBN, 2005), medicine had concentrated on certification and has current programs for maintenance of certification (MOC) using educational and self-assessment programs deemed necessary by member boards (American Board of Medical Specialties [ABMS], 2012). Other professions such as chiropractic medicine and physical therapy, to name a couple, both require **continuing education (CE)**, including a national clearinghouse to avoid duplication (Federations of Chiropractic Licensing Boards [FCLB], 2008; Federations of State Boards of Physical Therapy [FSBPT], 2013).

The NCSBN (2005) has analyzed the practices of experienced nurses to use as a beginning point in determining the best model of continuing competence to apply. In summary, it is not enough, the NCSBN argues, that nurses complete nursing education and pass the National Council Licensing Examination® (NCLEX®). Nurses must also show substantial strides in maintaining their licensure. Some suggested methods include CE and **professional portfolios**. In the meantime, NCSBN urges that nurses, educators, administrators, consumers, BONs, and all stakeholders offer suggestions and feedback regarding this vital issue.

Should mandatory portfolio and/or CE requirements for continued licensure become a reality, it is this author's earnest hope that all BONs will mandate a national standard CE for diversity and cultural competence. Standardization of culturally competent care as part of nursing education, licensure, and continuing competence of all nurses—and eventually for all health care professionals—will strengthen the preparedness of professionals to care for diverse clients, communities, and populations.

Continuing competence in the workplace, also referred to as **workplace learning** (WPL), would bridge the gaps between "the expected state and the actual state" (Schreiner, 2011, p. 254). For example, if the CTN has a goal of 100% utilization of the language access services (LAS) in an institution, planning for a series of workshops for nurses and allied health professionals would be a priority. The National Nursing Staff Development Organization (ANA & NNSDO, 2010) standards can be used in assessment, planning, implementation, and evaluation of this competence. (A review of Table 23.1, Chapter 23, is suggested.) Maintaining competence entails competence assessment and competence development, especially in the area of language, which is arguably essential in navigating client access to health services. Continuing competence may include mandatories and current clinical issues.

Life and safety issues required by The Joint Commission ([TJC], 2013) and the Occupational Safety and Health Administration (U.S. Department of Agriculture [USDA], OSHA, n.d.) are called **mandatories** (O'Shea & Smith, 2002). The *Hospital National Patient Safety Goals* include safety in patient identification, communication, infection control, medication administration, and surgery (TJC, 2013). Life and safety issues include fire, safety, and basic and advanced life support.

Other mandatory topics may include CE requirements for licensure or those required to renew and maintain certification. Some SBON—25 for registered nurses and 24 for licensed practical/licensed vocational nurses—require CE for renewal of licensure (NCSBN, 2005). The CE requirements, as well as the time period, vary from state to state. For example, California nurses need 30 CE every 2 years, whereas nurses from Nebraska only need 20 CE every 2 years (California State Board of Nursing, 2013; Nebraska Department of Health and Human Services, 2012; O'Shea & Smith, 2002). In California, diversity and cultural competence is one of the approved courses; in Nebraska, alternative therapy is among the approved courses.

Specialty certification—or certification in certain nursing specialties such as critical care, emergency, operating room, basic (CTN-B) and advanced (CTN-A)—as well as its role in nursing education, practice, administration, and research (Sagar, in press), must be included among the topics during orientation and continuing competence education. Only about 20% of nurses have specialty certification; in contrast, about 85% to 90% of physicians are certified (NCSBN, 2005). Chapter 26 contains a history of specialty certification in general and of CTN in particular, including research about staff nurses and managers' perceptions about the value of certification.

Some issues may arise in WPL, such as the modality of training, time of training, and pay for training (Schreiner, 2011). Nurses usually juggle personal and professional responsibilities; for example, required training must offer flexibility of time and easy computer access. In addition, electronic learning (e-learning) needs organizational support in areas of training time, ease of access to training, and technical support (Schreiner, 2011). For example, following training for completing online modules on cultural competence, a nurse can be compensated for completing 12 continuing education (CE) hours per year. This demonstrates that the organization values the nurse, holds lifelong learning as important, and ensures compliance with providing cultural competence training for staff.

INTEGRATING TCN CONCEPTS

Complying With Culturally and Linguistically Appropriate Services Standards

Documented disparities exist in health care access and quality in the United States, especially among African Americans, Hispanics, and Native Americans (Sullivan Commission, 2004) and Asian and Pacific Islanders (Agency for Health Care Policy and Research [AHRQ], 2012). The provision of culturally and linguistically appropriate services (CLAS) is one strategy to expedite the elimination of health inequities (USDHHS, OMH, 2013). Health professionals are in strategic points and have the power to assist in generating positive health outcomes for diverse populations through culturally and linguistically appropriate care. It is imperative that health equity be a top priority in health care (USDHHS, OMH, 2013) and that communication and linguistic care of clients and families be central to care as well (TJC, 2010a).

In compliance with CLAS, institutions must integrate this in the orientation of new staff as well as in all staff development and continuing competence requirements. In addition, they must carefully include important provisions in developing, revising, and updating policies and procedures. To reiterate the importance of language in navigating the health care system, a study of 14 hospitals in the state of Florida by The Joint Commission

(TJC, 2010b) revealed that, despite the presence of LAS resources, health care professionals were using family members or those accompanying the clients for interpretation. A review of Module 3.1 Culturally and Linguistically Appropriate Services (CLAS) Standards, Chapter 3, is suggested. During competence training or workshops, Sample Role Play Scenario 24.1 may be used.

APPLICATION: SAMPLE ROLE PLAY SCENARIO 24.1

Staff nurse: The nurse has been taking care of three acutely ill clients at the emergency department (ED). He or she is dressed in scrubs and is in the process of admitting a new client. The nurse proceeds to use the client's daughter as interpreter as she further assesses the client's difficulty in urination.

Serbian client: The client, a 50-year-old man from Serbia, has limited English proficiency (LEP) and is accompanied by his 14-year-old daughter.

Daughter: She looks at her father and appears unsure what to do or say. She speaks English fluently with no accent. She appears hesitant to ask her father about the difficulty of urination.

Nurse supervisor: The nurse supervisor is making rounds and comes into the ED as the staff nurse talks to the client's daughter. How will the supervisor help the ED nurse without embarrassing her? How will the supervisor ensure hospital compliance with CLAS standards and ensure that the client gets appropriate care?

Certified transcultural nurse: She will moderate the discussion following the role playing and will use the following questions as a guide:

1. Examine verbal and nonverbal communication issues in this scenario.
2. Have you ever used a family member or a nonprofessional hospital staff for interpretation and translation purposes? Describe the situation.
3. Discuss the possible applications of this role play in client situations.
4. Have you read The Joint Commission's (2009) linguistic care study among 14 hospitals in Florida? Do you think that study should be replicated? Why?

Staff Development Educator: Debriefing

1. Reflect on the action of the staff nurse. How did you feel?
2. Discuss what you learned. What other learning needs do you have? Explain.
3. Reflect on the changes needed in your own knowledge.
4. In client situations, why do you think interpreters or translators are necessary?

Tapping on Online Learning

Many websites offer unrestricted access to TCN resources, such as full-text research articles, essential reading, and in some cases even free CE credits. These could be assigned for orientation, staff development, maintenance of certification, and continuing competence. Table 24.1 has a sample listing of free online resources for continuing competence education of health care professionals. The **staff development specialist** must evaluate any recommended site for relevance, adequacy, and applicability to institutional and staff needs prior to assigning these learning resources.

TABLE 24.1   A Sample Listing of Free Online Resources for Continuing
Competence Education of Health care Professionals

Agency/Institution/ Owner	Link to Websites	Resources
American Public Health Association, Medical Care	http://journals.lww.com/lww-medicalcare/toc/2012/09002	Free copies of full-text research articles
Online Journal for Cultural Competence in Nursing and Healthcare, University of Michigan at Flint, Funding from U.S. Department of Health and Human Resources, Health Services Administration, Cultural Competence Program	www.ojccnh.org/2/3/index.shtml	Free journal subscription can be used for journal clubs Full-text articles–generally research—are available in print data file (PDF) format.
Transcultural Nursing Society	http://tcns.org	TCN curriculum for certification, standards of TCN practice, TCNS chapters, TCN scholar listing
USDHHS, Office of Minority Health, Think Cultural Health	https://www.thinkculturalhealth.hhs.gov/Content/clas.asp https://ccnm.thinkculturalhealth.hhs.gov	Think–Speak–Act Cultural Health: Part 1 (5 mins) Culturally. CLAS modules; culturally competent care education for nurses, physicians, etc.; free membership and CE; modules on dental health, disaster preparedness, specialty education
Unite for Sight	www.uniteforsight.org/cultural-competency	11 free modules on cultural competence
USDHHS, Health Resources Services Adminstration (HRSA)	www.hrsa.gov/publichealth/healthliteracy	Free modules on health literacy, universal precautions

Sources: All information retrieved September 1, 2013, from American Public Health Association Medical Care (2012); *Online Journal for Cultural Competence in Nursing and Health Care* (2013); Transcultural Nursing Society (2013); Unite for Sight (2013); USDHHS, Health Resources Services Adminstration (www.hrsa.gov/publichealth/healthliteracy); USDHHS, Office of Minority Health (2010).

Using Simulation in Staff Development

Due to decreasing clinical sites, simulation has been increasingly widespread in academic settings. Staff educators have also embraced simulation (Avillion, Holtscheider, & Puetz, 2010). Staff educators have embarked on using simulation for teaching new graduates and experienced nurses. Educators in academia and staff development must be facilitators on the side to enhance critical thinking and clinical judgment among learners. More discussion about the use of simulation in education can be found in Chapter 19.

The use of simulation is not confined to undergraduate nursing. Advanced nursing programs are employing simulation to teach advanced assessment, anesthesia administration and monitoring, communication, and role development (Avillion et al., 2010).

Collaborative Learning Between Hospital Nursing and Colleges and Universities

Ongoing staff development maintains and improves the quality of client care in institutional and community settings; this is of prime importance to strengthen the quality of clinical sites for students (Pugnaire-Gros & Young, 2007). A collaborative learning process between health systems and the university can be used, demonstrating and modeling innovationist ideas and fostering synergy between education and practice. The collaborative, learner-centered learning called the McGill method of education was used for staff education in this example. This collaboration between hospital nursing and university faculty reinforced the connection between the academic and practice settings (Pugnaire-Gros et al., 2007).

Exemplars like the above highlight the bridging of theory into practice and decrease the gap between the two realms. This bridging of theory to practice also dispels what some refer to as "the ivory tower of academia." Without this bridge, Schon (1987) alluded to this divide as the high ground of research and theory that does not solve the complex problems in the murky and swampy lowland of practice. It has been 26 years since Schon (1987) called attention to the lack of congruence between education and practice; however, there is still the huge lag of 8 to 15 years between the generation of new knowledge and its application in practice (Dobbins, Ciliska, Estabrooks, & Hayward, 2005). Indeed, professional curricula must prepare graduates to effectively care for diverse clients in a complex health care system. Partnerships such as this are mutually beneficial for health systems and colleges and universities. As the world's population becomes increasingly multicultural, there is a need to apply transcultural knowledge into client settings of care. The study by Taylor et al. (2011) about student and health care practitioners' intercultural knowledge and practical experiences exemplifies this (EBP 24.1).

EBP 24.1

Taylor et al. (2011) conducted a project to explore the perception of students and health care practitioners regarding intercultural theoretical knowledge and practical experiences as part of planning for employment in another European country or in a multicultural environment. For a conceptual framework, the researchers utilized the Papadopoulos, Tilki, and Taylor (1998, as cited in Taylor et al., 2011) *Model for the Development of Cultural Competence (MDCC)*. The MDCC describes 4 stages of progression to cultural competence: (1) cultural awareness; (2) cultural knowledge; (3) cultural sensitivity; and (4) cultural competence (Andrews et al., 2010; Taylor et al., 2011).

Background of the Study

The European Union is enlarging and Europe is increasingly becoming diverse. The IENE project supports the interchange and best practices between participating

(continued)

nations and aims to develop a model for intercultural education of professional health providers (Taylor et al., 2011). This project was started during the European Year of Intercultural Dialogue.

The health studies ethics subcommittee at Middlesex University approved the project. Participants were recruited from Belgium (10 nurses and other professionals), Bulgaria (23 health care professionals), Germany (19 nursing students in a course about the elderly), Romania (15 beginning nursing students and 25 students in the final year who recently returned from clinical placement in Italy), and the United Kingdom (19 final year students and 7 new professionals) and asked to respond to a questionnaire survey. Except for those recruits from Romania and Belgium, participants had diverse ethnicities. A total of 118 participant questionnaires were used for data analysis (Taylor et al., 2011).

The questionnaire centered on the participants' (1) perceptions of theoretical knowledge development and (2) participation in practical experiences that improve cultural awareness, knowledge, sensitivity, and competence. The questions were developed in English and translated into the particular languages of the participants; back translation verified the accuracy of the translation.

Findings indicated that practical experiences are vital when preparing for employment abroad or for work in a multicultural environment. Health care professionals need preparation and opportunities to learn about other cultures, values, and beliefs and to practice intercultural skills in a "safe environment of an education establishment, facilitated by skilled teachers" (Taylor et al., 2011, p. 188). The researchers pointed out that intercultural experience does not automatically result in knowledge development; the necessary integration of theory and cultural education programs were emphasized. Furthermore, the participants needed more information about regulation concerning diversity, equality, and human rights. No limitation of the study was suggested. As an offshoot of this study, the researchers received more funding from the EU for training nurse faculty for cultural competence education, the next step of their project.

Applications to Practice

■ Do you feel that you had enough theoretical knowledge and practical opportunities to enhance your cultural awareness, knowledge, sensitivity, and competence from your basic nursing program?

■ Discuss the benefits of continuing competence education and training in your ability to provide culturally congruent care to your clients.

■ Have you had cultural competence training this year? Is this required training for your employment, nurse registration, or both? Describe.

■ If you were to replicate this study, what would you do differently in terms of conceptual framework, sampling, and analysis of findings? Explain.

Sources: Taylor et al. (2011); and Papadopoulos (2010).

CRITICAL THINKING EXERCISES 24.1

Undergraduate Student
1. Does your school have a collaboration or partnership with a hospital staff development program? Describe.
2. Would you be in favor of having a collaboration as described in this chapter? If yes, why? If no, why not? Explain.
3. In this nursing program, how is your competence in a certain area reinforced and honed? Describe your optional plans for honing your competence after graduation.

Graduate Student
1. Does the collaboration or partnership between your school and an institution affect the quality of your didactic and clinical courses? Explain.
2. Do you feel that your education prepares you for the "real-world" practice? Are your feedback and suggestions incorporated into improvement of the program? Describe.
3. What continuing competence activities will you engage in on your own after completion of this program? Why?

Faculty in Academia
1. Is there a partnership between your school and a hospital? Describe the provisions of this partnership or collaboration.
2. Are you actively involved in this partnership or collaboration? Explain.
3. How does this partnership/collaboration affect the quality of learning experiences for your undergraduate and graduate students?

Staff Development Educator
1. Do you have a collaboration or partnership with an educational institution? Describe the nature of this collaboration.
2. What areas of continuing competence do you perform yearly for all nursing staff? For all certified nursing assistants? Describe.
3. Have you used free CE on competence? Do you provide incentives for staff to complete this online resource? Describe.
4. Do you provide a certain allowance for every staff nurse, nurse manager, and staff educator to pursue continuing competence education? How long has it been since you attended a workshop/conference on cultural diversity and promotion of cultural competence?

SUMMARY

Continuing competence has become a very vital issue that stakeholders—nurses, state boards, consumer advocates, and others—are analyzing for the most appropriate professional approach. Although 25 state boards of nursing already require CE credits for continued licensure for RNs, other SBONs still have no continuing competence requirements. On the other hand, physicians, physical therapists, and chiropractors—among others in the allied health field—have continuing competence requirements firmly in place. Diversity and cultural competence—if appropriately required among the CE credits topics for continued licensure—will be an effective way to deliver culturally congruent care and continue to eliminate health disparities. To foster continuing competence, it is the important responsibility of the SD specialist to rekindle the flame of lifelong learning among nurses; this has been firmly lighted in nursing schools.

REFERENCES

American Board of Medical Specialties. (2012a). *Maintenance of certification.* Retrieved April 14, 2013, from www.abms.org/Maintenance_of_Certification/ABMS_MOC.aspx

American Board of Nursing Specialties. (2012b). *ABNS endorses statement on continuing competence for nursing: A call to action.* Retrieved April 14, 2013, from www.nursingcertification.org/pdf/ABNS%20Press%20Release%20-%20Continued%20Competence%20Statement%20-%20Jan%202012.pdf

American Nurses' Association & National Nursing Staff Development Organization. (2010). *Nursing professional development: Scope & standards of practice.* Silver Spring, MD: Nursesbooks.org.

American Public Health Association Medical Care. (2012). *Medical Care: Official Journal of the APHA.* Retrieved September 1, 2013, from http://journals.lww.com/lww-medicalcare/toc/2012/09002

Avillion, A., Holtschneider, M. E., & Puetz, L. R. (2010). *Innovations in nursing staff development: Teaching strategies to enhance learner outcomes.* Marblehead, MA: HCPro.

California State Board of Nursing. (2013). *Continuing education for license renewal.* Retrieved August 22, 2013, from www.rn.ca.gov/licensees/ce-renewal.shtml#acceptable

Dobbins, M., Ciliska, D., Estabrooks, C., & Hayward, S. (2005). Changing nursing practice in an organization. In A. DiCenso, G. Guyatt, & D. Ciliska (Eds.), *Evidence-based nursing: A guide to clinical practice* (pp. 172–200). St. Louis, MO: Elsevier Mosby.

Federations of Chiropractic Licensing Boards. (2008). *Protecting the public by promoting excellence in chiropractic regulation.* Retrieved August 31, 2013, from www.fclb.org/AboutFCLB/Resolutions/2008Resolutions.aspx

Federations of State Boards of Physical Therapy. (2013). *The continuing competence model.* Retrieved August 31, 2013, from https://www.fsbpt.org/FreeResources/ContinuingCompetence/ContinuingCompetenceModel.aspx

Institute of Medicine. (2010, October 5). *The future of nursing: Leading change, advancing health.* Washington, DC: National Academies Press.

National Board for Certification of Hospice and Palliative Nurses. (2011). *Statement on continuing competence for nursing: A call to action.* Retrieved April 24, 2013, from www.nursingcertification.org/pdf/Statement%20on%20Continuing%20Competence%20for%20Nursing%20June%2011%20FINAL.pdf

National Council of State Boards of Nursing. (2005). *Meeting the ongoing challenge of continued competence.* Retrieved April 24, 2013, from Nursinghttps://www.ncsbn.org/Continued_Comp_Paper_TestingServices.pdf

Nebraska Department of Health and Human Services. (2011). *Registered nurse/licensed practical nurse renewal information.* Retrieved August 22, 2013, from http://dhhs.ne.gov/publichealth/Pages/crl_nursing_rn-lpn_renewal.aspx

Online Journal for Cultural Competence in Nursing and Healthcare. (2013). University of Michigan at Flint. Retrieved September 1, 2013, from http://ojccnh.org/v3n1.shtml

O'Shea, K. L., & Smith, L. (2002). The mandatories. In K. L. O'Shea (Ed.), *Staff development nursing secrets* (pp. 185–195). Philadelphia, PA: Hanley & Belfus.

Papadopoulos, I. (2010). The Papadopoulos, Tilki, and Taylor Model for the Development of Cultural Competence. In M. K. Douglas & D. F. Pacquiao (Eds.), *Core curriculum for transcultural nursing and health care.* Thousand Oaks, CA: Dual printing as supplement to *Journal of Transcultural Nursing, 21*(1), 116S–119S.

Pugnaire-Gros, C., & Young, L. E. (2007). Teaching the McGill model of nursing and client-centered care: Collaborative strategies for staff education and development. In L. E. Young & B. L. Paterson (Eds.), *Teaching nursing: Developing a student-centered learning environment* (pp. 189–220). Philadelphia, PA: Lippincott, Williams, & Wilkins.

Sagar, P. L. (in press). Transcultural nursing certification: Its role in nursing education, practice, administration, and research. In M. M. McFarland & H. Wehbe-Alamah (Eds.), *Culture care diversity and universality: A worldwide theory of nursing* (3rd ed.). Sudbury, MA: Jones & Bartlett.

Schon, D. A. (1987). *Educating the reflective practitioner.* San Francisco, CA: Jossey Bass.

Schreiner, B. (2011). Staff development and employee training. In T. J. Bristol & J. Zerwekh, *Essentials for e-learning for nurse educators* (pp. 241–256). Philadelphia, PA: F.A. Davis.

Sullivan Commission. (2004). *Missing persons: Minorities in the health professions: A report of the Sullivan Commission on diversity in the health care workforce.* Retrieved July 26, 2013, from http://health-equity.pitt.edu/40/1/Sullivan_Final_Report_000.pdf

Taylor, G., Papadopoulos, I., Dudau, V., Maerten, M., Peltegova, A., & Ziegler, M. (2011). Intercultural education of nurses and health professionals in Europe (IENE). *International Nursing Review, 58*, 188–195.

The Joint Commission. (2010a). *Advancing effective communication, cultural competence, and patient- and family-centered care: A roadmap for hospitals.* Oakbrook Terrace, IL: Author.

The Joint Commission. (2010b). *Cultural and linguistic care in area hospitals.* Oakbrook Terrace, IL: Author.

The Joint Commission. (2013). *Hospital: National patient safety goals.* Retrieved September 1, 2013, from http://www.jointcommission.org/assets/1/6/2013_HAP_NPSG_final_10–23.pdf

Transcultural Nursing Society. (2013). *TCN certification.* Retrieved September 1, 2013, from www.tcns.org

Unite for Sight. (2013). *Cultural competency online course.* Retrieved September 1, 2013, from www.uniteforsight.org/cultural-competency

U.S. Department of Health and Human Services, Office of Minority Health. (2010). *Think–speak–Act cultural health.* Retrieved September 1, 2013, from https://www.thinkculturalhealth.hhs.gov/Content/clas.asp and https://ccnm.thinkculturalhealth.hhs.gov

U.S. Department of Health and Human Services, Office of Minority Health. (2013). *Enhanced national CLAS standards.* Retrieved August 16, 2013, from https://www.thinkculturalhealth.hhs.gov/Content/clas.asp

U.S. Department of Labor, Occupational Health and Safety Administration. (n.d.). *OSHA laws and regulations.* Retrieved August 31, 2013, from https://www.osha.gov/law-regs.html

Preparing Policies and Procedure Guidelines

Priscilla Limbo Sagar

KEY TERMS

Consumers of research
Intranet
Mandates
Nursing clinical development units
Policies

Procedures
Producers of research
Standards of professional nursing practice
Staff development specialists

LEARNING OBJECTIVES

At the completion of this chapter, the learner will be able to

1. Review professional standards of nursing practice and code of ethics for integration in institutional policies and procedure guidelines.
2. Analyze guidelines and mandates for the inclusion of transcultural nursing (TCN) concepts in existing policies and procedures.
3. Develop new policies and procedures for culturally and linguistically appropriate services (CLAS).
4. Collaborate with interprofessional teams in integrating TCN concepts in individual and organizational policies.
5. Analyze methods to integrate accommodations/modifications for people from diverse cultures into existing policies and procedures.
6. Discuss strategies to enhance evidence-based practice (EBP) when developing, revising, or updating policies and procedure guidelines.

OVERVIEW

All nurses are accountable to practice in accord with "recognized **standards of professional nursing practice** and professional code of ethics" (American Nurses Association [ANA], 2010, p. 8). The education, skills, and experience of every nurse determine the level of application of these standards (ANA, 2010). In addition to professional standards, current mandates and guidelines from accrediting bodies and the government are essential when developing institutional policies and procedures. Moreover, it is imperative to use the best evidence available for culturally and linguistically appropriate client care.

Policies and procedures (P&Ps) guide professional practice (Ullrich & Haffer, 2009); these include standards for the nursing profession (ANA, 2010; and National Nursing Staff Development Organization [NNSDO], 2010), as well as directions for performance of specific procedures adopted by institutions. Whether P&Ps are located as hard copies in the units or departments, or are found in electronic formats on intranets (computer systems in an institution) and the Internet, they need to be handy references and resource materials and must be available for convenient access by the staff.

The hard copy format has the advantages of ready accessibility; unaffected by network or power failures; and requires no computer proficiency to access. Disadvantages of hard copies include the bulk of several binders, printing expenses, and only having a limited set of copies in the unit or department. Electronic copies offer the advantage of multiple users having simultaneous access, but is hampered by network and/or power failures and requires computer training. Therefore, having both formats is helpful for quick access. The staff development department usually exercises responsibility for making sure that P&Ps are current, accurate, and evidence-based.

Integration of TCN Concepts

It is vital that the staff development (SD) specialist first review all existing policies and procedures prior to planning concepts for integration. Although this integration is time-consuming and expensive, it can be planned ahead of time to best utilize staff resources. Staff nurses who are pursuing baccalaureate, master's, or doctoral education may need implementation of research utilization (RU) projects. A collaboration between the SD department and these nurses may yield projects for improvement of client outcomes, including those under the wide umbrella of the enhanced CLAS standards (U.S. Department of Health and Human Services [USDHHS], Office of Minority Health [OMH], 2013).

Partnerships with academic institutions enhance both academic and practice settings. In this instance, reviewing toolkits from the American Association of Colleges of Nursing (2008, 2011) and the National League for Nursing (NLN, 2009a, 2009b) is very helpful, since both have faculty toolkits for diversity and cultural competence that need to be incorporated in all levels of nursing curricula. It is imperative that the SD specialist ensure that policies and procedures are consistent with EBP guidelines such as current research, client preferences, and best practices.

Complying With Mandatories

It is imperative that the institution comply with the CLAS standards (USDHHS, OMH, 2013). Institutions receiving federal funding need to comply with CLAS standards 5, 6, 7, and 8 for language access services (LAS). A review of Module 3.1 in Chapter 3 is suggested.

The SD specialist must also monitor for current provisions as well as changes in the National Patient Safety Goals (NPSG) as specified by The Joint Commission (TJC, 2013); for mandates such as those for prevention of infection, and for other safety guidelines from the Occupational Safety and Health Administration (OSHA, 2001) and the Centers for Disease Control and Prevention (CDC, 2009). All these need prioritization and congruence with institutional policies and procedures. Careful documentation of policy and procedure development, updates, and revisions must be completed. Accuracy and comprehensiveness may take longer during the initial preparation of guidelines but may save a lot of time during updates and revisions.

Using Modules in Areas of Nursing Specialties

While awaiting full integration of CLAS standards, using modules for SD and integrating them into existing policies are suggested. Table 24.1 in Chapter 24 contains a listing of websites offering free resources for cultural competence, including continuing education (CE) credits. This book has four full-length SLMs, two in Chapter 3 (Culturally and Linguistically Appropriate Services, Generic Folk Practices: Theory of Hot and Cold); one in Chapter 10 (An Orthodox Child With Asthma); and one in Chapter 13 (Post-traumatic Stress Disorder in Women). Critical care nurses may use **unfolding case** scenario 18.1, depicting a Mexican migrant worker with Chagas disease; and community health nurses may find scenario 17.1, Use of the Purnell Model for Cultural Competence in Community Health Nursing, helpful. The SD specialist may assign any of the modules or unfolding case scenarios as needed.

Nursing specialty certification requires CE credits for continued renewal. Policies must be in place to reinforce motivation and recognition for certification. It is essential that these policies specify reimbursement for certification fees and other expenses incurred to take the examination, along with a paid workday on the day of the examination. Other motivational factors include pay differential, opportunities for advancement, and nonmaterial recognition such as a listing of certified nurses on unit bulletin boards, newsletters, or institutional press releases. Chapter 26 discusses specialty certification as part of credentialing. Nurses, with a specialty certification rate of 20%, lag behind medicine, with a certification rate of 85% to 90% (National Council of State Boards of Nursing [NCSBN], 2005).

Adding Accommodations, Modifications, or Implications for Diverse Clients Into Existing Policies and Procedure Guidelines

Many P&P guides do not contain accommodations for clients from different cultures, including different gender orientations. As the United States becomes increasingly more diverse, these accommodations are necessary. Adding these sections may be time-consuming, but there are strategies that may help. Staff members pursuing baccalaureate, master's, or doctoral degrees usually need to complete projects. These collaborations may be mutually beneficial to the student/staff; students are able to contribute and get recognition for contributing to enhancing nursing practice, and the staff realizes the applicability of theory to practice. The NPD specialist can partner with these staff in creating new policies, procedures, or research utilization (RU) projects. These projects usually have only a minimal cost to the institution.

Adopting Best Practices and Evidence-Based Practice

Although EBP has become a buzz word, there is still a considerable lag of 8 to 15 years between the discovery of new knowledge and its implementation in practice (Dobbins, Ciliska, Estabrooks, & Hayward, 2005). To decrease this time lag, staff can get ready for EBP through journal clubs and **nursing clinical development units (NCDUs)**.

Many practicing nurses do not have the background to use research in practice. Program completion of practicing nurses still shows the majority prepared at the diploma (45.4%) and associate (45.4%) levels, with baccalaureate preparation at 34.2% (USDHHS, HRSA, 2010). The body of TCN knowledge has expanded since Leininger's pioneering work with the Gadsup people in New Guinea (Andrews & Boyle, 2012). The research continuum has on one end all nurse **consumers of research,** or nurses who read research reports to keep updated with new findings that may affect client outcomes (Polit & Beck, 2010). The other end has the **producers of research,** or those who design and implement studies. At the middle of the continuum, Polit and Beck pointed out varied activities such as participation in journal clubs, attendance at research conferences, develoment of a clinical study idea assistance in recruitment of participants, and many others.

Journal clubs may include a critique of research studies, discussions about steps in EBP, or interpretation of findings about improvement of client outcomes in similar facilities and populations. Club meetings may be held during brown bag lunch hours or during change of shifts. For smaller institutions with no library or a librarian, the SD specialist can obtain full text research articles that are available online on websites, such as those listed in Table 24.1.

The use of NCDUs, or clinical development units (CDU), has been implemented in the United Kingdom since the 1980s; NCDUs utilize a team approach to foster SD, EBP, and quality practice (Happell & Martin, 2004). Employing a qualitative approach, Happell and Martin (2004) interviewed 14 NCDU participants from the 2000 and 2001 programs at Centre for Psychiatric Nursing Research and Practice at Victoria, Australia. The structured interview asked about impact, barriers, and outcomes of NCDU. Findings revealed changes in practice, increased positive attitudes of nurses, improved focus on research utilization and EBP, and an expansion in professional development activities inclusive of presentations at conferences (Happell & Martin).

Planning for Revision and Updates Ahead of Time

Planning for updates and revisions of P&Ps ahead of time saves a lot of time at the end. The NPD specialist can file research articles and best practices whether they are organized in hard copies such as folders and binders or in electronic filing systems as preparation for updates, revisions, or the development of new policies and procedures. As an example, the educator may come across a research article about CLAS initiatives at a similar hospital; this can be very beneficial when updating the policies and procedures for compliance with CLAS standards. Two vital sources in this area are documents from TJC titled *Advancing Effective Communication, Cultural Competence, and Patient- and Family-centered Care: A Roadmap for Hospitals* (2010a) and *Cultural and Linguistic Care in Area Hospitals* (2010b). The former is TJC's statement of commitment to CLAS; the latter is TJC's study of 14 Florida hospitals indicating that, even with the availability of LAS, health care workers use family members as interpreters. Aside from strongly suggesting replication of this study, NPD specialists must carefully integrate LAS provisions in all the institution's P&Ps.

These resources can be filed electronically or in hard copy in the folder specific to the policy and procedure. Hasty revision of policies when anticipating accreditation visits places undue pressure among **staff development specialists** in large institutions or requires a heavy burden on a team of one educator at small facilities. In either case, this heavy cost in time and resources may also lead to compromised overall quality of preparation for the visit.

Ensuring Availability of Enhancements for Health care Workers

Human resources are precious in any institution. As the nursing shortage worsens, overtime and short staffing may take its toll in terms of staff welfare and client safety. EBP 25.1 highlights the use of the Fatigue Severity Syndrome (FSS) questionnaire to determine its reliability and validity in measuring fatigue among nurses (Laranjeira, 2012). Policies must be in place regulating regular work hours, overtime (both optional and mandatory), and floating to other units.

The complexity of current health care settings require much clinical judgment, critical thinking, and thinking on one's feet from nurses and other health care workers; these individuals require consistent rest, recharging, and sustenance for body, mind, and spirit. Implications for these call for policies and procedures at the workplace that honor health care workers as human beings and provide benefits that include reimbursements for alternative therapies such as massage, tai chi, yoga, and acupuncture, among others. The availability of onsite classes in yoga, tai chi, meditation, and other disciplines can be promoted, along with gym and equipment facilities.

EBP 25.1

Laranjeira (2012) conducted a study among 424 Portuguese nurses to translate and examine the reliability and validity of the Portuguese version of the Fatigue Severity Syndrome (FSS) questionnaire. The FSS was selected for translation due to its wide use among fatigue scales; its brevity and simplicity; its cost-effectiveness; and its availability in several languages hence, leading to its global acceptance (Laranjeira, p. 213). The FSS was first translated into English; then the Portuguese version was back translated into English by a bilingual individual.

Prior to data collection, the researcher obtained approval from participating health care institutions. The 424 participants (283 females and 141 males) were invited to participate when they reported to the institution for physical examination. Other characteristics of the respondents included average age (30.9), hours of sleep (6), and overtime hours (6). The participants were assured of their voluntary and confidential participation; however, there was no mention of signing informed consents.

Along with the FSS in Portuguese, the researcher administered the Portuguese versions of the Maslach Burnout Inventory (MBI), Depression Anxiety Scale (DAS), and the Visual Analog Scale (VAS) to the 424 nurses. The survey was conducted over a 6-week period. Laranjeira used the Statistical Product and Service Solutions (SPSS) for data analysis.

Results showed the corresponding correlation coefficients between the FSS and the other instruments: with MBI, .55; with DAS, .62; with VAS, .68. These findings illustrate there is enough construct validity. Nurses with less sleep and more hours of work manifested more fatigue. In addition, nurses with less than 5 hours of sleep each night showed an increased tendency to sleep and beginning signs of a decline in cognitive performance.

(continued)

EBP 25.1 *(continued)*

Although nurse participants in this study were recruited from different hospitals, Laranjeira (2012) acknowledged the lack of representativeness of the Portuguese workforce. He suggested further research involving participants from other businesses and studies exploring other variables, such as the number of hours of sleep, overtime hours, and patterns of duty.

Applications to Practice

■ Differentiate between interpreters and translators.
■ Recall your classroom and clinical experiences. Have you had opportunities to use or observe translation services in terms of patient education materials?
■ Analyze the course you are taking/teaching. Is there integration of cultural concepts about translation of materials from one language to another? If yes, in what course? If not, in which course would you include this content?
■ Why is the study of fatigue, quality of work, and patient safety very important in health care?
■ If you were to replicate this study, how would you conduct it? What would you change in terms of conceptual framework, sampling, and analysis of findings?

Source: Laranjeira (2012).

CRITICAL THINKING EXERCISES 25.1

Undergraduate Student
1. Have you referred to P&Ps when checking standards and procedural guidelines during your clinical rotations? Were those P&Ps helpful in your clinical learning? In your integration of theory to practice?
2. Which format of P&Ps would you prefer, electronic or hard copies? Combination of the two? Why?
3. Did you find sections for accommodations of people from diverse cultures in those P&Ps? If you found information, is it up-to-date and evidence-based?
4. Do you think there is enough content of cultural diversity and promotion of cultural competence integrated in those P&Ps?

Graduate Student
1. Have you ever been involved in development, revisions, and updating of P&Ps either at your own institution or at another wherein you are pursuing your practice? Describe what areas, if any.
2. As a consumer of P&Ps, how helpful were those as a reference in clinical units or departments? Explain.
3. How would you rate P&Ps in your own institution in terms of accuracy, completeness, recency, and EBP content? Compare and contrast.
4. If you were to use a theory or model to guide P&Ps in your institution, which one would you select? Why?

(continued)

> **CRITICAL THINKING EXERCISES 25.1** *(continued)*
>
> **Faculty in Academia**
> 1. As a faculty, how would you rate the P&Ps at your SONs in terms of accuracy, completeness, recency, and EBP content? Compare and contrast.
> 2. As a faculty, how would you rate the P&Ps at affiliating institutions in terms of accuracy, completeness, recency, and EBP content? Compare and contrast.
>
> 3. Do you have a partnership with a health care institution? If you do, do you find more consistency in terms of what you teach at the school of nursing (SON) and the P&Ps at the partner institution? Explain.
> 4. Have you ever provided consultation in the development, revisions, and updating of P&Ps at your SON's affiliating institutions? At other facilities? Describe.
>
> **Staff Development Educator**
> 1. Analyze the system of staff development at your work setting. Are there similarities in your system and the NCDU discussed in this research? Are there differences between your system and the one described here?
> 2. How many staff development educators do you have in your institution? How many of you are responsible for the development, revision, and updating of P&Ps?
> 3. Do you have a systematic plan for developing, revising, and updating current P&Ps? Describe your systematic plan.
> 4. Do you plan ahead of accreditation visits to develop, revise, and update P&Ps? How do you ensure that you use current references for this development, revisions, and updates?
> 5. Have you collaborated with your staff who are currently pursuing further education in the preparation, revision, and updating of P&Ps? Describe.

SUMMARY

All nurses are duty bound to practice in accordance with professional nursing standards and the code of ethics. Policies and procedures (P&Ps) guide nursing services in institutions. As such, it is vital that P&Ps are consistent with CLAS standards and other available guidelines, mandates, and EBP. The NPD specialist is responsible for ensuring that these guidelines are updated, revised, evidence-based, and consistent with mandates from accrediting bodies and government regulating agencies. Strategies are discussed in planning ahead for P&P updates, revision, or development. The NPD specialist must keep abreast of new information from accrediting bodies and government regulating agencies. P&Ps need to include accommodation for clients with different cultures, gender, or sexual orientation.

REFERENCES

American Association of Colleges of Nursing. (2008). *Cultural competency in baccalaureate nursing education*. Washington, DC: Author.

American Association of Colleges of Nursing. (2011). *Toolkit for cultural competence in master's and doctoral nursing education*. Washington, DC: Author.

American Nurses Association. (2010). *Nursing's social policy statement: The essence of the profession.* Silver Springs, MD: Nursesbooks.org

American Nurses Association & National Nursing Staff Development Organization. (2010). *Nursing professional development: Scope & standards of practice.* Silver Spring, MD: Nursesbooks.org.

Andrews, M. M., & Boyle J. S. (2012). *Transcultural concepts in nursing care* (6th ed.). Philadelphia, PA: Wolters Kluwer/Lippincott Williams & Wilkins.

Centers for Disease Control and Prevention. (2009). *The direct medical costs of healthcare-associated infections in U.S. hospitals and the benefits of prevention.* Retrieved September 2, 2013, from www.cdc.gov/HAI/pdfs/hai/Scott_CostPaper.pdf

Dobbins, M., Ciliska, D., Estabrooks, C., & Hayward. (2005). Changing nursing practice in an organization. In A. DiCenso, G. Guyatt, & D. Ciliska (Eds.), *Evidence-based nursing: A guide to clinical practice* (pp. 172–200). St. Louis, MO: Elsevier Mosby.

Happell, B., & Martin, T. (2004). Exploring the impact of the implementation of a nursing clinical development unit program: What outcomes are evident? *International Journal of Mental Health Nursing, 13,* 177–184. Retrieved March 28, 2013, from http://0-content.ebscohost.com.opac.acc.msmc.edu/pdf14_16/pdf/2004/KLH/01Sep04/14359202.pdf?

Laranjeira, C. A. (2012). Translation and adaptation of the Fatigue Severity Scale for use in Portugal. *Applied Nursing Research, 25,* 212–217.

National Council of State Boards of Nursing. (2005). *Meeting the ongoing challenge of continued competence.* Retrieved April 24, 2013, from www.ncsbn.org/Continued_Comp_Paper_TestingServices.pdf

National League for Nursing. (2009a). *A commitment to diversity in nursing and nursing education.* Retrieved August 22, 2013, from NLN website: www.nln.org/aboutnln/reflection_dialogue/rfl_dial3.htm

National League for Nursing. (2009b). *Diversity toolkit.* Retrieved August 22, 2013, from www.nln.org/facultyprograms/Diversity_Toolkit/index.htm

Polit, D. F., & Beck, C. T. (2010). *Essentials of nursing research: Appraising evidence for nursing practice* (7th ed.). Philadelphia, PA: Wolters Kluwer/Lippincott, Williams, & Wilkins.

The Joint Commission. (2010a). *Advancing effective communication, cultural competence, and patient- and family-centered care: A roadmap for hospitals.* Oakbrook Terrace, IL: Author.

The Joint Commission. (2010b). *Cultural and linguistic care in area hospitals.* Oakbrook Terrace, IL: Author.

The Joint Commission. (2013). *Hospital: National patient safety goals.* Retrieved September 1, 2013, from www.jointcommission.org/assets/1/6/2013_HAP_NPSG_final_10–23.pdf

Ullrich, S., & Haffer, A. (2009). *Precepting in nursing: Developing an effective workforce.* Sudbury, MA: Jones & Bartlett.

U.S. Department of Health and Human Services, Office of Minority Health. (2013). *Enhanced national CLAS standards.* Retrieved August 16, 2013, from https://www.thinkculturalhealth.hhs.gov/Content/clas.asp

U.S. Department of Health and Human Services, Health Resources Services Administration. (2010). *The registered nurse population: Initial findings from the 2008 National Sample Survey of registered nurses.* Retrieved July 27, 2013, from http://bhpr.hrsa.gov/healthworkforce/rnsurveys/rnsurveyfinal.pdf

U.S. Department of Labor, Occupational Safety and Health Administration. (2001). *Bloodborne pathogens.* Retrieved August 26, 2013, from https://www.osha.gov/pls/oshaweb/owadisp.show_document?p_table=STANDARDS&p_id=10051

Preparing for Credentialing

26

Priscilla Limbo Sagar

KEY TERMS

Accreditation

Advanced transcultural nursing certification (CTN-A)

Basic transcultural nursing certification (CTN-B)

Certification

Credentialing

Credentials

Magnet recognition program (MRP)

Pathway to excellence (PEP)

Recertification

LEARNING OBJECTIVES

At the completion of this chapter, the learner will be able to

1. Examine transcultural nursing (TCN) concepts for inclusion in credentialing for nurses.
2. Collaborate with interprofessional teams in integrating TCN concepts at individual and organizational levels.
3. Discuss the evolution of certification in nursing in general and of TCN certification in particular.
4. Analyze factors preventing nurses from seeking certification or renewing certification.
5. Develop strategies for fostering specialty certification among nurses.
6. Evaluate transcultural concepts in magnet recognition program.

OVERVIEW

The International Council of Nurses (ICN, 2009) refers to **credentialing** as the processes used for designating achievement of standards set by governmental or nongovernmental agencies qualified to grant that approval to individuals, programs, or institutions. "Credentialing is a means of assuring quality and protecting the public" (ICN, 2009, p. 1); this is gaining prominence and importance as health systems endeavor to improve quality of services and enhance public safety.

As nurses earn academic degrees and certification **credentials**; these credentials, at times, could be difficult to list. According to Smolenski (2010), there are six types of credentials that can be used after a nurse's name: degree, licensure, state designation, national certification, awards or honors, and other certifications. Degree credentials are awarded upon completion of an educational program.

After completion of an educational program and passing of a national licensure exam such as the National Council Licensing Examination for registered nurses (NCLEX-RN®; National Council of State Boards of Nursing [NCSBN], 2013), a licensure credential is awarded. Required or state-designated credentials pertain to those beyond basic licensure and are entitlements to practice at a more advanced level statewide (Smolenski, 2010). A nationally acknowledged and accredited certifying body awards national certification after successful completion of an examination. Awards or honors are bestowed to nurses for outstanding service or accomplishments in a specific area. Other certifications may be awarded for additional skills acquired through education or testing (Smolenski, 2010). When nurses have more than one credential, Smolenski suggested adding the credentials to one's name in descending order, from the least likely to be "taken away" (p. 5). For example, "Katrina Henri, EdD, RN, ACNS-BC, CTN-A": EdD is least likely to be taken away. The RN license can be revoked; likewise, national certifications such as the board certification in adult health or in advanced transcultural nursing are subject to renewal.

Certification is a procedure whereby a nongovernmental agency or organization verifies "that an individual licensed to practice a profession has met certain predetermined standards specified by that profession for specialty practice" (ANA, 1979, as cited by American Nurses Credentialing Center [ANCC], 2009a, para 2). The purpose of certification is to assure the public that the professional individual has proficiency in a body of knowledge and has developed skills in a particular specialty. The Accreditation Board of Nursing Specialties (ABNS) Accrediting Council was founded in 1991 to foster consistency in nursing certification and to enhance public awareness of the value of certification (ABNSC, 2010). In 2009, in light of the need for an independent accreditation entity, the ABNS Accreditation Council became the Accreditation Board for Specialty Nursing Certification (ABSNC, 2010). ANCC was accredited by the ABNSC.

ANCC recently completed its journey toward International Organization for Standardization (ISO) 9001 certifications of all of its programs (ANCC, 2013c). The largest global designer of voluntary international standards was founded in 1947; with 164 national members, ISO (2013) offers "state of the art requirements for products, services and sound practice helping to make industry more efficient and effective" (para 1). By means of global consensus, national members alleviate barriers to international trade (ISO, 2013). ANCC (2013c) believes that the global quality management systems (QMS) that ISO bestows not only ensures uniform policies but also gives the assurance that products and services are the same quality worldwide; hence, all applicants from other parts of the globe have equal chances in the credentialing process. In going for the ISO certification, ANCC (2013c) emphasizes its valuing of the credentialing process and its willingness to undertake the same level of scrutiny that it requires of its clients.

There was the increasing need to maximize congruence among licensure, accreditation, certification, and education. To meet this need, representatives from each of these bodies established the organization *Licensure, Accreditation, Certification, and Education* (LACE); its members are made up of organizations that affect any of the four entities (ABNSC, 2010). In addition to congruency between each body, LACE aims to enhance the capacity of advance practice registered nurses (APRNs) to deliver safe and effective care.

Nursing practice and nursing education are intertwined. When discussing credentialing in practice, a similar process of ensuring quality and public protection occurs in academia. Box 26.1 outlines information about the two accrediting bodies available for programs

BOX 26.1   ACCREDITATION IN NURSING EDUCATION

Accreditation is "a process of peer evaluation of educational institutions and programs to ensure an acceptable level of quality" (CCNE, 2009, p. 11). Accreditation of higher education in the United States is a distinctive voluntary and nongovernment process. Individual states approve nursing programs based on meeting certain regulatory criteria. Accreditation reviews of nursing programs are performed by either the CCNE (2013) or the ACEN (2013a). Both AACN and NLN are committed to diversity and have faculty toolkits for integrating TCN concepts in nursing curricula (AACN, 2008, 2011; NLN, 2009a, 2009b).

AACN members established CCNE in 1998 as an accrediting body focused exclusively on baccalaureate and graduate degree nursing programs (CCNE, 2009). CCNE (2009), as an organization, believes that baccalaureate and graduate degree nursing programs "have unique goals and outcomes that should be supported and encouraged through an effective accrediting body" (p. 3). Officially recognized by the U.S. Secretary of Education as a national accreditation agency, CCNE is an independent accrediting agency devoted to the advancement of the health of the public. CCNE "ensures the quality and integrity of baccalaureate, graduate, and residency programs in nursing" (CCNE, 2013b, para 1).

The accreditation of nursing education programs started in 1893 with the establishment of the American Society of Superintendents of Training Schools for Nurses; its purpose was to establish standards for training of nurses (ACEN, 2013b). In 1912, this organization became the National League of Nursing Education (NLNE). In its effort to improve nursing school standards, the NLNE published *A Standard Curriculum for Schools of Nursing* in 1917 (ACEN, 2013b).

According to ACEN (2013b), the NLNE started accreditation of nursing programs in 1938. In 1996, NLN established the National League for Nursing Accreditation Commission (NLNAC) as a separate accreditation entity (ACEN, 2013b). NLNAC changed its name to ACEN in 2013. An independent subsidiary of the NLN, ACEN performs the accreditation of all levels of nursing programs both postsecondary and higher degree (ACEN, 2013a). ACEN is recognized by both the U.S. Department of Education (USDOE) and Council for Higher Education Accreditation (CHEA) as the only accrediting agency to offer accreditation for all six types of nursing programs: clinical doctorate, master's/postmaster's certificate, baccalaureate, associate, diploma, and practical (ACEN 2013a).

Information about application for accreditation can be found at the CCNE and ACEN websites at www.aacn.nche.edu/ccne-accreditation and http://acenursing.org/, respectively. Guidelines for preparation for self-study and site visit are also contained on those websites.

Both accrediting bodies implement peer review processes and examine the compliance with key elements under each accreditation standard. Similarly, CCNE and ACEN evaluate these areas: mission and governance; institutional support and resources; curriculum, teaching, and learning; and program effectiveness.

Integration of diversity and cultural competence in the self-study report may include essential elements such as vertical and horizontal curricular threads; classroom and clinical assignments; recruitment, retention, and engagement of

BOX 26.1 ACCREDITATION IN NURSING EDUCATION (*continued*)

minority students; academic support that includes those of English as a second language (ESL) students; and use of tools to measure student, faculty, and graduate cultural competence. Samples of evidence of curricular integration must be available to the site visitors.

in nursing: Commission on Collegiate Nursing Education (CCNE), a subsidiary of the American Association of Colleges of Nursing (AACN), and Accreditation Commission for Education in Nursing (ACEN), a subsidiary of the National League for Nursing (NLN).

SPECIALTY NURSING CERTIFICATION

Nursing curricula has embraced lifelong learning. While still students, nurses developed a keen awareness of the need to further their education beyond graduation. Many nurses aim to hone their knowledge and skills and to prepare to care for clients in the ever changing health care arena. *The Future of Nursing*, the Institute of Medicine's (2010) report, calls upon nurses, faculty, and student nurses "... to engage in lifelong learning to gain the competencies needed to provide care for diverse population across the life span" (IOM, 2010, p. 5). Certification is in line with lifelong learning.

Certification is aligned with lifelong learning; it is a process of awarding recognition for meeting criteria of specialty practice (Davis, 2011; Eisemon & Cline, 2006; Fights, 2012; Wolgin, 1998). Specialty certification started in 1946 when the American Association of Nurse Anesthetists (AANA) required certification for entrance into nurse anesthesia practice (Wolgin, 1998). In 1971, the American College of Nurse Midwives began requiring certification. Three years later, the ANA started offering specialty certification programs (Wolgin, 1998).

The American Nurses Credentialing Center (ANCC), a subsidiary of the ANA, is the largest and most prestigious credentialing organization in nursing. In addition to offering specialty certification in nursing, the ANCC also developed the **Magnet Recognition Program** (MRP), **Pathway to Excellence program** (PEP), and certification of continuing education programs (ANCC, 2009a, 2009b). In 1966, the ANCC reported that 111,164 nurses had obtained certification in 16 specialties; those figures included 2,078 nurses who held certification in staff development (Kelly-Thomas, 1998). Between 1990 and 2009, the ANCC certified more than 250,000 nurses and approximately 75,000 advanced practice nurses (ANCC, 2009a).

Piazza, Donohue, Dykes, Griffin, and Fitzpatrick (2006) conducted a descriptive comparative study among nurses in a 174-bed acute care hospital in Connecticut to validate the overall value of certification. A total of 103 (39%)—out of the 259 participants in this nurse empowerment study—had obtained national certification. The respondents worked as staff nurses (72.2%), administrators (12%), and advanced practice nurses (3.5%); 69% worked in the day shift (Piazza et al., 2006). The registered nurses (RNs) in the Piazza et al. study (2006) had a total CWEQ-II score of 21.28 out of 30, which indicated moderate levels of empowerment. There were high levels of scores of empowerment among administrators, while those of APRNs, like the staff nurses, indicated moderate empowerment. The findings of the Piazza et al. study showed a positive effect on the empowerment levels of the nurses resulting from specialty certification; this empowerment may then enhance work effectiveness.

The study by Kendall-Gallagher, Aiken, Sloane, and Cimiotti (2011) links nurse specialty certification among baccalaureate-prepared nurses with improved patient outcomes and higher proportions of baccalaureate-prepared nurses on staff. Kendall-Gallagher et al., used secondary data for this nurse survey, in combination with data from the American Hospital Association (AHA) and deidentified hospital abstracts of 1,283,241 surgical patients from 652 hospitals in California, Florida, New Jersey, and Pennsylvania. A noteworthy finding was the correlation of nurse specialty certification among baccalaureate-prepared nurses or higher degrees with decreased surgical mortality (Kendall-Gallagher et al., 2011). Studies similar to Piazza et al. (2006) and Kendall-Gallagher (2011) must be conducted in order to add to the body of knowledge regarding specialty certification and outcomes for both clients and nurses.

Maintaining certification is a further indication of commitment to lifelong learning, professional recognition, and refinement of skills (Davis, 2011; Eisemon & Cline, 2006). Commonly cited barriers to seeking certification include cost of examination, lack of support and reward system, and access to course materials to prepare for the exam (ABNS, 2006). EBP 26.1 contains the synopsis of the ABNS study on the value of certification.

EBP 26.1

Employing the Perceived Value of Certification Tool (PVCT), the ABNS conducted a *Value of Certification Survey (VCS)* among its 20 (83%) member organizations. The participant organizations used the online survey hosted by the Professional Examination Service from March 31 through June 10, 2005.

The PVCT, containing 18 value statements related to certification, has been proven as a reliable tool. Before the study, the ABNS Research Committee initially conducted a pilot study along with two representatives from each of the 20 organizations. Among the 20 participant organizations to the survey were the American Academy of Nurse Practitioners, American Board of Perianesthesia Nursing Certification, American Nurses Credentialing Center, National Certification Board for Diabetes Education, Oncology Nursing Certification Corporation, Orthopedic Nurses Certification Board, Pediatric Nursing Certification Board, and Rehabilitation Nursing Certification Board.

All 20 (83%) ABNS member organizations cooperated and encouraged their nurse members to participate in the survey. ABNS requested all organizations to also select a nurse manager sample in equal numbers to the certified and noncertified samples. Of the total 94,768 respondents to the VCS, 8,615 (75%) were certified nurses and 2,812 (25%) were noncertified nurses. Among the noncertified nurses, 1,608 (14%) were nurse managers. The educational preparation of the respondents was as follows: baccalaureate (43.4%), master's (21.5%), associate (20.4%), diploma (13.4%), and doctorate (1.3%). Most of the respondents were female (91.6%) and Caucasian (92.1%). The majority of the nurses with certification (72.5%) indicated that seeking certification was voluntary.

Findings indicate a high level of agreement on the value of certification among certified nurses, noncertified nurses, and nurse managers (ABNS, 2006). The main barriers cited by respondents who never held certification were cost of the exams and lack of institutional rewards and support. Respondents who allowed their certification to lapse cited reasons of not practicing in the specialty, inadequate compensation or no compensation for certification, and lack of recognition for certification. The rewards and benefits cited for certification were: reimbursement of certification

(continued)

cost, displaying of credentials, and reimbursement for continuing education. Only 18.6% of respondents indicated salary increase; 21.4% did not receive any incentive for certification. Two areas—absences in a 1-year period and nurse retention rates—did not show any differences between certified and noncertified nurses.

The ABNS (2006) enumerated three implications of this survey: (1) health care organizations need to support nurses in overcoming barriers to certification and must offer incentives for certification; (2) a specialty nursing certification board needs to promote appreciation of certified nurses and encourage minority nurses to obtain certification; and (3) nurses with no certification need to surmount barriers and pursue certification. Furthermore, it is crucial that nurses with specialty certification serve as role models and work in partnership with "professional nursing organizations, specialty nursing certification boards, and their employers to advocate for meaningful incentives and rewards that foster certification" (ABNS, 2006, p. 4).

Applications to Practice

■ Investigate the number of nurses with certifications at your work setting.
■ Discuss the benefits of certification. What incentives for certification do you have at your work setting?
■ Have you held any type of certification before? What was the reason you let it lapse? Are you planning to again seek certification? Would it be the same specialty area as before?
■ If you were never certified before, what are the three main reasons for not seeking certification? Explain

Source: American Board of Nursing Specialties (2006).

Certification in Transcultural Nursing

Founding the field of TCN in the 1950s, Dr. Madeleine Leininger inspired followers to contribute to the body of knowledge in caring for people from diverse cultures. Since that time, more than 400 scientific studies have been added to these vast and impressive collections (Glittenberg, 2004). As nurses struggled in the 1970s to care for immigrants, refugees, and other people from different cultures, it was evident that TCN certification was needed (McFarland & Leininger, 2002).

Evolution of CTN examination. Established in 1987, the Transcultural Nursing Certification Committee ([TCNCC], Transcultural Nursing Society, 2013) offered its initial examination in 1988 at the Transcultural Nursing Society (TCNS) annual conference and meeting in Edmonton, Alberta, Canada (Andrews & Boyle, 2012). According to McFarland and Leininger (2002), the main purpose of certification was to protect clients of various cultures from "...negligent, offensive, harmful, unethical, non-therapeutic, or inappropriate care practices" (p. 544). The certification examination—usually administered by the Certification Committee during the annual international TCNS conference—consisted of multiple choice questions and an oral examination (TCNS, 2013).

The TCNS Board of Trustees appointed a Certification Task Force (CTF) in 2004. The CTF's main goals were "...to review current certification practices and make recommendations for future directions in certification" (TCNS, 2013, para 1). The CTF completed its work in 2006. In the same year, the TCNS Board of Trustees established the Transcultural Nursing Certification Commission (TNCC) with Dr. Marilyn McFarland as chair. However, the TNCC was not chartered and hence it functioned as a committee with the following appointed as committee chairs: curriculum (Dr. Susan Mattson); evaluation (Dr. Mary Simpson); eligibility and credentialing (Dr. Priscilla Sagar); finance and grants (Dr. Patricia Vint); marketing and public relations (initially, Dr. Beth Rose; later, Dr. Hiba Wehbe-Alamah); and, **recertification** evaluation (Maj Helen Nyback).

Development of the certification exams. Based on an outline developed by the Core Curriculum Committee, Dr. Mary Simpson, Dr. Priscilla Sagar, Dr. Marilyn McFarland, and Dr. Hiba Wehbe-Alamah developed the advanced certification examination from 2007 to 2009. Test questions were requested from TCNS scholars and divided into seven domains. In 2011, an *ad hoc* committee of four—Dr. Marty Douglas, Dr. Dula Pacquiao, Dr. Melissa Scollan-Koliopolus, and Dr. Arlene Farren—developed the basic certification examination (Sagar, in press). The basic exam was based on the Core Curriculum for Transcultural Nursing and Health Care.

The TNCC abolished the oral examination and decided to base the examination on strictly multiple choice questions to be on par with other certification examinations (Sagar, 2012). In addition, the TNCC adopted online versus paper-and-pencil testing; the online examination was made available at various testing locations nationally during multiple test periods throughout the year (Andrews & Boyle, 2012; Sagar, 2012, in press).

Pilot exams. Consisting only of multiple choice questions, the first advanced certification pilot exams were offered in January and February 2009; the second exams were administered in June and July 2009 (TNCC, 2007). The new eligibility requirements for advanced certification examination went into effect in December 2009 and the basic certification examination was piloted in November 2011 (TCNS, 2013). In employing the basic certification, the TNCC acknowledged that all nurses must be prepared in cultural competence (Andrews & Boyle, 2012) and that all 3,063,163 RNs in the United States (USDHHS, HRSA, 2010) must heed the call for cultural knowledge, skills, and competencies in TCN and apply these in all settings of practice (Sagar, 2012).

TNCC received full support from a 3-year (2008–2011) project called *Developing Cultural Competencies for Nurses: Evidence-based Best Practices,* funded by a U.S. Department of Health and Human Services, Health Resources and Services Administration grant written and directed by Dr. Margaret Andrews, Director of Nursing, School of Health Professions Studies at the University of Michigan-Flint (Andrews et al., 2011) The project was codirected by Dr. Teresa Cervantez Thompson from Madonna University, Livonia, Michigan, and has subsequently been extended for an additional 2-year period (2012–2013). This grant-funded support enabled the TNCC to (1) employ statisticians to establish reliability and validity of both basic and advanced certification examinations; (2) support committee members' attendance at TNCC meetings; and (3) participate in preparatory precertification train-the-trainer workshops nationwide (Andrews et al., 2011).

Number of CTN-As and CTN-Bs. In 2002, there were approximately 100 certified and recertified nurses (McFarland & Leininger, 2002). The current TCNS (2013) listing has 22 transcultural nurses with **basic transcultural nursing certification (CTN-B)** and 59 with **advanced transcultural nursing certification (CTN-A)**. Of those with CTN-B, all are from the United States except one from Canada; the nurses with advanced certification are all from the United States except for one TCN nurse from each of these countries: Australia, Israel, and Saudi Arabia (TCNS, 2013). Recertification requires further pursuit of lifelong learning and enhancement of skills (Davis, 2011; Eisemon & Cline), maintenance of knowledge and competence (ABNS, 2012), and keeping updated with new trends and development in the field (McFarland & Leininger, 2002). Organizations must offer incentives for certification so nurses are more likely to recertify.

Eighty-one TCN nurses are too few, considering that there are 3,163,063 U.S. nurses (USDHHS, HRSA, 2010). Moreover, 81 nurses is like a drop in the bucket if we are to effectively "answer the need for caring, mentoring, and role modeling in the vast arena of nursing practice, education, administration, and research" (Sagar, in press). The growing diversity of the U.S. population and the increasing emphasis on both individual and organizational competence will boost the demand for CTNs in the near future, both at the basic and advanced levels.

MAGNET RECOGNITION PROGRAM

The ANCC (2009a) Magnet Recognition Program (MRP) "recognizes health care organizations that provide the best in nursing care, including high quality patient care, and the most supportive and innovative of working environments" (p. 8). Magnet recognition, a prestigious seal of excellence, began as a study conducted by McClure, Poulin, Sovie, and Wandelt (1983) for the American Academy of Nursing (AAN) Task Force on Nursing Practice. McClure et al. (1983) collected data from AAN fellows to identify attraction and retention factors contributing to both nurse professional and personal satisfaction. The second phase of the study entailed the collection of data from staff nurses and directors of nursing in 41 hospitals to explore the environments that appeal to well-qualified nurses, that foster nurse retention, and that promote quality client care.

The MRP was developed in 1990, an offshoot of the McClure et al. (1983) study, with the original 14 forces of magnetism. The new model has five components that contain the original 14 forces of magnetism: (1) transformational leadership; (2) structural empowerment; (3) exemplary professional practice; (4) new knowledge, innovation, and improvements; and (5) empirical quality results (ANCC, 2008).

Ludwig-Beymer (2012) illustrated the application of Leininger's CCT (2006) in the assessment of an organization; she pointed out the MRP's strong requirement for culturally and linguistically appropriate services (CLAS). These requirements are under "exemplary professional practice," whereby the MRP explicitly calls for identification and tackling of disparities between diverse populations; individual and organizational competence; nondiscriminatory practices; and resources to meet the unique needs of the client and families (ANCC, 2008).

Evidence of positive outcomes in magnet versus nonmagnet hospitals includes reduction in excess mortality rate (Aiken, Sloane, & Lake, 1999; Aiken, Smith, & Lake, 1994, as cited in Hanson & Spross, 2005), increased patient satisfaction (Cardner, Fogg, Thomas-Hawkins, & Latham, 2007), decreased pressure ulcer (Goode & Blegen, 2009), increased RN retention and lower burnout (Aiken et al., 1999), and increased RN satisfaction (Brady-Schwartz, 2005; Laschinger, Fingan, Shamian, & Wilk, 2004; Smith, Tallman, & Kelley, 2006), among many others. Presently, there are 397 hospitals with magnet designation: Australia (3), Lebanon (1), Saudi Arabia (1), Singapore (1), and United States (391). (ANCC, 2013d).

The MRP—conceived, started, and grown by nurses—is a testament to what nurses are capable of as leaders in achieving and bestowing recognition of excellence, in improving client outcomes, and in enhancing the nursing profession. It is noteworthy that the Gallup poll shows the public's view of nurses as the most trustworthy of all health care professionals for 11 years in a row (ANA, 2012). These are further testaments to the increasing public recognition of nurses as professionals and their contribution to enhancing client outcomes. Nurses must capitalize on this and continue their visibility in advocating for health reforms, in enticing young people to go into nursing as a rewarding profession, and in leading other professionals to eliminate disparities in health care.

PATHWAY TO EXCELLENCE PROGRAM

The Pathway to Excellence Program (PEP) acknowledges the essential elements of "an ideal nursing practice environment" (ANCC, 2009a, p. 11). The PEP program is available for acute and long-term care organizations. However, an organization must meet 12 practice standards that respect and support nurses and value their contribution. Six of the 12 practice standards are

■ nurses control practice of nursing;
■ work environment is safe and healthy;
■ systems are in place to address patient care and practice concerns;
■ orientation prepares new nurses for the work environment;
■ the chief nursing officer is qualified and participates in all levels of the organization; and
■ professional development is provided and used (ANCC, 2013a, para 2–7).

The above standards, though not implicitly mentioning diversity and cultural competence, lend themselves well to integration of CLAS as well as the processes and systems of professional nursing development. Currently, there are 109 PE-designated organizations throughout the United States (ANCC, 2013b).

The initial step in applying for PE recognition is self-assessment; the program has separate tools for acute and LTC facilities for self-assessment. Research studies that both quantify outcomes and explore lived experiences of nurses and patients in facilities designated as PE are vital to the effectiveness of the PEP.

ACCREDITATION OF CONTINUING NURSING EDUCATION

Continuing education (CE) is the most common method of assuring continuing competence; this is currently required in 25 states for RN and in 24 states for licensed practical or licensed vocational nurses (NCSBN, 2005). The ANCC accredits CE programs. One of ANCC's programs is the Nursing Skills Competency (NSC) program; the NSC offers skills training to new nurses or those reentering the work force (ANCC, 2009a). Programs such as these are very important in light of the persistent nursing shortage.

Acknowledging continued competence as a crucial issue for boards of nursing (BONs), the NCSBN (2005) has been examining this since 1985. Although medicine did not pursue the issue of continuing competence until 1998 (NCSBN, 2005), medicine has intensified the push for certification and has current programs for maintenance of certification (MOC)—implementing educational and self-assessment programs viewed necessary by member boards (American Board of Medical Specialties [ABMS], 2012). Chiropractic medicine and physical therapy both require CE, including a national clearinghouse to avoid duplication (Federations of Chiropractic Licensing Boards [FCLB], 2008; Federations of State Boards of Physical Therapy [FSBPT], 2013). If nurses will continue to be effective leaders of the multidisciplinary health care team, they must pursue continuing education and competence. Agencies preparing for accreditation of their CE programs can find resources at the ANCC's Institute for Credentialing Innovation ([ICI], ANCC, 2009a). Continuing competence is further discussed in Chapter 24.

CRITICAL THINKING EXERCISES 26.1

Undergraduate Student
1. Compare and contrast licensure and credentialing. What are their differences? What are their similarities?
2. How do you explain lifelong learning? Do you think there is enough critical thinking content integrated in your classes (theory) and in clinical to feed your curiosity and desire for lifelong learning?
3. Have you started thinking of pursuing a specialty in nursing? How would you go about your path to that specialty?
4. Do you have a professional timeline in 3, 5, 7 years? If yes, when do you plan to start graduate education? Where? Why?

Graduate Student
1. What is your view of lifelong learning? How is this sustaining you in your pursuit of the master's program? Of you obtaining specialty certification?
2. Do you plan to seek certification after completing the graduate program?
3. Are you an advanced practice nurse? Describe. What is the role of lifelong learning in AP nursing?
4. Discuss your professional timeline in 3, 5, 7 years. When do you plan to continue to pursue doctoral education?
5. If you have a plan to pursue doctoral education, which track are you planning to pursue, the clinical or the research track? Explain.

Faculty in Academia
1. Were you familiar with the history of specialty certification in nursing?
2. Do you hold any specialty certification? Would you be in favor of using certification as one of the criteria for promotion and tenure? Why? Why not?
3. Do you include lifelong learning as a professional goal for yourself? For your students?
4. How do you mentor students to pursue lifelong learning? Do you agree that role modeling is an important part of mentoring? How have you acted as a role model for lifelong learning? Describe.

Staff Development Educator
1. How do you motivate nurses to seek specialty certification in nursing?
2. What material rewards do you give certified nurses? Do you offer nonmaterial rewards for certification? Discuss.
3. Do you hold any specialty certification? Describe your motivation for seeking certification then. What motivates you to seek recertification now?
4. How do you foster lifelong learning among your staff nurses? How many nurses are back to school seeking the baccalaureate, master's, and doctoral program? Does your institution offer tuition reimbursement?

SUMMARY

Credentialing aims to protect the public and enhance quality and standard of services. Certification, magnet recognition, pathway to excellence, and accreditation of continuing education programs are some forms of credentialing. All these credentialing programs solidify the value of nursing as an ethical profession that has the most potential to influence health-client outcomes. As the largest group of health care providers and the most trusted by the public for over a decade, nurses are coming to the frontlines of leading health care globally in the 21st century.

There are increasing studies on the value of specialty certification. However, further studies need to be pursued regarding the value of certification, especially research about client satisfaction of care rendered by certified nurses compared with those without certification. Certification in TCN is 25 years old; yet to date the number of nurses with this specialty certification has not shown much growth. The gathering momentum between the converging of forces from academic and practice accreditation; governmental mandates and guidelines; consumer demand for culturally based care; and rapid, continuing population diversification will increase the demand for CTN certification. CTNs will lead in initiatives for culturally and linguistically congruent approaches in nursing education, practice, administration, and research.

REFERENCES

Accreditation Commission for Education in Nursing. (2013a). *Mission, purpose, and goals*. Retrieved September 1, 2013, from http://acenursing.org/mission-purpose-goals

Accreditation Commission for Education in Nursing. (2013b). *Accreditation manual*. Atlanta, GA: Author. Retrieved September 1, 2013, from www.acenursing.net/manuals/SC2013_BACCALAUREATE.pdf

Aiken, L. H., Sloane, S. M., & Lake, E. T. (1999). Organization and outcomes of inpatient AIDS care. *Medical Care, 37*, 760–772.

American Association of Colleges of Nursing. (2008). *Cultural competency in baccalaureate nursing education*. Washington, DC: Author.

American Association of Colleges of Nursing. (2011). *Toolkit for cultural competence in master's and doctoral nursing education*. Washington, DC: Author.

American Board of Medical Specialties. (2012). *Maintenance of certification*. Retrieved April 14, 2013, from www.abms.org/Maintenance_of_Certification/ABMS_MOC.aspx

American Board of Nursing Specialties. (2006). *Value of certification survey executive summary*. Retrieved March 6, 2013, from www.nursingcertification.org/pdf/executive_summary.pdf

American Board of Nursing Specialties. (2010). *Frequently asked questions about absnc accreditation*. Retrieved March 6, 2013, from www.nursingcertification.org/pdf/10–19-10%20Final%20FAQs.pdf

American Board of Nursing Specialties. (2012). *ABNS endorses statement on continuing competence for nursing: A call to action*. Retrieved March 6, 2013, from www.nursingcertification.org/pdf/ABNS%20Press%20Release%20-%20Continued%20Competence%20Statement%20-%20Jan%202012.pdf

American Nurses Association. (2012). *Nurses earn highest ranking ever, remain most ethical of professions in poll*. Retrieved September 1, 2013, from www.nursingworld.org/FunctionalMenuCategories/MediaResources/PressReleases/Nurses-Remain-Most-Ethical-of-Professions-in-Poll.pdf

American Nurses Credentialing Center. (2009a). *Nursing excellence. Your journey. Our passion*. [ANCC overview brochure] Retrieved January 6, 2013, from www.nursecredentialing.org/FunctionalCategory/AboutANCC/ANCC-Overview-Brochure.pdf

American Nurses Credentialing Center. (2009b). *Credentialing definitions*. Retrieved September 3, 2013, from http://www.nursecredentialing.org/FunctionalCategory/ANCC-Awards/Grants/Credentialing-Definitions.html

American Nurses Credentialing Center. (2013a). *Practice standards*. Retrieved September 3, 2013, from www.nursecredentialing.org/PracticeStandards

American Nurses Credentialing Center. (2013b). *Pathway designated organizations*. Retrieved September 3, 2013, from http://www.nursecredentialing.org/Pathway/DesignationOrganizations

American Nurses Credentialing Center. (2013c). *ISO journey at ANCC: ANCC earns prestigious international certification for operational excellence*. Retrieved October 10, 2013, from www.nursecredentialing.org/ISOJourney

American Nurses Credentialing Center. (2013d). *List of all magnet-recognized facilities*. Retrieved February 16, 2014, from www.nursecredentialing.org/Magnet/FindaMagnetFacility

Andrews, M. M., & Boyle, J. S. (2012). *Transcultural concepts in nursing care* (6th ed.). Philadelphia, PA: Wolters Kluwer/Lippincott Williams & Wilkins.

Andrews, M. M., Thompson, T. L., Wehbe-Alamah, H., McFarland, M. R., Hanson, P. A., Hasenau, S. M.,...Vint, P. A. (2011). Developing a culturally competent workforce through collaborative partnerships. *Journal of Transcultural Nursing, 22*(3), 300–306. doi:10.1177/1043659611404214

Brady-Schwartz, D. C. (2005). Further evidence on the Magnet Recognition program: Implications for nursing leaders. *Journal of Nursing Administration, 35*(9), 397–403.

Cardner J. K., Fogg, L., Thomas-Hawkins, C., & Latham, C. E. (2007). The relationships between nurses' perceptions of the hemodialysis work environment and nurse turnover, patient satisfaction, and hospitalization. *Nephrology Nursing Journal, 34*(3), 271–281.

Commission on Collegiate Nursing Education. (2009). *Achieving excellence in accreditation: The first 10 years of CCNE*. Washington, DC: Author. Retrieved September 26, 2013, from www.aacn.nche.edu/ccne-accreditation/about/mission-values-history

Commission on Collegiate Nursing Education. (2013). *Standards for accreditation of baccalaureate and graduate nursing program*. Washington, DC: Author. Retrieved September 26, 2013, from www.aacn.nche.edu/ccne-accreditation

Davis, J. (2011). What is the value of orthopaedic certification? [Guest editorial]. *Orthopaedic Nursing, 30*(2), 86–87.

Eisemon, N., & Cline, A. (2006). The value of certification [Guest editorial]. *Gastroenterology Nursing, 29*(6), 428–429.

Federations of Chiropractic Licensing Boards. (2008). *Protecting the public by promoting excellence in chiropractic regulation*. Retrieved August 31, 2013, from www.fclb.org/AboutFCLB/Resolutions/2008Resolutions.aspx

Federations of State Boards of Physical Therapy. (2013). *The continuing competence model*. Retrieved August 31, 2013, from https://www.fsbpt.org/FreeResources/ContinuingCompetence/ContinuingCompetenceModel.aspx

Fights, S. D. (2012). *Lippincott's 2012 nursing directory* [Supplement] (pp. 10–11). Retrieved September 17, 2013, from www.nursingcenter.com/pdf.asp?AID=1287263

Glittenberg, J. (2004). A transdisciplinary, transcultural model for health care. *Journal of Transcultural Nursing, 15*(1), 6–10.

Goode, C., & Blegen, M. (2009, October 1–3). *The link between nurse staffing and patient outcomes, 2009*. National Magnet Conference Abstract and presentation at the Magnet conference; Louisville, KY.

Hanson, C. M., & Spross, J. A. (2005). Collaboration. In A. B. Hamric, J. A. Spross, & C. M. Hanson (Eds.), *Advanced practice nursing: An integrative approach* (3rd ed., pp. 341–378). St. Louis, MO: Elsevier Saunders.

Institute of Medicine. (2010, October 5). *The future of nursing: Leading change, advancing health*. Washington, DC: National Academies Press.

International Council of Nurses. (2009). *Fact sheet: Nursing matters*. Retrieved September 2, 2013, from www.icn.ch/images/stories/documents/publications/fact_sheets/1a_FS-Credentialing.pdf

International Organization for Standardization. (2013). *About ISO*. Retrieved October 10, 2013, from www.iso.org/iso/home/about.htm

Kelly-Thomas, K. J. (1998). The nature of staff development practice: Theories, skill acquisition, and research. In K. J. Kelly-Thomas (Ed.), *Clinical and nursing staff development: Current competence, future focus* (2nd ed., pp. 54–72). Philadelphia, PA: Lippincott.

Kendall-Gallagher, D., Aiken, L. H., Sloane, D. M., & Cimiotti, J. P. (2011). Nurse specialty certification, inpatient mortality, and failure to rescue. *Journal of Nursing Scholarship, 43*(2), 188–194.

Laschinger, H. K. S., Fingan J. E., Shamian J., & Wilk, P. (2004). A longitudinal analysis of the impact of workplace empowerment on work satisfaction. *Journal of Organizational Behavior, 25*, 527–545.

Ludwig-Beymer, P. (2012). Creating culturally competent organizations. In M. M. Andrews & J. S. Boyle (Eds.), *Transcultural concepts in nursing care* (6th ed., pp. 211–242). Philadelphia, PA: Wolters Kluwer/Lippincott Williams & Wilkins.

McClure, M. L., Poulin, M. A., Souvie, M. D., & Wandelt, M. A. (1983). For the American Academy Task Force of Nursing Practice in Hospitals. *Magnet hospitals: Attraction and retention of professional nurses*. Kansas City, MO: American Nurses Association.

McFarland, M. R., & Leininger, M. M. (2002). Transcultural nursing: Curricular concepts, principles, and teaching and learning activities for the 21st century. In M. M. Leininger & M. R. McFarland (Eds.), *Transcultural nursing: Concepts, theories, research, and practice* (3rd ed., pp. 527–561). New York, NY: McGraw-Hill.

National Council of State Boards of Nursing. (2005). *Meeting the ongoing challenge of continued competence*. Retrieved April 24, 2013, from Nursinghttps://www.ncsbn.org/Continued_Comp_Paper_TestingServices.pdf

National Council of State Boards of Nursing. (2013). *NCLEX examination*. Retrieved October 7, 2013, from https://www.ncsbn.org/nclex.htm

National League for Nursing. (2009a). *A commitment to diversity in nursing and nursing education*. Retrieved August 22, 2013, from www.nln.org/aboutnln/reflection_dialogue/rfl _dial3.htm

National League for Nursing. (2009b). *Diversity toolkit*. Retrieved August 22, 2013, from www.nln.org/facultyprograms/Diversity_Toolkit/index.htm

Piazza, I. M., Donohue, M., & Dykes, P. (2006). Differences in perceptions of empowerment among nationally certified and noncertified nurses. *Journal of Nursing Administration, 36*(5), 277–283.

Sagar, P. L. (2012). *Transcultural nursing theory and models: Application in nursing education, practice and administration*. New York, NY: Springer Publishing.

Sagar, P. L. (in press). Transcultural nursing certification: Its role in nursing education, practice, and administration. In M. M. McFarland & H. Wehbe-Alamah (Eds.), *Culture care diversity and universality: A worldwide theory of nursing* (3rd ed.). Sudbury, MA: Jones & Bartlett.

Smith, H., Tallman, R., & Kelley, K. (2006). Magnet hospital characteristics and northern Canadian nurses' job satisfaction. *Canadian Journal of Nursing Leadership, 19*(3), 73–86.

Smolenski, M. C. (2010). *ANCC nurse certification: Playing the credentials game*. Silver Spring, MD: American Nurses Credentialing Center (ANCC Nurse Certification brochure).

Transcultural Nursing Certification Commission. (2007, March 23–25). *Transcultural nursing certification revision* [Personal archive of minutes from Transcultural Nursing Certification Committee meeting, Fenton, Michigan].

Transcultural Nursing Society. (2013). *Transcultural nursing certification*. Retrieved September 4, 2013, from www.tcns.org/Certification.html

U.S. Department of Health and Human Services, Health Resources Services Administration. (2010). *The registered nurse population: Initial findings from the 2008 National Sample Survey of registered nurses*. Retrieved April 15, 2013, from bhpr.hrsa.gov/healthworkforce/rnsurveys/rnsurveyinitial2008.pdf

Wolgin, F. (1998). Competence assessment systems and measurement strategies. In K. J. Kelly-Thomas (Ed.), *Clinical and nursing staff development: Current competence, future focus* (2nd ed., pp. 92–120). Philadelphia, PA: Lippincott.

Recruitment and Retention of Foreign-Educated Nurses

Priscilla Limbo Sagar

Acculturation
Brain drain
Brain hemorrhage
Circular migration
Commission on Graduates of Foreign
 Nursing Schools
Enfermeros
Ethical recruitment
Expatriate nurses
Foreign-educated nurses
Hospitallers

International Council of Nurses
Internationally educated nurses
Mentoring
Nurse drain
Nurse immigrants
Preceptor
Preceptorship
Receiving countries
Sending countries
Train-the-trainer
Twinning

At the completion of this chapter, the learner will be able to

1. Trace statistics and trends of the migration of foreign-educated nurses.
2. Analyze programs that facilitate adjustment, mentoring, and acculturation of foreign-educated nurses.
3. Develop an educational plan to promote cultural competence among foreign nurses and their employers.
4. Discuss evidence-based practice utilized by receiving institutions to reduce turnover and enhance retention of nurses.
5. Propose possible solutions to nurse migration and exodus of nurses from developing countries.

OVERVIEW

In the United States and in the international arena, nurses make up the largest group of health care workers. Generally, in every nation, nurses provide the bulk of health services; nursing services can be up to 80% of the total health services (International Council of Nurses [ICN], 2007a). Shortages of nurses adversely affect health services in any nation.

There is a current global nursing shortage affecting developed and developing countries. Developed countries that reported nurse shortages were: the United Kingdom, 22,000 nurses in 2000; the Netherlands, 7,000 in 2002; Australia, 40,000 in 2010; Canada, 78,000 in 2011; and the United States, 800,000 by 2020 (Arends-Kuenning, 2006). Nurse shortages in underdeveloped countries were also cited, with as much as a 72% shortage in Malawi in 2003 and 6% shortage in the Philippines in 2005; however, estimates are the shortage in the Philippines will worsen to 29% in 2020 (Arends-Kuenning, 2006).

One strategy that has been used to alleviate the persistent shortage of nurses in the United States and other countries is the recruitment of **foreign-educated nurses (FENs;** Ea, Griffin, L'Eplatenier, & Fitzpatrick, 2008; Jeffreys, 2010), or those nurses born and educated in schools of nursing outside U.S. jurisdiction. For the sake of consistency, *foreign born nurses,—* also referred to as *foreign trained nurses, expatriate nurses, internationally recruited nurses, and nurse immigrants* in literature—will be referred to in this book as FENs.

The mobility of nurses has been documented since early times. Nurse involvement in global causes was exemplified by Rufaida Al-Aslamia, who travelled with the prophet Muhammad throughout the Arab peninsula (Meleis & Glickman, 2012), and by Florence Nightingale, who made a great impact in the health outcomes of soldiers in the Crimean War. In recent times, nurses have moved from underdeveloped countries to more developed nations.

Although the ICN (2007a) believes that nurses from all nations have a right to migrate and acknowledges the benefits of migration, it has expressed grave concern about the negative effects of health care quality in countries so drained and exhausted of their nurses. According to the **International Council of Nurses (ICN)**, international migration and the continuing shortage of nurses creates an imperative mandate to prepare a self-sustainable nursing workforce in **receiving countries** and to improve the quality of work life in **sending countries** (ICN, 2007a, 2007b). In addition, the ICN (2007a, 2007b) calls for **ethical recruitment** of nurses; effective orientation and mentoring; and equal pay for work of equal value, among others. To provide a forum for global nursing education issues, the ICN (2013) has established the ICN Nursing Education Network (ICNEN).

Established in 1977, the **Commission on Graduates of Foreign Nursing Schools (CGFNS)** aimed at ensuring patient safety and preventing exploitation of nurses who completed their education outside of the United States (Davis & Nichols, 2002). CGFNS has a certification process for FEN postsecondary education and a requirement of passing of English proficiency and its own examination that widely predicts success in the NCLEX-RN® (Arends-Kuenning, 2006).

Sending and Receiving Countries

The Philippines, a country of about 105 million people (Central Intelligence Agency [CIA], 2013), is the world's largest exporter of nurses (Brush, 2008) and has been doing so for more than half a century (Choo, 2003; Choy, 2003). According to the Philippine Nurses Association (PNA, 2011), there are now approximately 350 nursing schools in the Philippines; all of these schools are regulated by the Commission on Higher Education (CHED). On an annual basis, the schools of nursing in the Philippines graduate an average of 13,000 new nurses (PNA, 2011). Box 27.1 contains an overview of the development of nursing education in the Philippines.

BOX 27.1 AN OVERVIEW OF NURSING EDUCATION: PHILIPPINES

The country. The Philippines—an archipelago of over 7,000 islands and islets—has a land surface of 114,830 square miles (Agoncillo, 1990). Its current population is approximately 105,720,644; vital statistics include life expectancy (72.2 for total population), maternal mortality rate (99/100,000 live births), infant mortality rate (18.9/1,000 live births), and with a ratio of 1.15 physicians per 1,000 population (Central Intelligence Agency [CIA] World Factbook, 2013). The ratio of nurses per 1,000 population is 485 (Arends-Kuenning, 2006).

The country had a civilization of Oriental texture—although there is a dearth of continuous documentation of this and its thriving relations with neighboring countries—before the coming of the Spaniards in 1521, a colonization that lasted until 1898. The earliest Europeans to come to the Philippines were from the Spanish expedition sailing around the globe directed by the Portuguese explorer Fernando Magallanes in 1521. Other Spanish expeditions ensued, including one from Mexico (then New Spain), commanded by Ruy López de Villalobos. It was Villalobos, who named the islands *Las Islas Filipinas* (the Philippine Islands) in 1542, in honor of then Prince Philip, later Philip II of Spain (De LaSalle University [DLSU], 2002).

Because of the continuing economic oppression, bigotry, and racial discrimination, the Filipinos revolted against Spain in 1896. That was shortly after the execution of Jose Rizal on December 30, 1896; Rizal later become a Philippine national hero (DLSU, 2002). With Spain's defeat in the Spanish-American War in 1898, the Philippines and Cuba were ceded to the United States, thus beginning the U.S. colonialism in the country. The Philippines gained independence from the United States on July 4, 1946.

During the Spanish colonization, there was not much information about nursing (Goodnow, 1928, as cited by Sotejo, 2001). Giron-Tupas (1952, 1961) accounted for some hospitals—mostly established by the Franciscans—such as the Hospital Real de Manila in 1577 for Spanish soldiers and civilians; San Lazaro in 1578 for lepers; and Hospital de Indios in 1586 for the "Indios." Giron-Tupas (1952) narrated a Fr. Juan Clemente, who tended to lepers and used some native herbs and medicines. Workers in the early hospitals mentioned **enfermero**, which referred to the religious as well as the native attendant caring for the sick under the direction of the **hospitallers**, or religious persons caring for the sick (Giron-Tupas, 1952). The Spaniards deemed themselves superior to the Indio (Filipino). For example, no Filipino was permitted to sit at the same table with a Spaniard, even though the Spaniard was visiting the Indio's house (Agoncillo, 1990). According to Agoncillo (1990), Friar M. L. Bustamante wrote in 1885 that the Filipino "could never learn the Spanish language and or be civilized" (p. 121).

Goodnow (1928), as cited by Sotejo (2001), narrated the abhorrent health conditions after the United States acquired the Philippines from Spain, including extremely high death and infant mortality rates. The U.S. army began a health program which was continued by American nurses. Thus, western medicine and nursing was introduced in the Philippines during the U.S. colonial rule from 1898 to 1946 (Agoncillo, 1990), including the formation of standards of professional nursing (Choy, 1998). Choy (2003) contends that the growth of nursing education in the Philippines "followed the patterns of American professional nursing" (pp. 50–51).

(continued)

BOX 27.1 AN OVERVIEW OF NURSING EDUCATION: PHILIPPINES *(continued)*

From pre-World War II to 1945, there were hospital-based 3-year programs (Divinagracia, 1996a) in the Philippines. Bachelor of Science in Nursing (BSN) supplemental completion programs were introduced in the late 1940s for graduates of these 3-year programs. The 63 initial graduates of the 4-year BSN programs in 1950 were from the University of Santo Tomas (Giron-Tupas, 1952) and the University of the Philippines (UP) in 1952 (Divinagracia, 1996a). Three-year programs converted to BSN programs in the late 1970s. Since the 1980s, baccalaureate nursing has been adopted as the entry level of nursing education in the Philippines. In the mid-1980s to the early 1990s, the BSN was not only adopted as the basic nursing program but the country also phased out all graduate nursing (GN) programs and BSN completion programs (Divinagracia, 1996a).

It is noteworthy to trace the proliferation of nursing schools in the Philippines as cited in literature: 170 in 1996 (Divinagracia, 1996b) and 175 in 1998 (Sison, 2002) to almost 300 in 2004 (Nakashima & Cody, 2004) and about 350 in 2011 (PNA, 2011). Of those colleges of nursing, 30 were accredited (Association of Deans of Philippine Colleges of Nursing (ADPCN), 1998). In an effort to make programs more relevant and comparable to other programs in other parts of the world, the ADPCN consistently revisits its curriculum. In addition, the ADPCN maintains alliances with key organizations such as CHED; Professional Regulation Commission, Board of Nursing; Department of Health; Association of Nursing Service Administrator of the Philippines (ANSAP); and the PNA (Divinagracia, 1998).

The Filipino Nurses Association (FNA) was founded at a meeting of 150 nurses on September 2, 1922; presiding was Anastacia Giron-Tupas. Incorporated in 1924, the FNA gained acceptance as one of the member organizations of the ICN during its congress held in Montreal, Canada, on July 8–13, 1929. The FNA converted its name to the PNA (Philippine Nurses Association) in 1966 (PNA, 2011). Another notable Filipino leader of nursing is Dr. Julita V. Sotejo, who was founder and long-time dean of the UP College of Nursing (UPCON). The UPCON was later named for this beloved nursing leader who is credited—among other Filipino nurse leaders—with professionalization of Philippine nursing (Tungpalan, 2001).

Nurse Drain: The Continuing Migration

There was a decrease in the Exchange Visitor Program in the late 1960s and early 1970s, giving way to a limited working permit or H-1 visa (Choy, 2003). Choy (2003) contends that Filipino nurse migration is "inextricably linked to the larger process of global restructuring" (p. 2) whereby the increased demand for services in developed countries and the export of manufacturing to developing countries account for higher global mobility. The outsourcing of industries has become more common in the last 10 years. Although the most common reason cited is economic, Choy (2003) eloquently reminded us of the hidden U.S. colonialism in the Philippines and the Americanized training hospital system that prepared Filipino nurses to work in the United States rather than in the Philippines. Two thirds of the world's population lives in developing countries, which only retain 15% of the

(continued)

BOX 27.1   AN OVERVIEW OF NURSING EDUCATION: PHILIPPINES *(continued)*

word's nurses; nurse migrations increase the severity of "empire of care" (Choy, 2003, p. 3) or the disparities of health services in those countries.

First migration wave. Graduate nurses from the Philippines began coming to the United States to study after 1948 as part of the exchange visitor program (EVP; Choy, 2003; Marquand, 2006). After World War II, the nursing shortage intensified and the United States recruited more Filipino nurses. Choy (2003) reported some nurse exploitation whereby nurses were assigned unfavorable job positions and shifts. In addition, nurses were paid stipends instead of full salaries. From 1956 to 1969, more than 11,000 nurses participated in the EVP (Choy, 2003).

Second migration wave. In 1965, U.S. laws changed, favoring migration from the Philippines and Asia and hence a large surge in nurse emigration. Postgraduate study in the United States allowed returning Filipino nurses to lead curricular revision in nursing education that are was consistent with educational trends in higher education (Choy, 2003).

The Philippines train more nurses than it can employ in its health care delivery system. While the average salary of nurses in the Philippines is 11,000 pesos a month ($200), some nurses may only earn 5,000 pesos (current exchange rate is 42 pesos for every dollar) a month (Sison, 2002). In the current economy, it is easy to see the struggle of making both ends meet with such meager salaries. Nurses, however, do not migrate just solely for economic reasons. Other reasons for migration include opportunities for professional advancement and travel.

Balancing Health Care Needs at Home

The Association of Deans of Philippine Colleges of Nursing (ADPCN) has focused its energies and resources to provide "globally competitive and excellent education, training, and research" (Ocampo, 1997, p. 14).

The increase of nursing schools amid the exodus of nurses is compromising the quality of education in the Philippines for these reasons: lack of qualified faculty; shortage of hospitals for clinical affiliation, and low passing rate in the state boards (Estella, 2005a, 2005b; Wong, 2006). There are now too many schools for eligible training hospitals across the country (Estella, 2005b). To address the issue of quality nursing education, CHED declared a moratorium on opening new schools, recommended closure of some accelerated programs, and planned to close programs with a 30% passing rate or less (Wong, 2006).

   Since experienced faculty members have also left for abroad, CHED plans to train deans and faculty of schools of nursing. CHED categorized nursing schools from high- to low-performance. To remain open, a school must have a minimum of 5% pass rate; CHED proposes an increase of this percentage from 5% to 30% (Estella, 2005b). In addition, a requirement to perform service for 2 years prior to going abroad has been effective since 2009 (Wong, 2006). In the late 1970s, a community service with stipend for 6 months was a requirement for all nursing graduates awaiting results of the board exam. Other suggestions included 'balik bayani" (Wong, 2006, para 12), or circular migration, as proposed by the ICN (2007a).

A fifth of the labor force in India might be lost to the United States, UK, Ireland, Singapore, New Zealand, Australia, and the gulf nations (Tiwari, Sharma, & Zodpey, 2013). Most hospitals in India pay nurses 2,500 to 3,000 Indian rupees (INRs)/month; whereas a nurse could earn as much as INR 40,000/month in one of the gulf states. Tiwari et al. cited two surveys whereby Indian nurses planned to emigrate because of dissatisfaction with working conditions and unhappiness with social attitudes toward nurses (Thomas, 2006) and better salary prospects (Khadria, 2004). The nurse drain from India to developed countries has been reported since the 1970s (Basuray, 1997). Medical and nursing care in colonial India, just like in the Philippines, were originally established for the colonists and selected Indian servants; hospital buildings were segregated between natives and colonists (Basuray, 1997).

The UK imported a total of 16,155 FENs in 2002, the most of any developed country that year (Arends-Kuenning, 2006). The UK Central Council for Nursing (UKCCN) registered 13,750 Filipino nurses in 2001; that is about 47% of UK's foreign nurses ("UK Draining Third World of Nurses, 2001"). In addition, the UKCC registration statistics also indicated a 63% and 127% of registration from the West Indies and South Africa, respectively.

What was called **brain drain** before is now termed "**brain hemorrhage**" (Nakashima & Cody, 2004, para 11), referring to 25,000 nurses leaving the Philippines in 2002 and 2003. Usually, the best and most experienced nurses leave, leaving novices to work the health care system (Sison, 2002). To illustrate this, 7,009 nurses came to the United States from 1994 to 2001, while a total of 5,535 Filipino nurses migrated to the UK from 1999 to 2001. In addition to the UK where Filipino nurses comprise the largest group of foreign nurses, Norway, Netherlands, and Ireland are among the other European countries recruiting Filipino nurses (Sison, 2002).

There has been an increase of FENs practicing professionally in the United States from 3.7% in 2004 to 5.6% in 2008 (USDHHS, HRSA, 2010). FENs originate from the Philippines (48.7%), Canada (11.5%), India (9.3%), United Kingdom (5.8%), Korea (2.6%), and Nigeria (2.0%) (Andrews & Ludwig-Beymer, 2012). Mason (2009) cited four reasons for nurse migration to the United States: (1) attain better living conditions, (2) work in complex U.S. nurse settings, (3) pursue graduate degrees, and (4) experience living in another nation. Meleis and Glickman (2012) stressed the challenges and opportunities facing FEN in their commentary about "expatriate nurses" (p. S24).

Some governments encourage migration of foreign laborers for the volume of remittances to the home country. Although the exact remittance from nurses is not available, Filipino migrant workers sent back approximately $7 and $8 billion in 2002 and 2003 (Arends-Kuenning, 2006; Nakashima & Cody, 2004); this helps keep the Philippine economy afloat. Indian nurses also help their economy through the remittances they send home (Tiwari et al., 2013).

Ethics of Recruitment

The **nurse drain** from developing countries to developed countries creates health care problems (Aiken, Buchan, Sochalski, Nichols, & Powell; ICN, 2007a, 2007b; Tiwari et al., 2013). The exodus of nurses from the country is compromising health care in the Philippines (Ea et al., 2008). Equally alarming are the indicators pointing to the decline in the quality of nursing education, such as lower pass rates in the nursing boards, decrease in the quality of nursing instructors, and inadequate clinical facilities (Estella, 2005b; Wong, 2006).

Another alarming trend in the Philippines is the loss of physicians from medicine to nursing (Estella, 2005a). There are some conflicting figures regarding physician's salaries in the country, but it appears to be between $300 to $800 per month (Choo, 2003; Clemente, 2003; Nakashima & Cody, 2004). As many as 4,000 physicians were taking up nursing in 2004 (Nakashima & Cody, 2004); they finish nursing in 2 years since they have already completed their prerequisite courses (Choo, 2003).

Globally, there are glaring inequities in the distribution of human resources for health. The World Health Organization (WHO, 2006) indicates that the United States and Canada only have 10% of the global burden of disease (GBD), yet it has 52% of the world's financial resources and 37% of global health workers (Sheer & Wong, 2008). Comparatively, Asia has 29 GBD, 1% financial resources, and 12% of the health workforce. Africa has 24 GBD with 3% of the health service. As of February 2005, there was a total of 368,589 licensed nurses in the Philippines (PNA, 2011).

The WHO suggests that underdeveloped countries maintain 1,000 nurses per 100,000 population. The UK and the United States have 847 and 782 nurses for every 100,000 population; comparatively, the ratio of registered nurses (RNs) per 100,000 population for some sending countries are: Philippines (485), Nigeria (66), and India (45; Arends-Kuenning, 2006).

The salaries of nurses in the United States are among the highest in the world. In comparison, nurses in the Philippines earn between $100 to $200 a month (Sison, 2002). Working in advanced health care areas in the United States enriches nurse clinical and leadership abilities. There are graduate programs offering advanced practice nursing (APN), education, administration, and research; completion of any of these increases a nurse's opportunity for advancement here and elsewhere in the globe (Mason, 2009). The opportunity to live in another country and be immersed in another culture is also attractive to some nurses.

Orientation of Foreign-Educated Nurses

The orientation of nurses recruited from foreign countries poses a more complicated challenge. Foreign nurses are not only adjusting to a new facility but also to a new culture and to a new country (Amerson, 2002). Common problems may include differences in language, communication style, education (Amerson, 2002), standards of practice, and culture of health care. Jeffreys and Karczewski (2010) urged that an employee orientation program be designed for a particular population and be evidence-based. In the case of the newly recruited FENs, profile and affective characteristics need to be assessed.

The **preceptor** is an experienced staff nurse who acts as a role model and educator and assists the orientee "in the process of socialization and role transition" (Amerson, 2002, p. 166). Preceptors are generally used in staff orientation to enhance socialization and role transition, to increase staff retention, and to reduce staff turnover. Criteria for preceptors include excellent communication skills, sound knowledge of adult learning theories, and competency in the areas where the orientee will be evaluated and validated (Amerson, 2002). Some institutions pay preceptors; others do not.

It is imperative that preceptors have the awareness and sensitivity regarding the difficult transition into professional U.S. nursing practice while also undergoing cultural transitions. Structured programs for FENs, preceptors, managers, and coworkers are likely to produce better outcomes (Pacquiao, 2007). Preceptors would be also be helpful if they studied organizational culture to assess employer-to-employee fit by identifying artifacts and by comparing observations with organizational mission and goals, policy and procedures, and promotional materials (Ullrich & Haffer, 2009). With assistance and guidance from the preceptor, the preceptee will be appropriately guided to socialize into the organization.

Retention Strategies

Preceptorship was already cited as the most helpful strategy in the transition phase to U.S. practice. The use of mentoring is another strategy used for the retention of FENs.

In 2007, Pacquiao conducted a 3-year outcome evaluation of an **acculturation** program for both FENs (from India, the Philippines, and Trinidad and Tobago) and their managers, preceptors, and educators. The program curriculum included effective written and verbal communication, leadership training, clinical judgment, and professional roles. The outcomes of the 5-day intervention for the FENs and 2-day session for managers, preceptors, and educators were positive: increased empathy for clients and coworkers, enhanced transition to organizational culture, and improved teamwork and organizational support for diverse workforce development (Pacquiao, 2007).

The Process of Acculturation

Nurse immigrants face obstacles and challenges while working in the host country and undergoing acculturation (Brunero, 2008; Choi, 2003; DiCicco-Bloom, 2004; Ullrich & Haffer, 2009). In a 2005 survey conducted among employers of FEN, the CGFNS (as cited in Nichols & Davis, 2009) cited **preceptorship** as the biggest factor in the transition process to U.S. nursing practice. As the FEN works toward transitioning to U.S. practice, there is the larger process of acculturation to the ways of life in the new country. Furthermore, the CGFNS survey indicated that the average length of time for FEN to acquire a sense of comfort and to demonstrate safe practice is 6 months (Nichols & Davis, 2009).

The Philippine Nurses Association of America (PNAA) was founded 30 years ago. The PNAA, with 35 chapters all over the United States, offers support and assistance such as review classes for the National Council Licensure Examination-Registered Nurse (NCLEX-RN), networking, and methods of addressing issues in the workplace (Conclara, 2002). The PNAA is in the process of collecting data about nurses' contracts with hospitals and the way they are treated once they have arrived in the United States (Wong, 2006). This database will help recommend agencies in the future and indicate those that the nurses need to avoid. Wong emphasized collaboration between the PNAA and both the United States and Philippines governments in this endeavor for a more ethical recruitment and retention of FENs.

Although they speak English back home and use mostly American textbooks during the duration of their nursing education, transitioning to work in the United States presents a cultural shock to many Filipino nurses. Programs such as those from the PNAA are helpful. However, they are not consistently implemented for every new group of nurse recruits. Orientation lengths vary from hospital to hospital. Furthermore, with the nursing shortage, many nurses find themselves facing a full assignment before having a chance to have full orientation and use of preceptors. In many instances, these new nurses are mandated to work evening and night shift positions that are more difficult to fill. The previously mentioned programs will be helpful. Although Ea et al. (2008) found a strong correlation between acculturation and job satisfaction among Filipino nurses, the study by Reyes and Cohen (2013) among nurses employed at skilled nursing facilities did not show this correlation. In light of this, it is imperative to offer comprehensive acculturation programs and cross-cultural workshops addressing the similarities and differences of Filipino culture from other cultural groups.

ALLEVIATING THE EFFECTS OF NURSE DRAIN, SHORTAGES, AND EXODUS

In the words of Meleis and Glickman (2012), "Nurses will continue to travel the world and make a difference in health care....Knowledge is power, being connected is empowering, and having a collective voice is transforming" (p. S25). To build on these powerful words, this author will use eclectic models in planning orientation and mentoring for FEN (Appendices 18, 19, and 20).

The nurse migration and exodus will probably get worse before it gets better. There are, however, measures that need to continue to regulate the processes for the benefit of global health, for ensuring quality and standards of nursing care, and for the welfare of FENs themselves. These measures include, but are not limited to, ethical recruitment and retention; train-the-trainer approach; and circular migration.

Ethical Recruitment

There are proposals that would mutually benefit both the receiving and sending countries. Nurses must lobby legislators for their support of more ethical policies on recruitment. Some proposals are twinning (Aiken, 2007), circular migration (ICN, 207a), foreign aid investment in the production of nurses (Aiken, 2007; Wong, 2006), and lobbying for policies in recruitment of FENs (Wong, 2006), to name a few.

In light of the huge salary differential between sending and receiving countries, Aiken (2007) proposed nonwage strategies such as **"twinning"** (p. 1316). With support from the U.S. Agency for International Development (USAID), the Nursing Quality Improvement Program matched U.S. hospitals with Magnet Recognition Programs with Russian and Armenian hospitals; these countries have historically not capitalized on professional nursing initiatives. According to Aiken (2007), during a 3-year intercountry exchange of nurses and hospital managers, the following outcomes were achieved in the participating Russian and Armenian hospitals: expansion of the professional roles of nurses; increase in nurses' satisfaction with their jobs; improvement in patients' satisfaction with their care; and reduction in adverse patient outcomes. Replication of this model needs to be done in countries experiencing more nurse emigration to assess whether enhanced job satisfaction would transform into more nurse retention in sending countries (Aiken, 2007). Interestingly, one of the reasons for emigrating cited by 63% of 448 Indian nurses was dissatisfaction with working conditions (Thomas, 2006, as cited in Tiwari et al., 2013).

Choo (2003) echoed the proposal by Galvez-Tan, Vice Chancellor for Research at the University of the Philippines, for bilateral negotiations between the receiving and sending countries whereby the receiving country will provide the sending country some form of aid for nurse training and development. Choo described a similar arrangement whereby Germany compensates Turkey for any human resource that they gain. An analogy of this is reforestation; to prevent deforestation and destructive, torrential flooding, a seedling is planted after cutting a full grown tree.

Assessment for multicultural support entails an examination of the community and its population prior to starting recruitment (Christmas, 2002). Is there ethnic group support? Ethnic minority professional nurses associations are available in various parts of the United States. TCN theory and models can be applied when planning retention programs for FENs. Sagar (2012) illustrated the application of Spector's Health Traditions Model (2013) in planning orientation for new nurse immigrants from India (Appendices 19 and 20). During orientation, it is important to include culturally and linguistically appropriate services

(CLAS) mandates and guidelines (ICN, 2013; USDHHS, OMH, 2013) when planning the curriculum.

Retention Strategies

Christmas (2002) emphasized careful planning when recruiting nurses: Analysis of retention strategies; assessment of cultural fit; and mentoring and other support. Retention strategies are very important, considering the time and money invested in recruitment and orientation.

FENs, in addition to dealing with professional adjustment in a new country, oftentimes have spouses and children to relocate. Housing, transportation, safety, banking, and credit cards are essential areas where FENs may need assistance (Alinsao, 2009). Orientation and precepting are helpful, but **mentoring** will provide the one-on-one support and coaching to help the FEN adjust socially and professionally; this includes assistance in relocating family members (Christmas, 2002). A period of transition makes people vulnerable and helpless; in these cases, knowledge and empowerment are essential (Alinsao, 2009; Meleis & Glickman, 2013).

Mentoring from a minority nurses association is invaluable. The PNAA has 37 chapters in the United States: east (10), west (8), north central (7), and south central (12); it has two international chapters, one in Austria and another in the UK. Connecting with professional organizations is imperative in empowering expatriate nurses; there is much strength in knowledge, in numbers, and in having a collective voice (Meleis & Glickman, 2013; Wong, 2006). Another possible source of mentorship is Filipino nurses working in the locality in the areas of academia, practice, or administration. Mentors can also be non-nurses who are interested in helping a new immigrant.

Train-the-Trainer Approach

An example of the **train-the-trainer** approach is the Global Scholarship Alliance (GSA) partnership with U.S. universities and health care organizations for the improvement of global nursing and a more just distribution of nurses worldwide ("Graduate Education," 2005).The GSA provides scholarships for nurses from India, Canada, and the UK. Recently, the program funded 28 nurse scholars from the Philippines to pursue MS in Nursing degrees at Xavier University in Cincinnati and Long Island University in New York. The scholars are required to go back to their own countries for a minimum of 2 years to function as leaders in nursing education or administration and develop the next generation of nurses.

The train-the-trainer approach has being used successfully in the Vietnam Friendship Bridge Nurses Group (FBNG). Through a collaboration between Friendship Bridge and the Nursing Education Development program from Teachers College Columbia University, classes for 2 weeks in professional nursing were offered to nurse leaders in education and administration (Sagar, 2010). FBNG has sent over 60 nurse educators from the United States; in partnership with the University of Medicine and Pharmacy in Ho Chi Minh City, Vietnam, FBNG has implemented a master's program in nursing with eight students in 2007 and 18 students in 2008 (Jarrett, Hummel, & Whitney, 2010).

Tapping the Foreign-Educated Nurses Themselves

The ICN (2007a) proposes **circular migration** and calls for programs to support nurses to return to their own countries. In line with the ICN proposal, this author suggests tapping

FENs who have pursued graduate education and gained considerable experience in Australia, Canada, UK, the United States, and other places to return home for a few months and collaborate with and mentor their counterparts in nursing education, practice, administration, and research. Part of this collaboration and mentoring can also be done from a distance. Wong (2006) called this process of giving back "balik bayani" (returning hero). Most FENs desire to give back, an open acknowledgment of having left colleagues behind.

The experience, knowledge, and expertise of expatriate nurses can enrich education, practice, administration, and research. It is a way of mentoring, of giving back and lending a hand—or many hands, hearts, and minds—to those who stayed behind and to the next generation of nurses.

Ea et al. (2008) studied levels of acculturation and job satisfaction among Filipino nurses in the United States (EBP 27.1). EBP 27.2 provides a sample of research conducted among FENs. More studies need to be pursued among FENs and acculturation, job satisfaction, and strategies that have been effective in transitioning to U.S. nursing practice.

EBP 27.1

Ea, Griffin, L'Eplattenier, and Fitzpatrick (2008) conducted a descriptive correlational study using a convenience sample of 96 Filipino nurses at a Philippine Nurses Association (PNA) convention in the northeast United States. This study was performed to measure levels of acculturation among Filipino nurses in the United States as well as their level of job satisfaction. Additionally, this study sought to identify a demonstrable relationship between acculturation and job satisfaction among the nurses surveyed (Ea et al., 2008).

The study was reviewed and approved by their respective institutional review boards (IRB). The criteria for participation in this study was that nurses were from the Philippines, had received their nursing education prior to emigrating, were currently employed as a registered nurse (RN), and were at least 18 years of age. Recruitment techniques of prospective participants included direct approach of attendees at the conference as well as the use of flyers providing information which described the goals of the study. Those meeting the requirements were provided with a packet containing a letter of introduction and data collection instruments used for the study. Those nurses who returned completed survey instruments were given a 5 dollar Starbucks gift card as an added incentive and were assumed to have consented to the study (Ea et al., 2008).

The researchers administered two instruments: Part B of the *Index for Work Satisfaction (IWS)* scale and *A Short Acculturation Scale for Filipino Americans (ASASFA)* scale. The IWS, a widely used survey that measures nurses' job satisfaction, is a 44-item Likert-type scale consisting of areas such as "pay, autonomy, task requirements, organizational policies, interaction, and professional status" (Ea et al., 2008, p. 48). The ASASFA is a 12-item tool that assesses language at home and in media programs, as well as the preferred ethnicity of persons in social relationships (de la cruz, Padilla, & Agustin, 2000).

(continued)

EBP 27.1   *(continued)*

Among the nurses participating in the study, the average length of residency in the United States was approximately 15.5 years; this correlates to the period of professional practice of 15 years in the United States. Furthermore, these nurses demonstrated a moderately high level of income, on average earning more than $60,000 annually. The survey findings demonstrated a level of acculturation closer to mainstream American culture than to Filipino culture and a moderate degree of job satisfaction. Furthermore, a moderately positive correlation between job satisfaction and acculturation was demonstrated (Ea et al., 2008).

The limitations of this study include its relatively small sample size as well as the method of convenience sampling used. Further studies are needed implementing random sampling techniques and larger sample sizes to definitively demonstrate a correlation between acculturation and job satisfaction (Ea et al., 2008). In addition, the researchers suggest studies involving other ethnic groups of FENs; these will provide similarities and differences in acculturation and job satisfaction.

Applications to Practice

1. Do you favor the envelopment of programs to assist FENs with preceptorship, mentoring, and acculturation in order to reduce the incidence of job turnover?
2. What kind of programs would staff nurses and managers need to promote a collaborative and harmonious working relationship with FENs? Describe.
3. If you were to replicate this study, what would you do differently in terms of design, participants, instruments, and analysis of findings?

Source: Ea, Griffin, L'Plattenier, & Fitzpatrick (2008).

EBP 27.2

Title of Study, Author, and Year	Method/Instruments	Participants	Findings
Expectations and Experiences of Recently Recruited Overseas Qualified Nurses in Australia (Brunero, Smith, & Bates, 2008)	Descriptive survey	56 overseas nurses: England, 27; Canada, 6; Scotland, 3; US, 2; Ireland, 3; Sweden, 3; Zimbabwe, 2; China, 1; Italy, 1; Philippines, 1; Finland, 2; South Africa, 2; New Zealand, 1; Fiji, 1; Singapore, 1.	Three major themes: career and lifestyle opportunities; differences in practice; homesickness
Job Satisfaction and Acculturation Among Filipino Registered Registered Nurses (Ea, Griffin, L'Eplattenier, & Fitzpatrick, 2008)	Descriptive, correlational design; 12-item Short Acculturation Scale for Filipino Americans; Part B of Index of Work Satisfaction	96 Filipino RNs at a Philippine Nurses Association of America convention	Moderate level of job satisfaction that is correlated to a level of acculturation nearer American than Filipino
The Racial and Gendered Experiences of Immigrant Nurses From Kerala, India (DiCicco-Bloom, 2004)		10 Indian nurses from Kerala, India	Themes: cultural displacement "a foot here, a foot there, a foot nowhere"; experience of racism and alienation; intersections of categories of being a female nurse, an immigrant, and non-White
Nursing in a New Land: Acculturation and Job Satisfaction Among Filipino Registered Nurses Working in Skilled Nursing Facilities (Reyes & Cohen, 2013)	Cross sectional, descriptive, correlational, quantitative design; 12-item Short Acculturation Scale for Filipino Americans; Part B of Index of Work Satisfaction	42 Filipino immigrant nurses	Participants had acculturation levels closer to American culture than Filipino. No relationship noted between acculturation and job satisfaction.

(continued)

EBP 27.2 *(continued)*

Title of Study, Author, and Year	Method/Instruments	Participants	Findings
Generic and Professional Care of Anglo-American (AA) and Philippine American Nurses (PA) (Spangler, 1993)	Ethnonursing method (Leininger)	Key informants:AA, 9; PA, 10. General informants: AA, 13; PA, 16.	Themes: AA: promotion of autonomous care, value for patient education, expectations that patients will comply, control of situations and conditions. PA: seriousness and dedication to work, attentiveness to patient's physical comfort, care as respect, care as patience.

Source: Brunero, Smith, & Bates (2008); DiCicco-Bloom (2004); Ea, Griffin, L'Eplattenier, & Fitzpatrick (2008); Reyes & Cohen (2013); and Spangler (1993).

CRITICAL THINKING EXERCISES 27.1

Undergraduate Student

1. How many foreign-educated nurses are employed in your current work setting? How many of these foreign nurses work with you in your unit/department?
2. Review and compare and contrast two research articles or other literature pertaining to foreign graduate nurses.
3. What solutions can you propose, other than recruitment of FENs, to the nursing shortage?
4. How would you encourage young people to consider nursing as a career?

Graduate Student

1. Interview a foreign nurse using the following guide: date of arrival in the United States, date of passing the NCLEX-RN, program for acculturation/adjustment in the United States, preceptorship, mentoring, and strategies to cope with culture shock and homesickness.
2. If you are a nurse administrator, have you participated in the orientation of FENs? Were there specific TCN concepts in the orientation plan?
3. Compare and contrast three research articles regarding recruitment and retention of FENs. Are there gaps in those research studies?
4. If you were to conduct research among FENs, what would be your research questions? Discuss.

Faculty in Academia

1. Do you have faculty members at your school who are FENs?
2. If you do, what are their current ranks? Are they tenured?
3. Trace the educational background of these faculty members. Which one of their degrees was completed in the United States?
4. Are these faculty members involved in outreach to their countries of origin? Describe their programs of involvement.

Staff Development Educator

1. What percentage of your registered nurse employees are FENs? What are the three main sending countries of origin of these nurses?
2. How are these nurses recruited? Are there support services such as housing, transportation, and English as a second language (ESL) classes available to these nurses upon arriving to the United States?
3. Do you offer additional orientation for FENs? If yes, how? How many additional days do these nurses get?
4. Do you have a mentoring program for FENs? How are mentors assigned to the nurses? Do you collaborate with minority nursing organizations in terms of networking and mentoring? How often do nurses meet? How are follow-up activities implemented?

SUMMARY

To offset global nursing shortages, developed countries are recruiting FENs. However, the nurse migration causes severe drain from the sending countries; this compromises health care and the education of future nurses in those nations. Some solutions include more ethical ways of recruitment; requiring a certain number of years of service prior to leaving for abroad; the train-the-trainer approach; and circular migration, to name just a few.

An overview of the development of nursing education in the Philippines is included to provide a starting point of the cultural background and ways of life of the Filipino nurse. After all, the Philippines is the country sending the most FENs abroad. The face of the Filipino nurse graces the hospitals in the Middle East, in Australia, in Europe, in Canada, in the United States, and in many other parts of the world.

Giving back, "balik bayani," is imperative. We must be mentors to these FENs, as we are mentors to students and colleagues; in fact, many of us are products of mentoring. This author also suggests tapping FENs who have pursued graduate education in Australia, Canada, UK, and the United States to return home for a few months and assist in nursing education, practice, administration, and research in their respective countries. We, indeed, are at the crossroads in history where global strategies, more than ever, are needed for ethical recruitment and retention of FENs.

REFERENCES

Agoncillo, T. A. (1990). *History of the Filipino people*. Quezon City, Philippines: Garotech.

Aiken, L. (2007). U.S. nurse labor market dynamics are key to global nurse sufficiency. *Health Research and Educational Trust*, 42(3 Pt. 2), 1299–1320. doi:10.1111/j.1475–6773.2007.00714. Retrieved October 15, 2013, from www.ncbi.nlm.nih.gov/pmc/articles/PMC1955371/pdf/hesr0042–1299.pdf

Aiken, L., Buchan, J., Sochalski, J., Nichols, B., & Powell, M. (2004). Trends in international nurse migration. *Health Affairs*, 23(3), 69–77.

Alinsao, V. C. (2009). Adjusting to a new community. In B. L. Nichols & C. R. Davis (Eds.), *What you need to know about nursing and health care in the United States* (pp. 235–254). New York, NY: Springer Publishing.

Amerson, R. (2002). The nuts and bolts of common nursing staff development programs: Orientation. In K. L. O'Shea (Ed.), *Staff development nursing secret* (pp. 161–174). Philadelphia, PA: Hanley & Belfus.

Andrews, M. M., & Ludwig-Beymer, P. (2012). Cultural diversity in the health care workforce. In M. M. Andrews & J. S. Boyle (Eds.), *Transcultural concepts in nursing care* (pp. 316–348). Philadelphia, PA: Wolters Kluwer/Lippincott Williams & Wilkins.

Arends-Kuenning, M. (2006, September). The balance of care: Trends in the wages and employment of immigrant nurses in the US between 1990–2000. *Globalizations*, 3(3), 333–348.

Association of Deans of Philippine Colleges of Nursing (ADPCN). (1998). ADPCN Five-year development plan revisited. *Philippine Journal of Nursing Education*, 8(1), 13–15.

Basuray, J. (1997, December). Nurse Miss Sahib: Colonial culture-bound education in India and transcultural nursing. *Journal of Transcultural Nursing*, 9(14), 14–19.

Brunero, S., Smith, J., & Bates, E. (2008). Expectations and experiences of recently recruited overseas qualified nurses in Australia. *Contemporary Nurse*, 28(1), 101–110.

Brush, B. L. (2008). Global nurse migration today. *Journal of Nursing Scholarship*, 40(1), 20–25.

Brush, B. L., Sochalski, J., & Berger, A. (2004). Imported care: Recruiting foreign nurses to US health care facilities. *Health Affairs*, 23(3), 78–87.

Central Intelligence Agency. (2013). *The world factbook: The Philippines*. Retrieved October 13, 2013, from https://www.cia.gov/library/publications/the-world-factbook/geos/rp.html

Choo, V. (2003). Philippines losing its nurses, and now maybe its doctors. *The Lancet*, 361, 1356.

Choy, C. C. (1998). *The export of womanpower: Oral history of Filipino nurse migration to the United States*. University of California at Los Angeles. Ann Arbor, MI: UMI.

Choy, C. C. (2003). *Empire of care: Nursing and migration in Filipino American history*. Durham, NC: Duke University Press.

Christmas, K. (2002). Invest internationally. *Nursing Management*, 33, 20–21.

Clemente, D. (2003). Nursing matters: More Filipino nurses now work in the US. *The Filipino Express*, 17(42), 13.

Conclara, J. P. (2002, July). Filipino nurses in the US down to a trickle. *Filipinas*, 11, 25–28.

Davis, C. R., & Nichols, B. L. (2002). Foreign educated nurses and the changing US workforce. *Nursing Administration Quarterly, 26*(2), 43–51.

de la cruz, F. A., Padilla, G. V., & Agustin, E. O. (2000). Adapting a measure of acculturation for cross-cultural research. *Journal of Transcultural Nursing, 11*(3), 191–198.

De LaSalle University. (2002). *History of the Philippines.* Retrieved October 13, 2013, from http://pinas.dlsu.edu.ph/history/history.html

DiCicco-Bloom, B. (2004). The racial and gendered experiences of immigrant nurses from Kerala, India. *Journal of Transcultural Nursing, 15*(1), 26–33.

Divinagracia, C. C. (1996a). Cutting edge issues: New dimensions in nursing. *Philippine Journal of Nursing Education, 6*(1), 44–47.

Divinagracia, C. C. (1996b). President's annual report. *Philippine Journal of Nursing Education, 6*(1), 2–6.

Divinagracia, C. C. (1998). President's annual report. *Philippine Journal of Nursing Education, 8*(1), 4–6.

Ea, E. E., Griffin, M., L'Eplattenier, N., & Fitzpatrick, J. J. (2008). Job satisfaction and acculturation among Filipino registered nurses. *Journal of Nursing Scholarship, 40*(1), 46–51.

Estella, C. (2005a). Lack of nurses burdens an ailing healthcare system. *Philippine Center for Investigative Journalism.* Retrieved July 11, 2013, from http://pcij.org/stories/lack-of-nurses-burdens-an-ailing-healthcare-system

Estella, C. (2005b). Substandard nursing schools sell dreams of a life abroad. *Philippine Center for Investigative Journalism.* Retrieved July 11, 2013, from http://pcij.org/stories/substandard-nursing-schools-sell-dreams-of-a-life-abroad

Giron-Tupas, A. (1952). *History of nursing in the Philippines.* Manila, Philippines: Filipino Nurses Association.

Giron-Tupas, A. (1961). *History of nursing in the Philippines.* Manila, Philippines: University Book Supply.

Graduate education to ease the global nursing shortage. (2005, May/June). *Nursing Education Perspectives, 26*(3), 143.

International Council of Nurses. (2007a). *Nurse retention and migration.* Retrieved July 11, 2013, from www.icn.ch/images/stories/documents/publications/position_statements/C06_Nurse_Retention_Migration.pdf

International Council of Nurses. (2007b). *Ethical nurse recruitment.* Retrieved July 11, 2013, from www.icn.ch/images/stories/documents/publications/position_statements/C03_Ethical_Nurse_Recruitment.pdf

International Council of Nurses. (2013). *Cultural and linguistic competence.* Retrieved September 6, 2013, from www.icn.ch/images/stories/documents/publications/position_statements/B03_Cultural_Linguistic_Competence.pdf

Jarrett, S., Hummel, F., & Whitney, K. (2010). Nurse educators who work in other countries: Vietnam. In J. J. Fitzpatrick, C. M. Schultz, & T. D. Aiken (Eds.), *Giving through teaching: How nurse educators are changing the world* (pp. 307–312). New York, NY: Springer Publishing.

Jeffreys, M. R. (2010). Overview of key issues and concerns. In M. R. Jeffreys (Ed.), *Teaching cultural competence in nursing and health care* (pp. 3–26). New York, NY: Springer Publishing.

Jeffreys, M. R., & Karczewski, C. (2010). Case exemplar: Linking strategies-spotlight on employee orientation programs to enhance cultural competence. In M. R. Jeffreys (Ed.), *Teaching cultural competence in nursing and health care* (pp. 285–302). New York, NY: Springer Publishing.

Marquand, B. (2006). Philippine nurses in the US—Yesterday and today. *Minority Nursing, 3*(1), 16–25. Retrieved October 14, 2013, from www.minoritynurse.com/article/philippine-nurses-us%E2%80%94yesterday-and-today

Mason, D. (2009). Foreword. In B. L. Nichols & C. R. Davis (Eds.), *What you need to know about nursing and health care in the United States.* New York, NY: Springer Publishing.

Meleis, A., & Glickman, C. G. (2012). Empowering expatriate nurses: Challenges and opportunities: A commentary. *Nursing Outlook, 60,* S24–S26. Retrieved May 19, 2013, from http://download.journals.elsevierhealth.com/pdfs/journals/0029-6554/PIIS0029655412000796.pdf

Nakashima, E., & Cody, E., *The Washington Post.* (2004, May 30). Filipinos leaving home in huge numbers from doctors and nurses to lounge singers and circus performers, they are seeking their fortunes abroad: [region Edition]. *Pittsburgh Post-Gazette,* p. A-5.

Nichols, B. L., & Davis, C. R. (2009). *What you need to know about nursing and health care in the United States.* New York, NY: Springer Publishing.

Ocampo, R. F. (1997). Nursing education in the next millennium. *Philippine Journal of Nursing Education, 8*(1), 13–15.

Pacquiao, D. (2007). The relationship between cultural competence education and increasing diversity in nursing schools and practice settings. *Transcultural Nursing, 18*(1), 28S–37S.

Philippine Nurses Association, Inc. (2011). *Brief history.* Retrieved September 13, 2013, from www.pna-ph.org/about_history.asp

Reyes, L. Q., & Cohen, J. (2013). Nursing in a new land: Acculturation and job satisfaction among Filipino registered nurses working in skilled nursing facilities. *Online Journal of Cultural Competence in Nursing and Healthcare, 3*(1), 16–25. doi:10.9730/ojccnh.org/v3n1a2

Sagar, P. L. (2010). Nurse educators who work in other countries: Vietnam. In J. J. Fitzpatrick, C. M. Schultz, & T. D. Aiken (Eds.), *Giving through teaching: How nurse educators are changing the world* (pp. 306–307). New York, NY: Springer. Publishing.

Sagar, P. L. (2012). *Transcultural nursing theory and models: Application in nursing education, practice, and administration.* New York, NY: Springer Publishing.

Sheer, B., & Wong, F. K. Y. (2008). The development of advanced nursing practice globally. *Journal of Nursing Scholarship, 40*(3), 204–211.

Sison, M. (2002, July). Exodus of nurses grows: Flight of the nightingales. *Filipinas, 11*, 26–27.

Sotejo, J. V. (2001). Part II. Vantage point. In L. B. Tungpalan (Ed.), *Action oriented leadership and J. V. Sotejo: A biography* (pp. 453–481). Manila, Philippines: University of the Philippines College of Nursing Foundation.

Spangler, Z. (1993). Generic and professional care of Anglo-American and Philippine American nurses. In D. A. Gaut (Ed.), *Global agenda for caring* (pp. 47–61). New York, NY: National League for Nursing.

Tiwari, R. R., Sharma, K., & Zodpey, S. P. (2013). Situational analysis of nursing education and work force in India. *Nursing Outlook*, 129–136. Retrieved May 19, 2013, from http://download.journals.elsevierhealth.com/pdfs/journals/0029-6554/PIIS0029655412001753.pdf

Tungpalan, L. B. (2001). *Action oriented leadership and J. V. Sotejo: A biography.* Manila, Philippines: University of the Philippines College of Nursing Foundation.

UK 'draining third world of nurses.' (2001, April 23). British Broadcasting Corporation News: Health. Retrieved October 2, 2002, from http://news.bbc.co.uk/1/hi/health/1292413.stm

Ullrich, S., & Haffer, A. (2009). *Precepting in nursing: Developing an effective workforce.* Boston, MA: Jones & Bartlett.

U.S. Department of Health and Human Services, Health Resources Services Administration. (2010). *The registered nurse population: Initial findings from the 2008 National Sample Survey of registered nurses.* Retrieved March 9, 2013, from http://bhpr.hrsa.gov/healthworkforce/rnsurveys/rnsurveyfinal.pdf

U.S. Department of Health and Human Services, Office of Minority Health. (2013). *The national standards for culturally and linguistically appropriate services in health and health Care* (the national CLAS standards). Retrieved July 16, 2013, from https://www.thinkculturalhealth.hhs.gov/pdfs/EnhancedNationalCLASStandards.pdf

Wong, C. S. (2006). [Editorial]. Protecting a legacy. *Philippine Nurses Association, 25*(1).

World Health Organization. (2006). *Working together for health: The WHO report 2006.* Geneva, Switzerland: Author. Retrieved June 9, 2013, from www.who.int/whr/2006/whr06_en.pdf

CHAPTER

Then, Now, and Beyond: Quo Vadis, TCN?

28

Priscilla Limbo Sagar, Caroline Camuñas, and Sheila O'Shea Melli

KEY TERMS

Brain drain
Certification
Collaborations
Consultation
International partnerships
Mentoring

Migration
Multicultural centers
Nurse drain
Organizational culture
Train-the-trainer approach
Trends

LEARNING OBJECTIVES

At the completion of this chapter, the learner will be able to

1. Describe international issues related to health and well-being.
2. Discuss the implications of increasingly diverse populations for nursing.
3. Analyze the importance of cultural competence in professional nursing care.
4. Trace the historical highlights of transcultural nursing (TCN).
5. Explore concepts in consultation, mentoring, international partnerships, and collaborations.
6. Articulate visions for TCN in terms of future prospects.

OVERVIEW

We, the nurses of today, need to look back and reflect on where the profession and the nurse pioneers have been in order to see where nursing is going. The past, the present, and the future are so interconnected. It is one way to realize our own responsibilities in shaping the future role of nurses in health care and in society. Dr. Madeleine Leininger pioneered the development of the field of TCN and its integration in nursing education, practice, administration, and research. It is worth while to look back at Leininger's efforts in the 1950s, then reflect about TCN a year after it lost its founder and most ardent supporter. It is only then that with a clear head we can envision the trends for this very important field of nursing and the whole of health care.

It has been 5 decades since Dr. Madeleine Leininger founded the field of TCN. Since that time, TCN knowledge and evidence-based practice (EBP) have grown. It is now time to minimize the lag between the generation of knowledge and its application in client care settings; this lag may be an unbelievable, yet documented range from 8 to 15 years (Dobbins, Ciliska, Estabrooks, & Hayward, 2005). In both academic and staff development settings, there is a vast body of TCN knowledge to be applied to practice. This application helps minimize the lag that Dobbins et al. quoted.

There is an immense untapped strength in numbers among registered nurses. We have yet to capitalize on this strength as the largest group of professional health care providers. As of 2010, nurses numbered 3,063,133 strong in the United States (U.S. Department of Health and Human Services [USDHHS], Health Resources Services Administration [HRSA], 2010a). We can all take the lead in this initiative for TCN and continue culturally and linguistically congruent care for our clients, students, colleagues, and coworkers.

These are challenging times as we face the continued nurse shortage. The faculty nurse shortage is already acute and is predicted to get worse in the coming years. Unless we call upon our youth and invite them to the wonderful profession of nursing, it may take a long while before we have a steady supply of nurses educated in the United States. Although these are challenging times, there are vast opportunities. Nurses—for 11 years in a row—have been voted as the most trusted of professions according to the Gallup poll that ranks professions for honesty and ethical standards (American Nurses Association [ANA], 2010). Trust is the foundation of therapeutic nurse–client relationships. When a client trusts, the nurse can effectively bridge generic and professional care for the best client outcomes.

EIGHT TRANSCULTURAL TRENDS TO WATCH

When looking into the future, many **trends**—direction of changes or developments–are worth watching: renewed interest in curricular integration and cultural competence among faculty and students; increasing demand for individual and organizational cultural competence; expanding demand for academic and staff development **consultation**; rising need and demand for TCN **certification**; growing need for the **train-the-trainer approach**; escalating professional migration; intensifying focus for the interprofessional approach; and expanding need for mentoring, partnerships, and **collaborations**.

#1. Renewed Interest: Curricular Integration and Cultural Competence Among Students and Faculty

The American Association of Colleges of Nursing ([AACN], 2008, 2011) and the National League for Nursing ([NLN], 2009a, 2009b) both have faculty toolkits to guide curricular integration of TCN concepts in all levels of nursing education. Their respective accrediting bodies, the Commission of Collegiate Nursing Education ([CCNE], 2013) and the Accreditation Commission for Education in Nursing ([ACEN], 2013), require the utilization of professional standards as well as diversity and promotion of cultural competence.

The renewed interest in curricular integration of diversity and cultural competence in all levels of nursing programs has a concomitant question on how schools of nursing prepare practitioners to care for increasingly diverse clients, families, and communities. Research has been conducted regarding student cultural competence (Kardong-Edgreen & Campinha-Bacote, 2008; Kardong-Edgreen et al., 2010); diverse student recruitment, retention, and success (Sutherland, Hamilton, & Goodman, 2007; McFarland, Mixer, Lewis, & Easley, 2006); faculty practices in teaching culture (Hughes & Hood, 2007; Kardong-Edgreen, 2007; Mixer, 2008, 2011); faculty and students (Sargent, Sedlak, & Martsoff, 2005); multidisciplinary course for students (Muñoz, DoBroka, & Mohammad, 2009); and university-wide endeavors to assess the magnitude of curricular integration (Kennedy, Fisher, Fontaine, & Martin-Holland, 2008) and practices relating to education, research, and administration (Sumpter & Carthon, 2011).

In nursing education, trends will continue to fully integrate TCN into all levels of nursing curricula. Seamless articulation between associate and baccalaureate programs will be instrumental in including TCN concepts early in the education of all nurses. It is imperative to implement seamless articulation; some types of articulation agreements do not carefully look at every course in the curriculum to ensure that the transition is truly "bridged" from the community college to the college or university baccalaureate curriculum. Certification in TCN will be encouraged for faculty and graduate students and for baccalaureate-, associate-, and diploma-prepared nurses.

There will be increasing numbers of **multicultural centers** (MCs) in many schools of nursing. MCs will spearhead these two main goals: contribute to the development of culturally competent health care workers, and facilitate delivery of culturally and linguistically appropriate services ([CLAS], USDHHS, Office of Minority Health [OMH], 2013). Specifically, MCs will (1) develop programs to enhance the ability of health care educators in teaching culturally diverse students; (2) offer face-to-face and online programs to increase cultural competence of health care practitioners; and (3) design curricula integrating evidence-based and best practices of culturally competent care. Many of these MCs will offer a postmaster's certificate in TCN and review for basic and advanced certification in TCN.

Some MCs will provide face-to-face and online programs with continuing education (CE) or academic credits. An increasing number of MCs will have the infrastructure to provide blended as well as totally online, revenue-generating programs that will sustain these kinds of programs long after the initial external funding is used up. Foreign-educated nurses (FENs) moving globally for work and professional opportunities—as well as their employers and coworkers—will be in need of this program. Online programs such as these will augment orientation and continuing competence of respective institutions hiring these nurses. A funded MC will be able to afford to invite TCN worldwide experts as resident scholars. After the funding runs out, the center will be able to generate income from these programs and sustain itself. Certification in TCN will add value to nurse credentials and enable the holder to lead initiatives for culturally competent care.

#2. Increasing Demands: Individual and Organizational Cultural Competence

There have been increasing demands for both individual and organizational cultural competence. When aiming for organizational cultural competence, it is a good idea to first look at the culture of the particular organization. **Organizational culture** refers to patterns of role-related beliefs, ideals, and outlooks shared by members of an organization. These patterns produce the rules and norms of behavior that strongly influence individual and group behavior within the organization (Camuñas, 2013, pp. 72–73).

The American Nurses Association (1991) emphasized that the interaction between a health care provider and a client involves three cultural systems, namely that of the client, the health care provider, and the organization. These interactions may cause conflict and barriers to care, thereby causing more disparities. Therefore, cultural competence must be fostered in organizational settings (Sagar, 2012a). Ludwig-Beymer (2012) illustrated the use of Leininger's Cultural Care Theory (CCT) in organizational assessment. Guidelines and mandates from the government (USDHHS, OMH, 2013) and from accrediting bodies such as The Joint Commission (TJC, 2010a, 2010b) and the sought after American Nurses Credentialing Center (ANCC, 2009) all require culturally competent organizations (Ludwig-Beymer, 2012). In addition, organizations must provide the environment and leadership that are conducive to treating those who are different with respect, beneficence, care, and justice.

All employees have roles in fostering culturally competent organizations (Ludwig-Beymer, 2012). A few people who are passionate about diversity and cultural competence cannot by themselves make a culturally competent organization. It must live in all organizational levels: policy making, administrative, management, and provider (Ludwig-Beymer, 2012, p. 239). Policy, procedure, and culture affect the quality of care provided and can increase or ameliorate disparities in care and outcomes. The following can enhance an organization's ability to provide culturally competent care. These conditions must be apparent at every level of an organization: high value placed on diversity; importance of cultural self-assessment; capacity to evaluate the dynamics inherent in cultural interaction; necessity of knowledge of institutional culture; and flexibility in adapting care with an understanding of cultural diversity. The absence of these conditions can lead to deep distrust of fellow citizens/professionals and can aggravate or intensify health disparities and poor outcomes.

The cultural diversity of society has various strengths but also provides many challenges. These challenges include differing values that impact on health practices and disease experiences. Minorities often have limited access to health care. These factors lead to well-documented disparities in health (Haiman et al., 2006; Smedley, Stith, & Nelson, 2003). However, it is stunning that when U.S. health, morbidity, and mortality are compared with 16 high-income democracies (Western Europe, Australia, Canada, and Japan) the United States does not fare well. U.S. men have the lowest and U.S. women have the second to lowest life-expectancy in comparison with the 16 nations in the research study (National Research Council & Institute of Medicine [NRC & IOM], 2013). Americans also fared worse in infant mortality and low birth weight, heart disease, chronic lung disease, obesity, diabetes, injuries, homicides, disabilities, and sexually transmitted diseases. A disturbing fact is that the United States spends more than twice as much on health care per capita as the other 16 peer countries.

#3. Expanding Demand for Consultation: Academia and Staff Development

The Nursing Professional Development (NPD) Specialist Practice (ANA and National Nursing Staff Development Organization [NNSDO], 2010) model of CE, career development and role transition, research and scholarship, academic partnership, orientation, competency program, and service, as well as its central focus of EBP and practice-based evidence, would be complimented by culturally and linguistically appropriate services (USDHHS, OMH, 2013). EBP is defined as "the conscientious, explicit, and judicious use of current best evidence in making decisions about the care of individual patients" (Porter, O'Halloran, & Morrow, 2011, p. 106). Best evidence is the result of random controlled trials. Proponents have asserted that the clinician's judgments and patient's values must be included. Additionally, communication of EBP changes must be communicated consistently.

Academic and staff development settings will make more headway to require CE programs in diversity and cultural competence. In academia, consultation will entail integration of diversity in its mission, philosophy, and goals, as well as vertical and horizontal threading of these concepts in nursing and allied health science courses. There will be widening demand for tools to measure cultural competence of students and faculty, as well as college- and university-wide initiatives to evaluate academic programs, research, and practice.

In staff development, consultation will require a review of the mission, philosophy, and objectives of facilities and organizations for compliance with accreditation and CLAS mandates and guidelines. Tools will be used to measure the cultural competence of staff nurses, allied health practitioners, employees, and organizations. TCN consultation should seek to improve patient care, improve the work environment, and assist in the eradication of health disparities and increased mortality among minorities. Consultation may be performed in relation to patients, staff, committees, and organizations.

#4. Rising Need and Demand: Transcultural Certification

The Transcultural Nursing Society began its work on certification in 1987, administering the first examination in 1988 at its international conference (McFarland & Leininger, 2002). Leininger (1995) envisioned that certification in TCN would be required by the year 2020. Although certification in basic (CTN-B) and advanced (CTN-A) transcultural nursing has not yet reached a requirement stage, the impetus for certification will increase for both advanced and basic levels (Sagar, in press). Reliability and validity studies are being conducted by the Transcultural Certification Commission (TNCC), a subsidiary of TCNS, in a continued effort to make the CTN certification on par with other specialty nursing certifications (Andrews et al., 2011). Chapter 26 discusses certification more thoroughly.

The trend to seek CTN certification will be influenced by requiring individual and organizational cultural competence by accrediting bodies in practice settings such as the TJC (2010a, 2010b) and in academia such as the Commission on Collegiate Nursing Education (CCNE) and the Accreditation Commission for Education in Nursing (ACEN, 2013). Formerly the National League for Nursing Accreditation Commission (NLNAC), ACEN specifies diversity among its standards under "curriculum." The number of CTN entrepreneurs may also increase as CE providers, consultants, and TCN experts.

More than ever, there is a need for leadership by certified transcultural nurses in nursing education, practice, administration, and research. According to the TCNS (2013), there are only 22 CTNs with basic certifications (21 from the United States and one from Canada) and 59 CTNs with advanced certification (56 from the United States and one each from Australia, Israel, and Saudi Arabia). These 81 CTNs are far too few people to answer the clarion call for caring, educating, mentoring, and role modeling in nursing education, practice, and administration (Sagar, 2012a, in press). Both advanced and basic certification are offered by the TNCC (TCNS, 2013). Information about the certification core curriculum, application, testing, and renewal are all available at the TCNS website at www.tcns.org.

#5. Teaching Them How to Fish: Train-the-Trainer Approach

A 3-year funded program—*Developing Cultural Competencies for Nurses: Evidence-Based Practices*—is directed by Dr. Margaret Andrews (University of Michigan at Flint) and codirected by Dr. Theresa Thompson (Madonna University). This project has a train-the-trainer program that uses online and face-to-face classes and workshops, print materials, and audiovisual resources as an opportunity to assimilate TCN knowledge, skills, and competencies;

this can serve as foundational preparation for TCN certification (Andrews et al., 2011). This educational program series employs national and international TCN experts, authors, and leaders. The *Online Journal of Cultural Competence in Nursing and Health care* (OJCCNHC) is an offshoot of this funded project (Andrews et al., 2011). OJCCNHC disseminates scholarly work and encourages dialogue from diverse perspectives; journal subscription is free from this website: www.ojccnh.org.

Allied health such as medicine, pharmacy, dentistry, and physical therapy will also continue to make diversity and cultural competence a priority. For example, Assemi, Mutha, and Suchanek Hudmon (2007) developed, implemented, and evaluated the impact of a 2-day cultural competence train-the-trainer workshop for pharmacy educators from all over the United States. A total of 50 faculty members with no training in teaching cultural competency attended. *Incorporating Cultural Competency in Pharmacy Education* (1.65 CEUs) was provided to pharmacy faculty from schools across the United States. Assemi et al. (2007) surveyed the participants' characteristics and self-efficacy in developing and teaching content before, the workshop at the end the workshop, and 9 months after the workshop. At baseline, 94% of faculty members reported no formal training in teaching cultural competence. The participants' ratings of "very good" or "excellent" rose from 13% to 60% after the training (Assemi et al., p. 1). Notably, participants reported that they used one or more components of the workshop to teach close to 3,000 students within 9 months after the training.

#6. Escalating Migration of Professionals: The Brain Drain

Worldwide, people move from place to place in order to make better lives for themselves and their families. **Migration** is the act of going from one country, region, or place to settle in another. Migration has implications for health care, especially regarding access to care, quality of care, and cost of care. Discussion of migration as a whole is beyond the scope of this chapter; this will focus on professional migration.

There are many issues related to migration. Although migration very often provides a better life for migrants, it can also have a negative impact on the countries they leave. This is especially true when health care professionals leave their countries and migrate to global wealth centers. Migration of health professionals from developing countries leaves those countries with a severe shortage of such professionals. This is referred to as **brain drain.**

In the United States, there has been an increase of FENs from 3.7% in 2004 to 5.6% in 2008 (USDHHS, HRSA, 2010). FENs practicing professionally in the United States originate from the Philippines (48.7%), Canada (11.5%), India (9.3%), United Kingdom (5.8%), Korea (2.6%), and Nigeria (2.0%; Andrews & Ludwig-Beymer, 2012). According to Mason (2009), reasons for nurse migration to the United States include (1) better living conditions, (2) working in complex U.S. nurse settings, (3) pursuing graduate degrees, and (4) experience living in another nation. Referred to as **"nurse drain,"** the migration of nurses from developing to developed nations is expected to continue, especially with the continuing global nursing shortage. For more discussion about foreign-educated nurses (FENs), see Chapter 27.

#7. Intensifying Focus: Transcultural Health Care as an Interprofessional Approach

The Institute of Medicine (IOM, 2010) has advocated for interprofessional and collaborative education for nurses and allied professionals. For better client outcomes and professional development, collaboration is imperative in the complex health care delivery systems. Interprofessional education will be a solid foundation in future practice collaborations; each allied professional brings a unique perspective in client care. The allied health professions such as medicine, pharmacy, dentistry, and physical therapy have also made diversity and cultural competence a priority.

In nursing, administration at all levels will make diversity and cultural competence part of their collaborative work with all hospital departments. Eustis, Alexander, and Plaster (2010) illustrated diversity and cultural competence at Fairview Health Services, a 22,000-employee integrated health care system in the Minneapolis-St. Paul, Minnesota area. Eustis et al. (2010) referred to six key areas—called *levers*—that served as the foundation of their initiative and gave all employees optional participation: leaders at every level; systematic collection of data; community participation; creation of the Office of Diversity as the central component; empowerment of volunteer diversity advocates; and expectations for performance and competency for all levels of employees (p. 46). Acknowledging similarities and differences, this health care system placed the client at the center of care, using *namaste* as a greeting and as a commitment. Used often in yoga, namaste denotes an acknowledgment of the soul, heart, or light of another.

#8. Expanding Need for Mentoring, International Partnerships, and Collaborations

Mentoring has varied definitions. Huang and Lynch (1995) evoke grace, mutuality, and strength in their definition of mentoring as a two-way spherical dance that offers chances to individuals to experience giving and receiving of each other's gifts without limits and fears. **Mentoring** occurs in a one-to-one relationship; for example, a senior and a junior freely enter into an agreement where the senior instructs and guides the junior's career choices over a sustained period of time, oftentimes throughout a career (Vance, 2002, 2011; Vance & Olson, 1998).

Professional socialization includes such issues as development of skills of critical thinking, problem solving, and decision making; priority setting; understanding and adopting goals and norms of professional practice; and development of self-confidence. Career guidance is valuable for achievement. Mentors and preceptors are important to this end. It is important to remember that mentorship and preceptorship are different. Precepting, although also a one-to-one relationship that is sustained over time, it is usually short term, such as a school semester or a year. Preceptorships, with definite goals and objectives, generally are contractual or informally arranged. The person who is precepted is often called an apprentice (Barnum, 2006).

There are **international partnerships** and collaborations between schools all over the world. These partnerships and collaborations entail some exchange of faculty and students, sharing of curricula, and transnational research. In the process of mentoring international colleagues, mentors need to reflect on the question of whether the initiative is reflective of its people's culture. Will it grow and function in harmony with its people and environment? An example is a nursing curriculum being developed in a foreign nation. It has to be a curriculum for nurses in that nation, for professionalism of its nurses, for the health outcomes of its own people, and not an export of a U.S. curriculum.

In the United States, research addressing disparities in health care, generic folk healing, effects of alternative treatments, navigating the health care system, and client and family satisfactions with health care will increase. Emphasis on ethnic-specific research—instead of "lumping" groups together—is essential (EBP 28.1). There will be renewed community participation and involvement in keeping healthy communities as envisioned by *Healthy People 2020* (USDHHS, 2010b).

EBP 28.1

Problem: An assumption often found in the literature is that acculturation is a wanted health-related result of immigration. However, research does not support this idea. There is a need for clarification, explication, and development of evidence-based, ethnic specific cancer pain theories to improve nursing care and facilitate research.

Background: Im conducted this study to clarify reports that Asian Americans are less likely to experience severe pain than other ethnic groups. The perceived wisdom is that Asians, including Asian Americans, most often do not seek help until they have severe pain. The following have been used to account for this: (1) stoicism is highly valued by Confucianism and Taoism, philosophies prevalent in many Asian cultures; (2) cultural belief that pain helps build strong character; (3) patients want to be seen as "good" by providers; (4) many may have erroneous ideas about the use of opioid analgesics (e.g., They shorten life and are addictive).

Method: Im presents a situation-specific, midrange transition theory that explains the cancer pain experience of Asian Americans. The theory was developed on the basis of evidence. She used an integrative approach with diverse sources. Im began with the transition theory developed by Meleis et al. (2000), Chick and Meleis (1986), and Schumacher and Meleis (1994), all as cited in Im (2008). An integrative literature review was conducted.

Results: The literature review demonstrated that while some studies have been conducted with Asian Americans, these studies did not differentiate among ethnic groups such as Vietnamese, Korean, or Thai. Indeed, each ethnic group of Asian Americans has its own specific culture, beliefs, values, and attitudes.

Im conceptualized the response patterns to (1) tolerance—overcoming pain demonstrates strength and being a "good" patient; (2) natural—believing pain is a natural consequence of cancer; (3) normal—seeing pain as natural, resulted in trying to live normal lives and avoid the stigma of cancer; and (4) mind control—attempting to control cancer by positive thinking that would decrease pain and increase hope (Im, 2008, p. 320).

Discussion: There is a growing emphasis on the need for theory and evidence-based translational studies for the improvement of patient care and research. Specificity is easily translated into research and can provide a thorough view of nursing practice. Because this approach is evidence-based and anchored in extant theory, it is applicable to both research and nursing practice with Asian American cancer patients as well as other ethnic minorities.

Application to Practice

■ Investigate the pain assessment guidelines used in your clinical rotation. Is it inclusive of adaptations for culturally diverse clients?

■ In a scenario where you are the nurse educator about to revise the above tool, what would you add?

■ If you were to replicate this study, how would you conduct it? What would you change in terms of conceptual framework, sampling, and analysis of findings?

Source: Im (2008).

VISIONS FOR THE FUTURE

Culture is a large measure in quality. Cultural differences in beliefs (including health beliefs), practices, and standards can vary and can be profound. All of this has ethical implications. The Code for Nurses strongly emphasizes that the need for health care is universal, regardless of all individual differences; the nurse is duty-bound to implement nursing services without prejudice and with the utmost respect for human needs and for the client as a person (American Nurses Association [ANA], 2001, p. 9).

Behavior and decision making must be understood as outcomes or reflections of culture. Diversity is enriching; it broadens our sense of the human condition. The United Nations Educational Scientific and Cultural Organization (UNESCO, 2001) Universal Declaration on Cultural Diversity states:

> Culture takes diverse forms across time and space. This diversity is embodied in the uniqueness and plurality of the identities of the groups and societies making up humankind. As a source of exchange, innovation and creativity, cultural diversity is as necessary for humankind as biodiversity is for nature. In this sense, it is the common heritage of humanity and should be recognized and affirmed for the benefit of present and future generations. (UNESCO, 2001, para 26)

All indicators bode well for a future of growing cultural diversity. Historically, nurses have led others in demonstrating a deep, enduring concern for ethics. Cultural diversity brings new facets to the issues surrounding the provision of competent, effective care. However, while at first sight these issues may seem alien, it does not mean that they are so different that they pose insurmountable realities. The underlying precepts for solving these issues remain the same. That is, they are the same issues in different guise, and as such, they are amenable to the application of basic nursing skills. Although cultural diversity carries with it many challenges, it also brings a wide worldview—and new knowledge and expertise—that are both exciting and fulfilling.

In a closing poem tribute to Leininger's pioneering work, Sagar (2012b) alluded to TCN as a vital water supply that needs to reach and be piped into villages. Prior to the poem, Sagar (2012a) exhorted all nurses—all 3,063,133 in number (USDHHS, 2010a)—to heed the call to political activism and to meet the cultural and linguistic needs of individuals, families, communities, and organizations.

CRITICAL THINKING EXERCISES 28.1

Undergraduate Student

1. When referring to the total number of nurses in the United States, what does the phrase "strength in numbers" mean to you?
2. What examples of collaboration, partnerships, and mentoring connections have you observed in your clinical rotations? Discuss.
3. As a student of today and a nurse of tomorrow, what do you envision about TCN in the next 5 years? Next 10 years?

Graduate Student

1. How would you exercise political activism in terms of providing for the cultural and linguistic needs of all clients in your capacity as a graduate student nurse?
2. Who among your current mentor, nursing leader, or historical figure has exercised political activism? Explain.
3. Have you been a preceptor or mentor to students and fellow nurses?
4. As a graduate student of today and a nurse leader of tomorrow, what do you envision about TCN in the next 5 years? Next 10 years?

Faculty in Academia

1. How would you exercise political activism in terms of providing for the cultural and linguistic needs of all clients in your capacity as a faculty member?
2. In what examples of collaboration, partnerships, and mentoring connections have you been involved? Discuss.
3. Would you be in favor of mandating CTN certification for faculty teaching diversity and cultural competence? Why?
4. How do you integrate TCN concepts in your National Council Licensing Examination® (NCLEX®)-type questions?
5. Do you have certification in TCN? Are you planning to obtain CTN certification in the next 2 years?

Staff Development Educator

1. What examples of collaboration, partnerships, and mentoring connections have you initiated, maintained, and evaluated with the community? Discuss.
2. Would you be in favor of mandatory continuing education (CE) for nurses and allied professionals in your organization? Why? Discuss?
3. Would you be in favor of mandatory CE for nurses and allied professionals in your state for renewal of registration? Why? Discuss?
4. As a large teaching hospital, you employ a very large number of nurses. A great many of them are foreign-educated immigrants. How do you help them overcome the culture shock encountered in their work with a multicultural staff and patients?
5. Do you have certification in TCN? Are you planning to obtain CTN certification in the next 2 years?
6. How many nurses in your organization have basic (CTN-B) and advanced (CTN-A) certification in TCN? Are there incentives for these nurses in seeking certification and in renewing and maintaining certification?

SUMMARY

In this chapter, the authors envisioned eight TCN trends that bear watching as the United States becomes increasingly more diverse. In addition to being a required human right, there are mandates and guidelines for CLAS for all, not just a select few. Nurses, as the largest group of health care professionals—and voted as the most trusted for over a decade—have untapped potential as change agents. Nurses, from all settings of education, practice, administration, and research, are the logical choice to lead the endeavor for culturally and linguistically appropriate health care.

REFERENCES

Accreditation Commission for Education in Nursing. (2013). *ACEN standards and criteria: Baccalaureate.* Retrieved August 22, 2013, from www.acenursing.net/manuals/SC2013_BACCALAUREATE.pdf

American Nurses Association. (1991). *Position statement on cultural diversity in nursing practice.* Kansas City, MO: Author.

American Nurses Association. (2001). Code of ethics for nurses with interpretive statements. Silver Spring, MD: Author.

American Nurses Association. (2010). *Public ranks nurses as most trusted profession: 11th year in number one slot in Gallup poll.* Kansas City, MO: Author. Retrieved August 6, 2013, from http://nursingworld.org/FunctionalMenuCategories/MediaResources/PressReleases/2010-PR/Nurses-Most-Trusted.pdf

American Nurses Association & National Nursing Staff Development Organization. (2010). *Nursing professional development: Scope and standards of practice.* Silver Spring, MD: Nursesbooks.org

Andrews, M. M., & Ludwig-Beymer, P. (2012). Cultural diversity in the health care workforce. In M. M. Andrews & J. S. Boyle (Eds.), *Transcultural concepts in nursing care* (pp. 316–348). Philadelphia, PA: Wolters Kluwer/Lippincott Williams & Wilkins.

Andrews, M. M., Thompson, T. L., Wehbe-Alamah, H., McFarland, M. R., Hanson, P. A., Hasenau, S. M.,... Vint, P. A. (2011). Developing a culturally competent workforce through collaborative partnerships. *Journal of Transcultural Nursing, 22*(3), 300–306. doi:10.1177/1043659611404214

Assemi, M., Mutha, S., & Suchanek Hudmon, K. (2007). Evaluation of a train-the-trainer program for cultural competence. *American Journal of Pharmaceutical Education, 71*(6), 1–8.

Barnum, B. S. (2006). Precepting, not mentoring or teaching: Vive la difference. In J. P. Flynn & M. C. Stack (Eds.), *The role of the preceptor: A guide for nurse educators and clinician* (pp. 1–14). New York, NY: Springer Publishing.

Camuñas, C. (2013). Culture and decision-making. In S. B. Lewenson & M. Truglio-Londrigan (Eds.), *Decision-making in nursing* (pp. 71–87). Boston: Jones & Bartlett.

Commission on Collegiate Nursing Education. (2013). *CCNE accreditation.* Retrieved July 4, 2013, from www.aacn.nche.edu/ccne-accreditation

Dobbins, M., Ciliska, D., Estabrooks, C., & Hayward, S. (2005). Changing nursing practice in an organization. In A. DiCenso, G. Guyatt, & D. Ciliska (Eds.), *Evidence-based nursing: A guide to clinical practice* (pp. 172–200). St. Louis, MO: Elsevier Mosby.

Eustis, M., Alexander Jr., G., & Plaster, E. (2010). Our experience: Strong foundations accelerate change in diversity and cultural competence. *Frontiers of Health Services Management, 26*(3), 45–51.

Haiman, C. A., Stram, D. O., Wilkins, L. R., Pike, M. C., Kolonel, L. N,... LeMarchand, L. (2006). Ethnic and racial differences in smoking-related risk of lung cancer. *New England Journal of Medicine, 354*(4), 333–342.

Huang, C. A., & Lynch, J. (1995). *Mentoring: The Tao of giving and receiving wisdom.* New York, NY: Harper.

Im, E. O. (2008). The situation-specific theory of pain experience for Asian American cancer patients. *Advances in Nursing Science, 31*(4), 319–331.

Institute of Medicine. (2010, October 5). *The future of nursing: Leading change, advancing health.* Washington, DC: National Academies Press.

Kardong-Edgreen, S. (2007). Cultural competence of baccalaureate nursing faculty. *Journal of Nursing Education, 46*(8), 360–366. Patients. *Advances in Nursing Science, 31*(4), 319–331.

Kardong-Edgreen, S., Cason, C. L., Walsh Brennan, A. M., Reifsnider, E., Hummel, F., Mancini, M., & Griffin, C. (2010). Cultural competency of graduating BSN students. *Nursing Education Perspectives, 31*(5), 278–285.

Kennedy, H. P., Fisher, L., Fontaine, D., & Martin-Holland, J. (2008) Evaluating diversity in nursing education. *Journal of Transcultural Nursing, 19*(4), 363–370. doi:10.1177/104.3659608322500

Leininger, M. M. (1995). *Transcultural nursing: Concepts, theories, research, and practice.* New York, NY: McGraw-Hill.

Mason, D. (2009). Foreword. In B. L Nichols & C. R. Davis (Eds.), *What you need to know about nursing and health care in the United States.* New York, NY: Springer Publishing.

McFarland, M. R., & Leininger, M. M. (2002). Transcultural nursing: Curricular concepts, principles, and teaching and learning activities for the 21st century. In M. M. Leininger & M. R. McFarland (Eds.), *Transcultural nursing: Concepts, theories, research, and practice* (3rd ed., pp. 527–561). New York, NY: McGraw-Hill.

McFarland, M., Mixer, S., Lewis, A. E., & Easley, C. (2006). Use of the culture care theory as a framework for the recruitment, engagement, and retention of culturally diverse nursing students in a traditionally European American baccalaureate nursing program. In M. M. Leininger & M. R. McFarland (Eds.), *Culture care diversity and universality: A worldwide nursing theory* (2nd ed., pp. 239–254). Sudbury, MA: Jones & Bartlett.

Mixer, S. J. (2008). Use of the culture care theory and ethnonursing method to discover how nursing faculty teach culture care. *Contemporary Nurse, 28*, 23–36.

Mixer, S. (2011). Use of the culture care theory to discover nursing faculty care expressions, patterns, and practices related to teaching culture care. *Online Journal of Cultural Competence in Nursing and Healthcare, 1*(1), 3–14.

Muñoz, C. C., DoBroka, C. C., & Mohammad, S. (2009). Development of a multidisciplinary course in cultural competence for nursing and human service professions. *Journal of Nursing Education, 48*(9), 495–503.

National League for Nursing. (2005). *Core competencies of nurse educators with task statements.* New York, NY: Author. Retrieved January 26, 2011, from www.nln.org/aboutnln/core_competencies/cce_dial3.htm

National League for Nursing. (2009a). *A commitment to diversity in nursing and nursing education.* Retrieved January 26, 2011, from www.nln.org/aboutnln/reflection_dialogue/rfl _dial3.htm

National League for Nursing. (2009b). *Diversity toolkit.* Retrieved January 26, 2013, from www.nln.org/aboutnln/reflection_dialogue/rfl _dial3.htm

National Research Council and Institute of Medicine. (2013). *United States health in international perspective: Shorter lives, poorer health.* S. H. Woolf & L. Aron (Eds.). Washington, DC: National Academies Press.

Porter, S., O'Halloran, P., & Morrow, E. (2011). Bringing values back into evidenced-based nursing: The role of patients in resisting empiricism. *Advances in Nursing Science, 34*(2), 106–118.

Sagar, P. L. (2012a). *Transcultural nursing theory and models: Application in nursing education, practice, and administration.* New York, NY: Springer Publishing.

Sagar, P. L. (2012b)....and the river flows. *Transcultural nursing theory and models: Application in nursing education, practice, and administration.* New York, NY: Springer Publishing.

Sagar, P. L. (in press). Transcultural nursing certification: Its role in nursing education, practice, administration, and research. In M. M. McFarland & H. Wehbe-Alamah (Eds.), *Culture care diversity and universality: A worldwide theory of nursing* (3rd ed.). Burlington, MA: Jones & Bartlett.

Sargent, S. L., Sedlak, C. A., & Martsoff, D. S. (2005). Cultural competence among nursing students and faculty. *Nurse Education Today, 25*(3), 214–221.

Smedley, B. D., Stith, A. Y., & Nelson, A. R. (2003). Unequal treatment: Confronting racial and ethnic disparities in health care. Washington, DC: National Academies Press.

The Joint Commission. (2010a). *Advancing effective communication, cultural competence, and patient- and family-centered care: A roadmap for hospitals.* Oakbrook Terrace, IL: Author.

The Joint Commission. (2010b). *Cultural and linguistic care in area hospitals.* Oakbrook Terrace, IL: Author.

Transcultural Nursing Society. (2013). *Transcultural nursing certification*. Retrieved June 15, 2013, from www.tcns.org/Certification.html

United Nations Educational Scientific and Cultural Organization. (2001). *Universal declaration on cultural diversity*. New York: United Nations.

U.S. Department of Health and Human Services, Health Resources Services Administration. (2010a). *The Registered Nurse population: Initial findings from the 2008 National Sample Survey of registered nurses*. Retrieved December 26, 2012, from bhpr.hrsa.gov/healthworkforce/rnsurveys/rnsurveyinitial2008.pdf - 2011–05-06

U.S. Department of Health and Human Services, Office of Minority Health, (2010b). *National partnership for action to end health disparities*. Retrieved February 2, 2013, from www.healthypeople.gov/2020/about/DisparitiesAbout.aspx

U.S. Department of Health and Human Services, Office of Minority Health. (2013). *Enhanced national CLAS standards*. Retrieved August 16, 2013, from https://www.thinkculturalhealth.hhs.gov/Content/clas.asp

Vance, C. (2002). Leader as mentor. *Nursing Leadership Forum, 7*(2), 83–90.

Vance, C. (2011). *Fast facts for career success in nursing: Making the most of mentoring in a nutshell*. New York, NY: Springer Publishing.

Vance, C., & Olson, R. K. (1998). *The mentor connection in nursing*. New York, NY: Springer Publishing.

Independent Study Syllabus

NUR 497—Filipino Americans and Filipino Nurse Migration to the United States

Credit Allocation: 1 credit: 15 hours   Class: as arranged
Prerequisites: GPA of 2.75 or above (see undergraduate catalog)
Faculty:

COURSE DESCRIPTION

This course will focus on Filipino Americans and their generic folk and healing practices. In addition, the student will explore Filipino nurse migration to the United States and the ethical issues surrounding "nurse drain" when migrating from developing to developed countries. Furthermore, this course will explore the available research regarding Filipino nurses and the history of migration, acculturation, and job satisfaction. Available literature will be examined. The student will develop a review of literature in a specific area of interest.

COURSE OBJECTIVES

At the completion of this course, the learner will be able to

1. Discuss Filipino folk practices.
2. Describe folk health practices in the community.
3. Analyze the history of nursing in the Philippines and nurse migration to the United States.
4. Investigate the ethical implications of nurse recruitment by developed countries from developing countries.

SUGGESTED READINGS: ANY ONE OR MORE OF THE FOLLOWING BOOKS OR JOURNAL RESEARCH ARTICLES OF YOUR CHOICE

de la Cruz, F. A., Padilla, G. V., & Agustin, E. O. (2000). Adapting a measure of acculturation for cross cultural research. *Journal of Transcultural Nursing, 11*(3), 191–198.

de la Cruz, F., McBride, M., Compas, L. B., Calixto, P., & VanDerveer, C. P. (2002). White paper on the health status of Filipino Americans and recommendations for research. *Nursing Outlook, 50*(7), 7–15.

Ea, E. E., Griffin, M., L'Eplattenier, N., & Fitzpatrick, J. J. (2008). Job satisfaction and acculturation among Filipino registered nurses. *Journal of Nursing Scholarship, 40*(1), 46–51.

International Council of Nurses. (2007). *Ethical nurse recruitment position paper.* Retrieved September 17, 2012, from www.icn.ch/psrecruit01htm#ftn1

TEACHING-LEARNING METHODS

Discussions
Meetings with instructor
Written and oral assignments

EVALUATION/COURSE GRADING

Assignments	Points	Due Date
Journals (2)	50	
Paper	50	
Meetings with the professor	P/F	As agreed upon

Journals (2)

Each journal entry needs to be a minimum of 2 pages. Be reflective. Kindly include answers to the following questions:

- What are you learning in this independent study that you did not know before? What else would you like to learn? Why?
- How do you feel as you go through this literature search about Filipino Americans and their folk and healing practices? Discuss.
- What are your thoughts about Filipino nurse migration to the United States? Is this a solution to the nursing shortage here? What are the ethical considerations when developed countries recruit nurses from developing countries? Explain.

Paper

Develop a paper using the following component headings. Each paper should be between 1,500 and 1,600 words (approximately 4–6 double-spaced pages excluding references).

Unmarked copies of the research articles used need to be submitted with the paper. **Grading will be based upon the attached rubrics.**

COMPONENT HEADINGS

■ Introduction
■ Filipino Nurse Migration to the United States
  ● History
  ● Acculturation
  ● Job satisfaction
  ● Other
■ Critique of Research Studies
  ● Did you like the research studies? Why? Why not?
  ● How is one study different from the other? Similar?
  ● If you were to replicate the studies, how would you do it? Discuss.
■ Conclusion

  Use a minimum of eight (8) references as outlined:

At least five (5) journal research articles dated between 2002 and 2013
At least two (2) books/chapters of books of student's choice
Others.

Rubrics for Oral Presentation

NUR 5000—Transcultural Nursing
Rubrics for Oral Presentation

Presenter: _____   Date: _____

Topic: _____

	Possible Points	Points Achieved
Professional dress and demeanor	5	
Maintains eye contact with audience. Uses notes or slides as reference but explains important points. Voice is clear, audible, has appropriate speaking rate	10	
Use of technology and visual aids to enhance teaching. Electronic slides use bullets, not "too busy." Has maximum of 8 lines, no extraneous information	10	
Organization and flow (Followed suggested headings and discussed appropriately) ■ Brief history of migration to the United States and associated economic factors (5) ■ Cultural communication patterns (5) ■ Biologic variations and risk factors for diseases (5) ■ Healthcare practices (including folk medicine, lay practitioners) (5) ■ Discuss a minimum of two (2) research studies involving this group. Compare and contrast the research studies. Discuss strengths and limitations. Despite the weaknesses and limitations, are these research studies helpful in your case study and in your development of a culturally competent care plan? (10) ■ Discuss culturally competent nursing interventions utilizing one transcultural conceptual model and findings from research studies (10)	40	

(continued)

	Possible Points	Points Achieved
Knowledgeable about subject (Including references, citations)	15	
Originality—creativity of presentation	10	
Clarifies points and solicits questions from audience	5	
Submitted all appropriate materials (PowerPoint handout, bibliography, etc.) to instructor and other seminar participants on or before presentation date	5	

Comments: (Use back for additional comments)

Module Evaluation Form

Title of Module:_____   Date: _____

Circle the best answer:

1. This module is
   Very informative
   Informative
   Somewhat informative
   Not informative

2. This module is
   Very easy to navigate
   Easy to navigate
   Somewhat easy to navigate
   Not easy to navigate

3. The content of this module is
   Very helpful in my practice
   Helpful in my practice
   Somewhat helpful in my practice
   Not helpful in my practice

4. The pre- and posttests were
   Very helpful in learning the concepts
   Helpful in learning the concepts
   Somewhat helpful in learning the concepts
   Not helpful in learning the concepts

5. If I were to revise this module, I would add the following:

6. If I were to revise this module, I would delete the following:

7. List other areas of interest to you for which a module can be developed:

Pretest. Module 3.1. Culturally and Linguistically Appropriate Services (CLAS) Standards

A. TRUE OR FALSE (PLEASE ENCIRCLE YOUR ANSWER)

1. The CLAS standards are primarily directed to organizations; individuals are not encouraged to use the standards.
   True/False

2. CLAS guidelines are activities recommended by the Office of Minority Health (OMH) for adoption as mandates by federal, state, and national accrediting agencies (Standards 1, 2, 3, 4, 9, 10, 11, 12, 13, 14, and 15).
   True/False

3. The 15 CLAS standards are organized into four themes: The standards are divided into the **Principal standard** (Standard 1); **Governance, Leadership, and Workforce** (Standards 2, 3, and 4); **Communication and Language Assistance** (Standards 5, 6, 7, and 8); **Engagement, Continuous Improvement, and Accountability** (Standards 9–15).
   True/False

4. Though health inequities are directly related to the existence of historical and current discrimination and social injustice, one of the most modifiable factors is the lack of culturally and linguistically appropriate services, broadly defined as care and services that are respectful of and responsive to the cultural and linguistic needs of all individuals.
   True/False

5. Health care organizations should ensure that conflict and grievance resolution processes are culturally and linguistically sensitive and capable of identifying, preventing, and resolving cross-cultural conflicts or complaints by patients/consumers.
   True/False

B. MULTIPLE CHOICE (PLEASE ENCIRCLE THE BEST ANSWER)

1. Which one of the following offices of the U.S. Department of Health and Human Services (USDHHS) developed the CLAS standards?
   A. Office of Minority and Women
   B. Office of Minority Health
   C. Office of Budget
   D. Office of Population Affairs

2. Which of the following CLAS standards are mandated for agencies receiving federal funding?
   A. Standard 1
   B. Standards 2 to 4
   C. Standards 5 to 8
   D. Standards 9 to 15

3. The main difference between translators and interpreters is that **translators**
   A. Deal with the written word.
   B. Deal with the spoken word.
   C. Deal with both the written and the spoken words.
   D. Deal with neither the written nor the spoken word.

4. The main difference between interpreters and translators is that **interpreters**
   A. Deal with the written word.
   B. Deal with the spoken word.
   C. Deal with both the written and spoken words.
   D. Deal with neither the spoken nor the written word.

5. A newly hired certified transcultural nurse with advanced certification (CTN-A) is appraising the hospital's compliance with CLAS standards. Which of the following steps will be the transcultural nurse's priority?
   A. Examine if the hospital receives state funding and if language access services are appropriately used.
   B. Examine if the hospital receives federal funding and if language access services are appropriately used.
   C. Examine if the hospital receives private funding and if language access services are appropriately used.
   D. Examine if the hospital has nonprofit status and if language access services are appropriately used.

Posttest. Module 3.1. Culturally and Linguistically Appropriate Services (CLAS) Standards

A. TRUE OR FALSE (PLEASE ENCIRCLE YOUR ANSWER)

1. The CLAS standards are primarily directed to organizations; individuals are not encouraged to use the standards.
True/False

2. CLAS guidelines are activities recommended by the OMH for adoption as mandates by federal, state, and national accrediting agencies (Standards 1, 2, 3, 4, 9, 10, 11, 12, 13, 14, and 15).
True/False

3. The 15 CLAS standards are organized into four themes: The standards are divided into the **Principal standard** (Standard 1); **Governance, Leadership, and Workforce** (Standards 2, 3, and 4); **Communication and Language Assistance** (Standards 5, 6, 7, and 8); **Engagement, Continuous Improvement, and Accountability** (Standards 9–15).
True/False

4. Though health inequities are directly related to the existence of historical and current discrimination and social injustice, one of the most modifiable factors is the lack of culturally and linguistically appropriate services, broadly defined as care and services that are respectful of and responsive to the cultural and linguistic needs of all individuals.
True/False

5. Health care organizations should ensure that conflict and grievance resolution processes are culturally and linguistically sensitive and capable of identifying, preventing, and resolving cross-cultural conflicts or complaints by patients/consumers.
True/False

B. MULTIPLE CHOICE (PLEASE ENCIRCLE THE BEST ANSWER)

1. Which one of the following offices of the U.S. Department of Health and Human Services (USDHHS) developed the CLAS standards?
   A. Office of Minority and Women
   B. Office of Minority Health
   C. Office of Budget
   D. Office of Population Affairs

2. Which of the following CLAS standards are mandated for agencies receiving federal funding?
   A. Standard 1
   B. Standards 2 to 4
   C. Standards 5 to 8
   D. Standards 9 to 15

3. The main difference between translators and interpreters is that **translators**
   A. Deal with the written word.
   B. Deal with the spoken word.
   C. Deal with both the written and the spoken words.
   D. Deal with neither the written nor the spoken word.

4. The main difference between interpreters and translators is that **interpreters**
   A. Deal with the written word.
   B. Deal with the spoken word.
   C. Deal with both the written and spoken words.
   D. Deal with neither the spoken nor the written word.

5. A newly hired certified transcultural nurse with advanced certification (CTN-A) is appraising the hospital's compliance with CLAS standards. Which of the following steps will be the transcultural nurse's priority?
   A. Examine if the hospital receives state funding and if language access services are appropriately used.
   B. Examine if the hospital receives federal funding and if language access services are appropriately used.
   C. Examine if the hospital receives private funding and if language access services are appropriately used.
   D. Examine if the hospital has nonprofit status and if language access services are appropriately used.

Key to Pretest and Posttest. Module 3.1. Culturally and Linguistically Appropriate Services (CLAS) Standards

ANSWERS ARE INDICATED IN BOLD

1. The culturally and linguistically appropriate services (CLAS) standards are primarily directed to organizations; individuals are not encouraged to use the standards.
    True/**False**

2. CLAS guidelines are activities recommended by the Office of Minority Health (OMH) for adoption as mandates by federal, state, and national accrediting agencies (Standards 1, 2, 3, 4, 9, 10, 11, 12, 13, 14, and 15).
    True/False

3. The 15 culturally and linguistically appropriate services (CLAS) standards are organized into four themes: The standards are divided into the **Principal standard** (Standard 1); **Governance, Leadership, and Workforce** (Standards 2, 3, and 4); **Communication and Language Assistance** (Standards 5, 6, 7, and 8); **Engagement, Continuous Improvement, and Accountability** (Standards 9–15).
    True/False

4. Though health inequities are directly related to the existence of historical and current discrimination and social injustice, one of the most modifiable factors is the lack of culturally and linguistically appropriate services, broadly defined as care and services that are respectful of and responsive to the cultural and linguistic needs of all individuals.
    True/False

5. Health care organizations should ensure that conflict and grievance resolution processes are culturally and linguistically sensitive and capable of identifying, preventing, and resolving cross-cultural conflicts or complaints by patients/consumers.
    True/False

B. ANSWERS ARE INDICATED IN BOLD

1. Which one of the following offices of the U.S. Department of Health and Human Services (USDHHS) developed the CLAS standards?
   A. Office of Minority and Women
   B. Office of Minority Health
   C. Office of Budget
   D. Office of Population Affairs

2. Which of the following CLAS standards are mandated for agencies receiving federal funding?
   A. Standard 1
   B. Standards 2 to 4
   C. Standards 5 to 8
   D. Standards 9 to 15

3. The main difference between translators and interpreters is that **translators**
   A. Deal with the written word.
   B. Deal with the spoken word.
   C. Deal with both the written and the spoken words.
   D. Deal with neither the written nor the spoken word.

4. The main difference between interpreters and translators is that **interpreters**
   A. Deal with the written word.
   B. Deal with the spoken word.
   C. Deal with both the written and spoken words.
   D. Deal with neither the spoken nor the written word.

5. A newly hired certified transcultural nurse with advanced certification (CTN-A) is appraising the hospital's compliance with CLAS standards. Which of the following steps will be the transcultural nurse's priority?
   A. Examine if the hospital receives state funding and if language access services are appropriately used.
   B. Examine if the hospital receives federal funding and if language access services are appropriately used.
   C. Examine if the hospital receives private funding and if language access services are appropriately used.
   D. Examine if the hospital has nonprofit status and if language access services are appropriately used.

Pretest. Module 3.2. Generic Folk Practices: Theory of Hot and Cold

TRUE OR FALSE. PLEASE ENCIRCLE YOUR ANSWER

1. The hot and cold theory is based on the four concepts of body humors.
   True/False

2. Categorization of illnesses or disharmony and the corresponding remedies are uniform in all cultures.
   True/False

3. To restore balance during illness or disharmony, these two opposing forces—referred to as **yin** (female aspect, negative, dark, and empty) and **yang** (male aspect, positive, full, warm)—need to be adjusted to restore body functioning.
   True/False

4. Illnesses deemed cold are treated with hot remedies, diseases classified as hot are treated with cool or cold remedies.
   True/False

5. Because childbirth is considered a cold condition, the postpartum woman should avoid cold drinks; cool air; cool, uncooked fruits and vegetables; and showers, since most of the heat has already been lost during the birthing process.
   True/False

6. Clients, families, and communities may be more receptive to health promotion from knowledgeable and respectful transcultural nurses and other healthcare providers who incorporate generic folk practices in nursing care across the life span.
   True/False

7. The nurse's knowledge about hot and cold theory is beneficial when planning, implementing, and evaluating patient education.
   True/False

Posttest. Module 3.2. Generic Folk Practices: Theory of Hot and Cold

TRUE OR FALSE. PLEASE ENCIRCLE YOUR ANSWER

1. The hot and cold theory is based on the four concepts of body humors.
   True/False

2. Categorization of illnesses or disharmony and the corresponding remedies are uniform in all cultures.
   True/False

3. To restore balance during illness or disharmony, these two opposing forces—referred to as **yin** (female aspect, negative, dark, and empty) and **yang** (male, positive, full, warm)—need to be adjusted to restore body functioning.
   True/False

4. Illnesses deemed cold are treated with hot remedies, diseases classified as hot are treated with cool or cold remedies.
   True/False

5. Because childbirth is considered a cold condition, the postpartum woman should avoid cold drinks; cool air; cool, uncooked fruits and vegetables; and showers, since most of the heat has already been lost during the birthing process.
   True/False

6. Clients, families, and communities may be more receptive to health promotion from knowledgeable and respectful transcultural nurses and other healthcare providers who incorporate generic folk practices in nursing care across the life span.
   True/False

7. The nurse's knowledge about hot and cold theory is beneficial when planning, implementing, and evaluating patient education.
   True/False

Key to Pretest and Posttest. Module 3.2. Generic Folk Practices: Theory of Hot and Cold

ANSWERS ARE INDICATED IN BOLD

1. The hot and cold theory is based on the four concepts of body humors.
   True/False

2. Categorization of illnesses or disharmony and the corresponding remedies are uniform in all cultures.
   True/**False**

3. To restore balance during illness or disharmony, these two opposing forces—referred to as **yin** (female aspect, negative, dark, and empty) and **yang** (male aspect, positive, full, warm)—need to be adjusted to restore body functioning.
   True/False

4. Illnesses deemed cold are treated with hot remedies, diseases classified as hot are treated with cool or cold remedies.
   True/False

5. Because childbirth is considered a cold condition, the postpartum woman should avoid cold drinks; cool air; cool, uncooked fruits and vegetables; and showers, since most of the heat has already been lost during the birthing process.
   True/**False**

6. Clients, families, and communities may be more receptive to health promotion from knowledgeable and respectful transcultural nurses and other healthcare providers who incorporate generic folk practices in nursing care across the life span.
   True/False

7. The nurse's knowledge about hot and cold theory is beneficial when planning, implementing, and evaluating patient education.
   True/False

Lesson Plan: Applying Leininger's Culture Care Theory and Other Models in Nursing Education

Objectives	Content (Topics)	Time Frame	Presenter	Teaching Methods/ Categories of Evaluation
List learner's objectives in behavioral terms At the completion of this workshop, the learner will be able to:	Provide an outline of the content for each objective. It must be more than a restatement of the objective.	State the time frame for each objective.	List the faculty for each objective.	Describe the teaching methods, strategies, materials, and resources for each objective.
1. Describe cultural competence	I. Diversity and cultural competence Some definitions a. Diversity b. Cultural competence c. Linguistic competence d. Other terms	10 minutes	Dr. Priscilla Sagar	Lecture, slides, handout Check category of evaluation to be used: ▪ Learner satisfaction ▪ Knowledge enhancement ▪ Skill and attitude change

(continued)

Objectives	Content (Topics)	Time Frame	Presenter	Teaching Methods/ Categories of Evaluation

2. Discuss guidelines, mandates, and standards for integrating cultural diversity and promotion of cultural competence in nursing curricula	II. Guidelines, mandates, standards
	a. American Nurses Association (ANA)
	b. National League for Nursing (NLN)
	  i. Diversity toolkit
	  ii. Position on diversity
	  iii. ACEN standards curriculum
	c. American Association of Colleges of Nursing (AACN)
	  i. Essentials for baccalaureate
	  ii. Essentials for master's
	  iii. Essential for doctoral education
	  iv. Diversity toolkits
		20 minutes
		
		20 minutes
			Dr. Priscilla Sagar	Lecture, slides, handout
				
				Check category of evaluation to be used:
				■ Learner satisfaction
				■ Knowledge enhancement
				■ Skill and attitude change

3. Apply the Cultural Care Theory (CCT) in student assignments in NUR courses	d. Culturally and Linguistically Appropriate Services (CLAS)
	  i. Standards
	  ii. Mandates
	  iii. Guidelines
	e. The Joint Commission (TJC)
	  i. Patient- and family-centered care
	  ii. Linguistic care in area hospitals
	2. CCT theory
	a. Seven cultural and social structural dimensions
	  i. Cultural values and ways of life
	  ii. Political/legal
	  iii. Kinship/social
	  iv. Religious/ philosophical
		50+ minutes
		
		15-minute workgroup
		20 minutes group presentation
			Dr. Priscilla Sagar
			
			Dr. Priscilla Sagar
				Lecture, slides, handout
				
				Check category of evaluation to be used:
				■ Learner satisfaction
				■ Knowledge enhancement
				■ Skill and attitude change

(continued)

Objectives	Content (Topics)	Time Frame	Presenter	Teaching Methods/ Categories of Evaluation

	v. Technological
	vi. Economic
	vii. Educational
	b. Diverse health systems
	  i. Generic or folk care
	  ii. Nursing care
	  iii. Professional care
	c. Nursing care decisions and actions
	  i. Preservation/ maintenance
	  ii. Accommodation/ negotiation
	  iii. Repatterning/ restructuring			

4. Discuss the constructs of Campinha-Bacote's Model	d. Some applications of CCT in CSM NUR courses
	  i. Fundamentals
	  ii. Community/psych
	  iii. Maternity
	  iv. Pediatrics
	  v. Adult health
		15 minutes	Dr. Priscilla Sagar	Lecture, slides, handout
				Check category of evaluation to be used:
				◼ Learner satisfaction
				◼ Knowledge enhancement
				◼ Skill and attitude change

5. Describe overview of Purnell Model of Cultural Competence	e. Some student assignments/projects
	  i. Assessment tool
	  ii. NCP Unfolding case scenarios
	  iii. Reflective journals
	  iv. Role playing
		15 minutes	Dr. Priscilla Sagar	Lecture, slides, handout
				Check category of evaluation to be used:
				◼ Learner satisfaction
				◼ Knowledge enhancement
				◼ Skill and attitude change

(continued)

Objectives	Content (Topics)	Time Frame	Presenter	Teaching Methods/ Categories of Evaluation

6. Discuss the Giger and Davidhizar Transcultural Assessment Model	Overview of some other TCN models
	
	a. Campinha-Bacote's Model, the process of cultural competence in the delivery of health care services: The five constructs:
	
	   i. Cultural awareness
	   ii. Cultural knowledge
	   iii. Cultural skill
	   iv. Cultural encounter
	   v. Cultural desire
		15 minutes	Dr. Priscilla Sagar	Lecture, slides, handout
				
				Check category of evaluation to be used:
				
				■ Learner satisfaction
				■ Knowledge enhancement
				■ Skill and attitude change

	Brief overview : PMCC
	6 of 12 domains
	
	   i. Communication
	   ii. Nutrition
	   iii. Biocultural ecology
	   iv. Health care practices
	   v. Pregnancy and childbearing
	   vi. Family roles and organization
	
	TAM brief overview
	Six cultural phenomena
	
	   i. Communication
	   ii. Time
	   iii. Biological variation
	   iv. Environmental control
	   v. Space
	   vi. Social organization
	
	Wrapping up
	Next steps
	Questions and answers
		15 minutes	Dr. Priscilla Sagar	

Pretest. Self-Learning Module 10.1. An Orthodox Jewish Child With Asthma

MULTIPLE CHOICE (PLEASE ENCIRCLE YOUR ANSWER)

1. A prohibition concerning electrical and mechanical devices on the Sabbath is based on what religious rule?
   A. Electricity is a modern convenience and therefore prohibited.
   B. The Torah forbids women from using mechanical devices.
   C. Any activity associated with work is to be avoided on the Sabbath.
   D. Pregnant women are forbidden to operate machinery on the Sabbath.

2. Toddlers in ultra-Orthodox households are not expected to understand English because
   A. Yiddish is the primary language spoken at home.
   B. Toddlers are sent to day care centers early and rarely hear English.
   C. Hearing problems are common in this group of toddlers.
   D. Young children spend a lot of time with their Yiddish-speaking grandparents.

3. The nurse can start to establish a trusting relationship with a toddler who does not understand English by entering the room and
   A. Hugging the child.
   B. Offering a sticker or cookie.
   C. Using a high-pitched tone to tell the child how cute she is.
   D. Sitting near the child and smiling.

4. In the process of patient education, which of the following is the most therapeutic statement for the nurse to say?
   A. "Using electricity is not considered work. Your daughter is ill and needs her medication."
   B. "There is the potential for a life-threatening effect of not having the medication. with Consult your rabbi for an exemption."

C. "The physician ordered this medication. Your child needs to take it."

D. "Your child is ill. There usually are religious exemptions that your rabbi could clarify."

5. For observant Orthodox Jews, when does the Sabbath begin and end?
    A. Begins during sunset on Friday and ends after sunset on Saturday
    B. Begins after sunset on Friday and ends after sunset on Saturday
    C. Begins during the morning on Friday and ends after sunset on Friday
    D. Begins before sunset on Friday and ends after sunset on Saturday

Posttest. Self-Learning Module 10.1. An Orthodox Jewish Child With Asthma

MULTIPLE CHOICE (PLEASE ENCIRCLE YOUR ANSWER)

1. A prohibition concerning electrical and mechanical devices on the Sabbath is based on what religious rule?
   A. Electricity is a modern convenience and therefore prohibited.
   B. The Torah forbids women from using mechanical devices.
   C. Any activity associated with work is to be avoided on the Sabbath.
   D. Pregnant women are forbidden to operate machinery on the Sabbath.

2. Toddlers in ultra-Orthodox households are not expected to understand English because
   A. Yiddish is the primary language spoken at home.
   B. Toddlers are sent to day care centers early and rarely hear English.
   C. Hearing problems are common in this group of toddlers.
   D. Young children spend a lot of time with their Yiddish-speaking grandparents.

3. The nurse can start to establish a trusting relationship with a toddler who does not understand English by entering the room and
   A. Hugging the child.
   B. Offering a sticker or cookie.
   C. Using a high-pitched tone to tell the child how cute she is.
   D. Sitting near the child and smiling.

4. In the process of patient education, which of the following is the most therapeutic statement for the nurse to say?
   A. "Using electricity is not considered work. Your daughter is ill and needs her medication."
   B. "There is the potential for a life-threatening effect of not having the medication. Consult with your rabbi for an exemption."

C. "The physician ordered this medication. Your child needs to take it."

D. "Your child is ill. There usually are religious exemptions that your rabbi could clarify."

5. For observant Orthodox Jews, when does the Sabbath begin and end?
   A. Begins during sunset on Friday and ends after sunset on Saturday
   B. Begins after sunset on Friday and ends after sunset on Saturday
   C. Begins during the morning on Friday and ends after sunset on Friday
   D. Begins before sunset on Friday and ends after sunset on Saturday

Key to Pretest and Posttest. Self-Learning Module 10.1. An Orthodox Jewish Child With Asthma

ANSWERS ARE INDICATED IN BOLD

1. A prohibition concerning electrical and mechanical devices on the Sabbath is based on what religious rule?
   A. Electricity is a modern convenience and therefore prohibited.
   B. The Torah forbids women from using mechanical devices.
   C. Any activity associated with work is to be avoided on the Sabbath.
   D. Pregnant women are forbidden to operate machinery on the Sabbath.

2. Toddlers in ultra-Orthodox households are not expected to understand English because
   A. Yiddish is the primary language spoken at home.
   B. Toddlers are sent to day care centers early and rarely hear English.
   C. Hearing problems are common in this group of toddlers.
   D. Young children spend a lot of time with their Yiddish-speaking grandparents.

3. The nurse can start to establish a trusting relationship with a toddler who does not understand English by entering the room and
   A. Hugging the child.
   B. Offering a sticker or cookie.
   C. Using a high-pitched tone to tell the child how cute she is.
   D. Sitting near the child and smiling.

4. In the process of patient education, which of the following is the most therapeutic statement for the nurse to say?
   A. "Using electricity is not considered work. Your daughter is ill and needs her medication."
   B. "There is the potential for a life-threatening effect of not having the medication. Consult with your rabbi for an exemption."

C. "The physician ordered this medication. Your child needs to take it."

D. "Your child is ill. There usually are religious exemptions that your rabbi could clarify."

5. For observant Orthodox Jews, when does the Sabbath begin and end?

A. Begins during sunset on Friday and ends after sunset on Saturday

B. Begins after sunset on Friday and ends after sunset on Saturday

C. Begins during the morning on Friday and ends after sunset on Friday

D. Begins before sunset on Friday and ends after sunset on Saturday

Pretest. Module 13.1. Posttraumatic Stress Disorder (PTSD) in Women

MULTIPLE CHOICE (PLEASE ENCIRCLE YOUR ANSWER)

1. You are planning care for a woman with PTSD. Which of the following statements is accurate about what a woman experiences with PTSD?
   A. Depression with coexisting anxiety
   B. Panic attacks after experiencing a life-threatening traumatic event
   C. A mental health disorder occurring after exposure to life-threatening events

2. You are planning care for a woman with PTSD. Which of the following feelings are manifested by someone with PTSD as a response to a traumatic event?
   A. Extreme fear
   B. Sadness
   C. Helplessness
   D. Horror
   E. A, C, & D
   F. All of the above

3. Which of the following reasons indicate women are at a higher risk than men to experience PTSD?
   A. Combat exposure
   B. Natural disasters
   C. Physical and sexual assault
   D. All of the above

4. While assessing a woman for PTSD, you identify which of the following to be risk factors for PTSD?
   A. Childhood abuse
   B. Depression
   C. Intimate partner violence
   D. Childbirth
   E. A, C, & D
   F. All of the above

5. As a nurse caring for a woman with PTSD, you recognize which of the following to be the three main cluster symptoms of PTSD?
   A. Reexperiencing, depression, hyperarousal
   B. Reexperiencing, avoidance, hyperarousal
   C. Reexperiencing, anxiety, hyperarousal

6. While assessing a woman for PTSD, you recognize which of the following is not a symptom of PTSD?
   A. Flashbacks
   B. Mania
   C. Irritability
   D. Detachment

7. You are planning care for a woman with PTSD. Which of the following is not a treatment for PTSD?
   A. Eye Movement Desensitization and Reprocessing Therapy
   B. Hypnosis Therapy
   C. Cognitive Processing Therapy
   D. Prolonged Exposure Therapy

8. You are providing medication education to a woman with PTSD. Which of the following are medications used to treat PTSD?
   A. Prozac
   B. Paxil
   C. Inderal
   D. Zoloft
   E. A, B, & D
   F. All of the above

9. Which of the following assessment tools may be used by a nurse to screen women for trauma exposure and PTSD?
   A. Clinician-Administered PTSD Scale
   B. The Primary Care PTSD Screen
   C. The Impact of Event Scale

10. You are caring for a woman dealing with a traumatic childbirth experience. Which of the following is not an appropriate nursing intervention?
    A. Consideration of cultural beliefs related to pregnancy.
    B. Explaining to a woman that negative feelings about her childbirth experience are normal and will go away in a few weeks.
    C. Asking open-ended questions about a woman's childbirth experience.

11. Which of the following is not an appropriate nursing intervention when caring for women with PTSD?
    A. Educating women, family, and friends about risk factors, symptoms, and treatments for PTSD.
    B. Discouraging women from repeating the story of the trauma to family and friends because it is detrimental for the healing process.
    C. Providing a community resource pamphlet for PTSD treatment and supportive services.
    D. Encouraging women to talk about their feelings related to the trauma with family and friends.

Posttest. Module 13.1. Posttraumatic Stress Disorder (PTSD) in Women

MULTIPLE CHOICE (PLEASE ENCIRCLE YOUR ANSWER)

1. You are planning care for a woman with PTSD. Which of the following statements is accurate about what a woman experiences with PTSD?
   A. Depression with coexisting anxiety
   B. Panic attacks after experiencing a life-threatening traumatic event
   C. A mental health disorder occurring after exposure to life-threatening events

2. You are planning care for a woman with PTSD. Which of the following feelings are manifested by someone with PTSD as a response to a traumatic event?
   A. Extreme fear
   B. Sadness
   C. Helplessness
   D. Horror
   E. A, C, & D
   F. All of the above

3. Which of the following reasons indicate women are at a higher risk than men to experience PTSD?
   A. Combat exposure
   B. Natural disasters
   C. Physical and sexual assault
   D. All of the above

4. While assessing a woman for PTSD, you identify which of the following to be risk factors for PTSD?
   A. Childhood abuse
   B. Depression
   C. Intimate partner violence
   D. Childbirth
   E. A, C, & D
   F. All of the above

5. As a nurse caring for a woman with PTSD, you recognize which of the following to be the three main cluster symptoms of PTSD?
   A. Reexperiencing, depression, hyperarousal
   B. Reexperiencing, avoidance, hyperarousal
   C. Reexperiencing, anxiety, hyperarousal

6. While assessing a woman for PTSD, you recognize which of the following is not a symptom of PTSD?
   A. Flashbacks
   B. Mania
   C. Irritability
   D. Detachment

7. You are planning care for a woman with PTSD. Which of the following is not a treatment for PTSD?
   A. Eye Movement Desensitization and Reprocessing Therapy
   B. Hypnosis Therapy
   C. Cognitive Processing Therapy
   D. Prolonged Exposure Therapy

8. You are providing medication education to a woman with PTSD. Which of the following are medications used to treat PTSD?
   A. Prozac
   B. Paxil
   C. Inderal
   D. Zoloft
   E. A, B, & D
   F. All of the above

9. Which of the following assessment tools may be used by a nurse to screen women for trauma exposure and PTSD?
   A. Clinician-Administered PTSD Scale
   B. The Primary Care PTSD Screen
   C. The Impact of Event Scale

10. You are caring for a woman dealing with a traumatic childbirth experience. Which of the following is not an appropriate nursing intervention?
    A. Consideration of cultural beliefs related to pregnancy.
    B. Explaining to a woman that negative feelings about her childbirth experience are normal and will go away in a few weeks.
    C. Asking open-ended questions about a woman's childbirth experience.

11. Which of the following is not an appropriate nursing intervention when caring for women with PTSD?
    A. Educating women, family, and friends about risk factors, symptoms, and treatments for PTSD.
    B. Discouraging women from repeating the story of the trauma to family and friends because it is detrimental for the healing process.
    C. Providing a community resource pamphlet for PTSD treatment and supportive services.
    D. Encouraging women to talk about their feelings related to the trauma with family and friends.

Key to Pretest and Posttest. Module 13.1. Posttraumatic Stress Disorder (PTSD) in Women

ANSWERS ARE INDICATED IN BOLD

1. You are planning care for a woman with PTSD. Which of the following statements is accurate about what a woman experiences with PTSD?
   A. Depression with coexisting anxiety
   B. Panic attacks after experiencing a life-threatening traumatic event
   C. A mental health disorder occurring after exposure to life-threatening events

2. You are planning care for a woman with PTSD. Which of the following feelings are manifested by someone with PTSD as a response to a traumatic event?
   A. Extreme fear
   B. Sadness
   C. Helplessness
   D. Horror
   E. A, C, & D
   F. All of the above

3. Which of the following reasons indicate women are at a higher risk than men to experience PTSD?
   A. Combat exposure
   B. Natural disasters
   C. Physical and sexual assault
   D. All of the above

4. While assessing a woman for PTSD, you identify which of the following to be risk factors for PTSD?
   A. Childhood abuse
   B. Depression
   C. Intimate partner violence
   D. Childbirth
   E. A, C, & D
   F. All of the above

5. As a nurse caring for a woman with PTSD, you recognize which of the following to be the three main cluster symptoms of PTSD?
   A. Reexperiencing, depression, hyperarousal
   B. Reexperiencing, avoidance, hyperarousal
   C. Reexperiencing, anxiety, hyperarousal

6. While assessing a woman for PTSD, you recognize which of the following is not a symptom of PTSD?
   A. Flashbacks
   B. Mania
   C. Irritability
   D. Detachment

7. You are planning care for a woman with PTSD. Which of the following is not a treatment for PTSD?
   A. Eye Movement Desensitization and Reprocessing Therapy
   B. Hypnosis Therapy
   C. Cognitive Processing Therapy
   D. Prolonged Exposure Therapy

8. You are providing medication education to a woman with PTSD. Which of the following are medications used to treat PTSD?
   A. Prozac
   B. Paxil
   C. Inderal
   D. Zoloft
   E. A, B, & D
   F. All of the above

9. Which of the following assessment tools may be used by a nurse to screen women for trauma exposure and PTSD?
   A. Clinician-Administered PTSD Scale
   B. The Primary Care PTSD Screen
   C. The Impact of Event Scale

10. You are caring for a woman dealing with a traumatic childbirth experience. Which of the following is not an appropriate nursing intervention?
    A. Consideration of cultural beliefs related to pregnancy.
    B. Explaining to a woman that negative feelings about her childbirth experience are normal and will go away in a few weeks.
    C. Asking open-ended questions about a woman's childbirth experience.

11. Which of the following is not an appropriate nursing intervention when caring for women with PTSD?
    A. Educating women, family, and friends about risk factors, symptoms, and treatments for PTSD.
    B. Discouraging women from repeating the story of the trauma to family and friends because it is detrimental for the healing process.
    C. Providing a community resource pamphlet for PTSD treatment and supportive services.
    D. Encouraging women to talk about their feelings related to the trauma with family and friends.

Separate TCN Course

HLT 3000: Transcultural Health Care

Credit Allocation: 3 credits
Prerequisites: English 101

COURSE DESCRIPTION

This course focuses on culture and its relationship to health. It introduces culture care beliefs, values, and practices of specific cultures and subcultures. Contemporary issues about diversity will be identified to assist students in analyzing problem areas related to culture care practices. Students will explore culture care differences and similarities as a basis for planning, implementing, and evaluating culturally competent care. The course includes current guidelines, mandates, and standards with regard to cultural diversity and promotion of cultural competence. Students will apply transcultural healthcare theory and models in the care of multicultural patients. Furthermore, students will utilize transcultural healthcare research findings to improve health care.

COURSE OBJECTIVES

At the completion of this course, the learner will be able to

1. Identify reasons for the trends, development, and importance of transcultural health care in improving care to multicultural patients.
2. Analyze generic (folk) and professional care practices of selected cultures.
3. Demonstrate strategies to provide culturally competent care to individuals, families, and communities.
4. Utilize selected models in the care of multicultural patients.
5. Apply the knowledge gained in the course concerning the culture–health relationship to the design of a domestic or global health promotion intervention.
6. Utilize transcultural healthcare findings in diverse health settings.

CURRICULUM OUTLINE AND COURSE CALENDAR

Module 1. Basic Concepts: Health, Culture, and Diversity (Weeks 1–2)

At the completion of this module, the learner will be able to

I. Analyze the meaning of health in different cultures.
II. Compare and contrast values, beliefs, and practices between two cultural groups across the life span.
III. Discuss the importance of transcultural health care
  A. Some Basic Concepts
    1. Culture
    2. Cultural shock
    3. Race
    4. Ethnicity
    5. Stereotyping
    6. Acculturation
  B. Cultural Competence: A Journey
    1. Self-reflection
    2. Self-awareness
  C. The Meaning of Health
    1. WHO definition
    2. Sampling of meaning of health
      a. Native Americans
      b. Native Hawaiians
      c. Urban Senegalese
      d. Thailand
  D. Importance of Transcultural Health Care
    1. Increase in migration
    2. Rise in multicultural identities
    3. Cultural conflicts and clashes
    4. Increased demand for culturally based health care
  E. Disparities in Health and Health Care
    1. Institute of Medicine Report: Unequal Treatment
    2. Sullivan Report: Missing Persons.

Module 2. Cultures, Healers, Rituals of Healing, and Institutions of Health

At the completion of this module, the learner will be able to

I. Discuss the role of folk healers in specific cultures.
II. Compare and contrast similarities and differences in the use of folk healing across cultures.
III. Enumerate strategies in preventing clashes between cultures.
IV. Provide examples of treatment-seeking behaviors and expectations of care among racial and ethnic groups
  A. Social Institutions of Healing
  B. Types of Healers and Rituals of Healing

1. Non-biomedical and spiritual healers
2. Folk healing and generic folk care
   a. Espiritismo
   b. Santerismo
C. Alternative Healing
D. Some Health Belief Systems
E. Treatment-seeking Behaviors of Some Cultures
   1. Mexicans
   2. Haitians
   3. Native Americans
   4. Southern Blacks
F. Cultural Clash: The Story of Lia Lee.

Module 3. Cultural Assessments Relevant to Health Care (Weeks 5–6)

At the completion of this module, the learner will be able to

I. Explore health, health-seeking behavior, and coping strategies of diverse individuals, families, communities, and institutions.
II. Discuss the use of at least one cultural assessment tool, instrument, or guideline.
III. Explain cultural nuances and their relevance to particular racial/ethnic groups.
IV. Discuss the concept of racial and ethnic disparities in health care.
V. Analyze important biological variations among clients that will affect care.
VI. Apply concepts of language, communication patterns, sexual orientation, and health literacy factors when caring for clients
   A. Exploring Cultural Nuances
   B. Some Assessment Tools, Instruments, Guidelines
      1. Leininger's Sunrise Model
      2. Spector's Heritage Assessment Tool
      3. Purnell Model of Cultural Competence
      4. Campinha-Bacote's Biblical Model of Cultural Competence
      5. Giger and Davidhizar Transcultural Assessment Model
      6. Andrews and Boyle's Transcultural Nursing Assessment Guide for Individuals, Families, and Communities
      7. Health Belief Model
      8. Other models specific to medicine, physical therapy, and others
   C. Guidelines for Assessment of Persons from Different Cultures (Ways to interview people, i.e., the concept of respect, birth order, sexual orientation, and gender issues)
   D. Methods for Conducting Assessment (Gathering Data)
   E. One-to-One Interview (although some cultures do not like to be interviewed alone and another person may be included during the process).

Module 4. Guidelines, Requirements, and Perspectives on Accreditation (Weeks 7–8)

At the completion of this module, the learner will be able to

I. Discuss the importance of the culturally linguistically and appropriate services (CLAS) standards in the care of clients.
II. Explain mandates among the CLAS standards.

III. Discuss accreditation guidelines pertinent to the practice arena.
IV. Delineate key accrediting organizations and their requirements/perspectives on cultural competence
    A. CLAS Standards
        1. Development
        2. Standards 1–3: Culturally Competent Care
        3. Standards 4–7: Language Access Services
        4. Interpretation
        5. Translation
        6. Standards 8–14: Organizational Supports for Cultural Competence
    B. Guidelines, Requirements, and Perspectives on Accreditation
        1. Commission on Accreditation of Healthcare Management Education
        2. The Joint Commission
        3. Nursing Education
           a. CCNE
           b. NLNAC
        4. Nursing Practice
           a. ANA
        5. Institute of Medicine.

Module 5. Using Evidence-Based Practice in Health Promotion (Weeks 9–10)

At the completion of this module, the learner will be able to

I. Compare and contrast current public health challenges such as obesity and human immunodeficiency virus (HIV)/acquired immunodeficiency syndrome (AIDS).
II. Apply concepts of language, communication patterns, and health literacy factors when caring for clients.
III. Analyze interactions of culturally diverse families with health professionals.
IV. Apply research findings when planning care for a specific ethnic/racial group
    A. Research and the Element of Trust: Some Unethical Studies
        1. Tuskegee syphilis study
        2. Ivory Coast, Africa: ADS/AZT case
        3. San Antonio contraceptive study
    B. A Sampling of Current Public Health Challenges
        1. Obesity
           a. Definitions of overweight and obesity for adults
           b. Obesity and cultural factors
        2. HIV/AIDS
    C. Evidence-Based Practice
        1. Some important research studies
        2. Lag time between new knowledge and practice
        3. Strategies to minimize lag
    D. Cultural Competence in Client Care
        1. Applying research in caring for culturally diverse clients.

Module 6. Creating a Culturally Competent Organization (Weeks 11–12)

At the completion of this module, the learner will be able to

I. Discuss some cultural origins of conflict.
II. Analyze strategies to promote conflict resolution.
III. Apply linguistically appropriate approaches with coworkers.
IV. Discuss insight about experiences unique to a special population
    A. Diversity in the Workforce
        1. Promoting multicultural harmony and teamwork
        2. Resources for staff development
        3. Performance evaluation incorporating culturally competent care
    B. Some cultural origins of conflict
        1. Cross cultural communication
        2. Time orientation
        3. Interpersonal relationships
        4. Gender and sexual orientation
    C. Strategies to prevent conflict
        1. Mission statement about diversity
        2. Zero tolerance for discrimination
        3. Effective cross cultural communication
        4. Commitment to multiculturalism at all levels of management.

Module 7. Journey to Cultural Competence (Weeks 13–14)

At the completion of this module, the learner will be able to

I. Describe one's own journey to cultural competence.
II. Discuss activities that will further enhance one's cultural competence.
III. Explain the relevance of measuring attitudes and skills of healthcare providers.
IV. Discuss the importance of establishing reliability and validity of cultural assessment tools
    A. Cultural Competence as a Journey
        1. Developmental process: Individuals and organization
            a. Organizations
                i. Diversity among board members
                ii. Enhanced data collection
                    a) Internal assessment
                    b) External assessment
                iii. Effective interpretation and translation services
                iv. Incorporation of cultural competence into organizational policy
    B. Cultural Assessment
        1. Individual
        2. Organization.

Lesson Plan: Use of Leininger's Culture Care Theory and Components Across Models

Objectives	Content (Topics)	Time Frame	Presenter	Teaching Methods
Learner-oriented with one measurable behavioral verb per objective	Outline of the content to be covered that will enable the learners to meet their objectives	State the time frame for each objective	List the faculty or content expert for each objective	Describe the teaching methods, strategies, materials, and resources for each objective.

At the completion of this workshop, the learner will:
 	
1. Identify challenges and opportunities of a growing multicultural population and workforce.
	Pretest
	
	I. Cultural diversity in the healthcare workforce
	  a. Cultural perspectives on the meaning of work
	    i. Individualism
	    ii. Collectivism
	
	II. Cultural diversity among our patients, their families/significant others
	  a. Cultural competence: A process
		5 minutes
		
		20 minutes
			Dr. P. Sagar	Pretest
				
				PowerPoint presentation
				
				Question and answer audiovisuals (AVs)
				
				Discussion
				
				Case studies/scenarios

(continued)

Objectives	Content (Topics)	Time Frame	Presenter	Teaching Methods
	III. History of transcultural nursing a. Transcultural nursing society b. Journal of Transcultural Nursing Society c. Challenges ahead IV. Cultural assessment guide a. Individual b. Organizational			
2. Use Leininger's action strategies in the care of multicultural clients.	I. Leininger's Sunrise Model Three action strategies a. Preservation/ maintenance/ b. Accommodation negotiation c. Repatterning/ restructuring Application of model to care of African Americans Some research Filipino Americans Some research Mexican Americans Some research Italian Americans Some research Arab Americans	20 minutes	Dr. P. Sagar	Case studies/ scenarios Nursing care plan Role playing PowerPoint presentation Case studies/ scenarios: African Americans Mexican Americans AVs

3. Apply cultural standards guiding equitable care.	I. Guidelines: Cultural standards
	 a. Nursing practice
	  i. American Nurses Association
	  ii. Office of Minority Health
	  iii. Culturally and linguistically appropriate services (CLAS) standards
	  iv. The Joint Commission (TJC) standards
	  v. Magnet criteria
	 b. Critique: Are we in compliance with these standards?
		15 minutes		Role playing
				
				Clinical examples
				
				Question and answer AVs

(continued)

Objectives	Content (Topics)	Time Frame	Presenter	Teaching Methods

4. Identify barriers and facilitators when promoting harmony in the multicultural workforce.
5. Enumerate culturally competent approaches in dealing with coworkers, patients, families, and/ or significant others.
	IV. Cultural Competence: Dealing with coworkers, patients, families, and/or significant others
	a. Cross-cultural communication
	  i. Touch
	  ii. Etiquette
	b. Clothing and accessories
	c. Time orientation
	d. Interpersonal relationships
	e. Gender and sexual orientation
	f. Moral and religious beliefs
	g. Creating a culturally competent organization: An ongoing process
	h. Promoting harmony in the multicultural workforce
	  i. Barriers
	  ii. Facilitators
	Follow-up activities
	Ongoing approaches to cultural competence
	Evaluation and posttest
		25 minutes
		5 minutes
			Dr. P. Sagar	Case studies/ scenarios
				Role playing
				PowerPoint presentation
				Question and answer
				Posttest
				Evaluation

Source: Originally published in *Transcultural Nursing Theory and Models: Application in Nursing Education, Practice, and Administration*, 2012, by Priscilla L. Sagar. Reprinted with permission of Springer Publishing Company.

Case Study: Evidence-Based Practice: Recruitment and Retention of Foreign-Educated Nurses From India

Visionary Hospital (VH), Anytown, USA, is in the process of hiring 35 new nurses from India. The Chief Nurse Officer (CNO) of VH traveled to Mumbai and personally interviewed and selected the nurses; the nurses will arrive in a month. All 35 nurses took the National Council Licensure Examination® (NCLEX®) in Mumbai and passed. Out of the 35 nurses, 25 scored more than 500 on the Test for English as a Foreign Language (TOEFL), whereas the remaining 10 obtained scores between 400 and 475. English as a second language classes are contracted with the community college nearby; classes will be given onsite at the VH. Although the nurses scored high in TOEFL, it is anticipated that slang, colloquialism, and other factors will be areas of concern.

The CNO of the hospital contacted the National Association of Indian Nurses of America (NAINA), in a city 300 miles away. The NAINA president and other officers plan to come to the hospital and welcome the nurses. The NAINA is planning to conduct one-on-one mentoring with the new nurses, although their membership numbers present a problem, as the NAINA has only 20 members. Belonging to the National Coalition of Ethnic Minority Nurses Association (NACEMNA), they enlisted the help of the other associations under the coalition. The Philippine Nurses Association of America (PNAA) regional chapter has already offered to help in the mentoring process. The NAINA plans to accept the PNAA's offer of assistance in the mentoring process, believing that although there is much differences between Asian Indian and Filipino American cultures, there are significant are similarities in the experience of being foreign nurses who immigrate to a new country and work as professional nurses. Furthermore, neither group had mentoring when they arrived 10 to 25 years ago. Individually, these nurses recalled the intense homesickness, painful process of acculturation, and difficulty with the English language, despite having been able to speak the language back home as part of their educational process.

Note: Originally published in *Transcultural Nursing Theory and Models: Application in Nursing Education, Practice, and Administration,* 2012, by Priscilla L. Sagar. Reprinted with permission of Springer Publishing Company.

Each nurse was surveyed with Appendix 20 in Mumbai during the time of contract-signing and immigration processing. The Director of Nursing Education (DNE) is collating the findings and will be using these to plan how to meet the nurses' needs, as well as other retention activities. The DNE and her staff are using the best evidence available regarding alleviation of the nursing shortage, acculturation of foreign nurses, retention strategies, and promotion of cultural competence among healthcare workers. Appendix 20 illustrates the use of the model in the orientation of the new nurses from India.

Survey Form: Use of Spector's Heritage Assessment Model in the Orientation of New Nurses From India

Name: _____   Survey Form: A

Directions: Please take time to answer this survey. Your thoughtfulness and thoroughness will assist us in planning to make resources available for you as you make your adjustment as professional nurses in the United States. Many thanks for your time.

	Physical	Mental	Spiritual
Communication	What is your native language? How long have you spoken English? TOEFL Score _____	How comfortable are you in speaking English? Very comfortable____ Comfortable____ With some discomfort____	What language or dialect do you use to pray?
Social organizations	Do you participate in ethnic activities? Yes ___ No ___ Specify: Singing _____ Dancing _____ Other ____	Do you anticipate homesickness? When you start feeling homesick, how would you alleviate it?	Do you have any family in this area? Friends? In any part of the United States? Do you know any of the other nurses who you came with from India?

(continued)

	Physical	Mental	Spiritual
Health maintenance	Do you have preferences in terms of healthcare providers? Where and how would you access health care? Are there any dietary limitation(s)? Explain.	What do you do for recreation? Do you have games, books, tapes, magazines, or television programs that are culture-specific?	Are there resources that you need to meet your spiritual needs? Explain. Do you belong to any temple or church? Are there any special holidays that you need to observe?
Health protection	Do you have special clothes worn for protection? Where can you obtain them from?	What activities do you need to avoid? Are there places that you need to visit? Places that you need to avoid?	Where do you get special amulets? What for and when do you wear those? Do you have special spiritual practices?
Health restoration	Who are the traditional healers in the community? If they are not available in the immediate community, where would you go? Do you use any traditional remedies? Where do you buy them from? Are you able to grow herbs or other remedies?	Are there special teas, other drinks, or food that you use? Where would you obtain them from? Are there any dietary limitation(s)?	Do you use folk healers? If they are not available in the community face-to-face, is there a way to contact them by phone or online?

Source: Adapted from Spector (2004). Originally published in *Transcultural Nursing Theory and Models: Application in Nursing Education, Practice, and Administration*, 2012, by Priscilla L. Sagar. Reprinted with permission of Springer Publishing Company.

Listing of Research Studies in EBP Boxes by Chapters

Chapter	Research
1-NURSING EDUCATION	Kennedy, H. P., Fisher, L., Fontaine, D., & Martin-Holland, J. (2008). Evaluating diversity in nursing education. *Journal of Transcultural Nursing, 19*(4), 363–370. doi: 10.1177/104.3659608322500.
2-INTEGRATION	Mixer, S. (2011). Use of the culture care theory to discover nursing faculty care expressions, patterns, and practices related to teaching culture care. *Online Journal of Cultural Competence in Nursing and Healthcare, 1*(1), 3–14.
4-SEP COURSE	Muñoz, C. C., DoBroka, C. C., & Mohammad, S. (2009). Development of a multidisciplinary course in cultural competence for nursing and human service professions. *Journal of Nursing Education, 48*(9), 495–503.
5-NCLEX	Sutherland, J. A., Hamilton, M. J., & Goodman, N. (2007). Affirming at-risk minorities for success (ARMS): Retention, graduation, and success on the NCLEX-RN®. *Journal of Nursing Education, 46*(8), 347–353.
6-INTRO	Mixer, S. J. (2008). Use of the culture care theory and ethnonursing method to discover how nursing faculty teach culture care. *Contemporary Nurse, 28*, 23–36.
7-SKILLS	Hughes, K. H., & Hood, L. J. (2007). Teaching methods and an outcome tool for measuring cultural sensitivity in undergraduate nursing students. *Journal of Transcultural Nursing, 18*(1), 57–62. doi: 10.1177/1043659606294196
8-ASSESS	Gay, Lesbian, & Straight Education Network. (2011). *The 2011 national school climate survey: Key findings on the experiences of lesbian, gay, bisexual, and transgender youth in our nation's school.* Retrieved May 15, 2013, from www.glsen.org/binary-data/GLSEN_ATTACHMENTS/file/000/002/2106–1.pdf

(continued)

Chapter	Research
9-CHILDBEARING	Anuforo, P. O., Oyedele, L., & Pacquaio, D. F. (2004). Comprative study of meanings, beliefs, and practices of female circumcision among three Nigerian tribes in the United States and Nigeria. *Journal of Transcultural Nursing, 15*(2), 103–113.
10-CHILD-REARING	Choi, H., Meininger, J. C., & Roberts, R. E. (2003). Ethnic differences in adolescents' mental distress, social stress, and resources. *Adolescence, 41*(162), 263–283.
11-ADULT	Tsugawa, Y., Mukamal, K. J., Davis, R. B., Taylor, W. C., & Wee, C. C. (2012). Should the Hemoglobin A1c diagnostic cutoff differ between Blacks and Whites? A cross-sectional study. *Annals of Internal Medicine, 157*(3), 153–159.
12-OLDER ADULT	Li, Y., Yin, J., Cai, X., Temkin-Greener, H., & Mukamel, D. (2011). Association of race and sites of care with pressure ulcers in high-risk nursing home residents. *Journal of the American Medical Association, 306*(2), 179–186.
13-MENTAL	Chandra, A., & Batada, A. (2006). Exploring stress and coping among urban African American adolescents: The Shifting the Lens study. *Preventing Chronic Disease: Public Health Research and Policy, 3*(2), 1–10.
14-PHARMACOLOGY	Keohane, C. A., Bane, D. A., Featherstone, E., Hayes, J., Woolf, S., Hurley, A., . . . Poon, E. (2008). Quantifying nursing workflow in medication administration. *Journal of Nursing Administration, 38*(1), 19–26.
15-NUTRITION	Fung, C., Kuhle, S., Lu, C., Purcell, M., Schwartz, M., Storey, K., & Veugelers, P. J. (2012). From "best practice" to "next practice": The effectiveness of school-based health promotion in improving healthy eating and physical activity and preventing childhood obesity. *International Journal of Behavioral Nutrition and Physical Activity, 27*, 1–9. Retrieved July 23, 2013, from www.ijbnpa.org/content/pdf/1479–5868-9–27.pdf
16-RESEARCH	Rew, L., Baker, H., Cookston, J., Khosropour, S., & Martinez, S. (2003). Measuring cultural awareness in nursing students. *Journal of Nursing Education, 42*(6), 249–257.
17-COMMUNITY HEALTH NURSING	Schuessler, J. B., Wilder, B., & Byrd, L. W. (2012). Reflective journaling and development of cultural humility in students. *Nursing Education Perspectives, 33*(2), 96–99.
18-PROFESSIONAL NURSING TRANSITION COURSE	Kardong-Edgreen, S., Cason, C. L., Walsh Brennan, A. M. Reifsneider, E., Hummel, F., Mancini, M., & Griffin, C. (2010). Cultural competency of graduating BSN students. *Nursing Education Perspectives, 31*(5), 278–285.
19-SIMULATION	Reising, D. L., Carr, D. E., Shea R. A., & King, J. M. (2011). Comparison of communication sleep outcomes in traditional versus simulation strategies in nursing and medical students. *Nursing Education Perspectives, 32*(5), 322–327.

(continued)

Chapter	Research
20- UNDERGRADUATE	Kardong-Edgreen, S. (2007). Cultural competence of baccalaureate nursing faculty. *Journal of Nursing Education, 46*(8), 360–366.
21-GRADUATE	Sumpter, D. C., & Carthon, J. M. B. (2011). Lost in translation: Student perceptions of cultural competence in undergraduate and graduate nursing curricula. *Journal of Nursing Scholarship, 27*(1), 43–49. doi: 10.10.16/j.profnurs.201009.005
22-FACULTY ORIENTATION and MENTORING	Hassouneh, D., & Lutz, K. F. (2013, June). Having influence: Faculty of color having influence in schools of nursing. *Nursing Outlook, 61*(3), 153–163. Retrieved July 29, 2013, from http://dx.doi.org/10.1016.j.outlook.2012.10.002
23-ORIENTATION	Narayanasamy, A. (2003). Transcultural nursing: How do nurses respond to cultural needs? *British Journal of Nursing, 12*(3), 185–194.
24-CONTINUING COMPETENCE	Taylor, G., Papadopoulos, I., Dudau, V., Maerten, M., Peltegova, A., & Ziegler, M. (2011). Intercultural education of nurses and health professionals in Europe (IENE). *International Nursing Review, 58*, 188–195.
25-POLICY AND PROCEDURE	Laranjeira, C. A. (2012). Translation and adaptation of the Fatigue Severity Scale for use in Portugal. *Applied Nursing Research, 25*, 212–217.
26-CREDENTIALING	American Board of Nursing Specialties. (2006). *Value of certification survey executive summary.* Retrieved March 6, 2013, from www.nursingcertification.org/pdf/executive_summary.pdf
27-FOREIGN-EDUCATED NURSES	Ea, E. E., Griffin, M., L'Eplattenier, N., & Fitzpatrick, J. J. (2008). Job satisfaction and acculturation among Filipino registered nurses. *Journal of Nursing Scholarship, 40*(1), 46–51.
28-VISION	Im, E. -O. (2008). The situation-specific theory of pain experience for Asian American cancer patients. *Advances in Nursing Science, 31*(4), 319–331.

Sample Syllabus

Culturally Congruent Care: Nursing Skills

Credit Allocation: 4 credits
Prerequisites:

COURSE DESCRIPTION

The focus of this course is culturally congruent care when performing foundational procedures for clients across the life span. Students will learn procedures in the college laboratory and will have opportunities to practice them in select clinical settings. There is emphasis on the psychomotor skills development in the areas of personal hygiene, medication administration, maintenance of safety, and meeting mobility, energy, and elimination needs. The *Healthy People 2020*; nursing process; application of research findings; and transcultural nursing are the framework for clinical decision making.

COURSE OBJECTIVES

At the completion of this course, the learner will be able to

1. Provide culturally congruent care to clients in a variety of settings.
2. Incorporate culturally and linguistically congruent care in clinical and in the learning resource center.
3. Utilize therapeutic communication techniques.
4. Provide nursing care that respects clients' culture, values, and beliefs.
5. Demonstrate a beginning sense of professionalism.
6. Collaborate with members of the healthcare team including peers to promote the welfare and well-being of clients.
7. Discuss the influence of legal, ethical, and societal issues affecting nursing practice.
8. Apply selected research findings as applicable to procedures.

MODULAR TOPICS

Module 1. Culturally and Linguistically Appropriate Services: Application in Nursing Skills	Weeks 1 to 2
Module 2. Proving Culturally Congruent Care: Hygiene	Weeks 3 to 4
Module 3. Culturally Congruent Care: Safety	Weeks 5 to 6
Module 4. Culturally Congruent Care: Energy Needs	Weeks 7 to 8
Module 5. Culturally Congruent Care: Nutrition	Weeks 9 to 10
Module 6. Culturally Congruent Care: Mobility and Elimination	Weeks 11 to 12
Module 7. Culturally Congruent Care: Medication Administration	Weeks 13 to 14
Module 8. Culturally Congruent Care: Intravenous Medication Administration	Weeks 15
Final Examination	Weeks 16

Teaching-Learning Methods

Anyone, or a combination of some, of the following methods may be integrated into class-room and clinical learning.

1. Demonstration and return demonstration of skills
2. Review of audio-visuals (AVs) of specific procedures
3. Storytelling and narratives about specific cultural traditions, values, and beliefs that may affect procedures
4. Group presentations about specific cultures and modifications added to procedures

Sample Syllabus

Culturally Congruent Care of the Childbearing Family

Credit Allocation: 5 credits

COURSE DESCRIPTION

The focus of this course is culturally congruent care of the childbearing family. Included are the processes of normal pregnancy, labor and delivery, the postpartum experience, and the care of the normal healthy newborn. Disorders and other health problems experienced by the childbearing family during these processes are also presented. Cultural patterns, family phenomena, and lifestyles are examined as they relate to and affect nursing interventions. Nursing process, health patterns, theories of growth and development, and transcultural nursing are the framework for clinical decision making and application of research findings.

COURSE OBJECTIVES

At the completion of this course, the learner will be able to

1. Provide culturally congruent care to childbearing families in a variety of settings.
2. Incorporate knowledge from nursing theories, the humanities, sciences, and transcultural nursing in the provision of nursing care.
3. Utilize the nursing process in a dependent/interdependent manner to provide nursing care to the childbearing family.
4. Apply selected research findings in professional nursing practice settings.
5. Articulate conflicts in moral, legal, and ethical aspects of nursing practice.
6. Analyze emerging nursing roles needed to meet the health needs of the childbearing family in a diverse, changing society.
7. Demonstrate an evolving growth of professionalism.

MODULAR TOPICS

Module 1. Partnering with Childbearing Families	Weeks 1–2
Module 2. Cultural Influences in Childbearing	Weeks 3–4
Module 3. Relevance of Genetics and Genomics in Childbearing	Weeks 5–6
Module 4. Health Promotion and Maintenance: Perinatal Period	Weeks 7–8
Module 5. Concepts of Growth and Development	Weeks 9–10
Module 6. Obstetrical Emergencies	Weeks 11–12
Module 7. Newborn Assessment and Nursing Care	Weeks 13–14
Module 8. Family-Centered Care	Week 15
Final Examination	Week 16

TEACHING–LEARNING METHODS

Anyone, or a combination of some, of the following methods may be integrated into class-room and clinical learning.

1. Transcultural nursing audio-visuals (AVs)
2. Story-telling and narratives about specific cultural traditions, values, and beliefs
3. Group presentations about specific cultures and childbearing practices
4. Lecture discussion about health disparities in access and quality of care

Sample Syllabus

Culturally Congruent Care: Nutrition

Credit Allocation: 3 credits
Prerequisites:

COURSE DESCRIPTION

The focus of this course is culturally congruent care in the context of the nutritive value of foods, nutritional requirements of various age groups, meaning of food in different ethnic groups and cultures, and the national epidemic of obesity. The nutritional therapy required in selected major health problems is explored. This course includes the processes of planning health promotion programs about good nutrition. Cultural patterns, economic factors, and lifestyles are examined as they relate to and affect nutritional nursing interventions. The *Healthy People 2020*, nursing process, theories of growth and development, application of research findings, and transcultural nursing are the framework for clinical decision making.

COURSE OBJECTIVES

At the completion of this course, the learner will be able to

1. Provide culturally congruent care to clients and families in a variety of settings.
2. Incorporate transcultural nursing in dietary client education.
3. Apply selected research findings in combating obesity.
4. Discuss the role of nutrients in health and illness, including nursing care of clients on enteral and parenteral nutrition.
5. Analyze the meaning of food for selected ethnic and cultural groups.
6. Explain common food-drug interactions including use of herbal preparations.
7. Develop a nutritionally adequate diet for an individual, considering height, weight, age, culture, health status, and economic factors.

MODULAR TOPICS

Module 1. Meaning of Food Among Selected Ethnic and Cultural Groups	Weeks 1 to 2
Module 2. Cultural, Social, and Economic Influences in Food Selection and Preparation	Weeks 3 to 4
Module 3. Biological Variations: Relevance of Genetics and Genomics in Nutrition	Weeks 5 to 6
Module 4. Planning Health Promotion Programs	Weeks 7 to 8
Module 5. Nutrition and Growth and Development	Weeks 9 to 10
Module 6. Obesity: The Epidemic	Weeks 11 to 12
Module 7. Therapeutic Diets: Culturally Congruent Care	Weeks 13 to 14
Module 8. Family-Centered Care: Nutrition	Week 15
Final Examination	Week 16

TEACHING-LEARNING METHODS

Anyone, or a combination of some, of the following methods may be integrated into classroom and clinical learning.

1. Transcultural nursing audio-visuals (AVs)
2. Review of some research studies
3. Stories and narratives about specific cultural traditions, values, and beliefs associated with food
4. Group or individual presentations about specific cultures and nutrition practices
5. Lecture discussion about health disparities in access and quality of care

Sample Syllabus

Educational Organization and Faculty Role Development

Credit Allocation: 3 credits
Prerequisites: none

COURSE DESCRIPTION

This course focuses on postsecondary education and organizational patterns in higher education and health agency staff development. Integration of diversity and cultural competence will be threaded through, using transcultural nursing (TCN) concepts, theories, and models; government mandates and guidelines such as the culturally and linguistically appropriate services (CLAS); academic accreditation from both the Commission on Collegiate Nursing Education (CCNE) and the Accreditation Commission for Education in Nursing (ACEN); and practice accreditation such as The Joint Commission (TJC). Multiple aspects of the faculty role, faculty socialization and development, and faculty/student issues will be addressed. Students will analyze the impact of healthcare reform as it relates to the role of nurse faculty in higher education and healthcare agencies.

COURSE OBJECTIVES

At the completion of this course, the learner will be able to

1. Analyze issues affecting contemporary higher education.
2. Examine the relationship between organizational structure, mission and governance of American colleges and universities, and the roles of faculty.
3. Integrate transcultural concepts in the mission, goals, and program outcomes of the school of nursing.

4. Apply a TCN theory or model in teaching cultural competence in any nursing curricula: associate, baccalaureate, master's, or doctoral.
5. Thread the CLAS standards in curricular development.
6. Develop a 5-year plan for professional growth as a new faculty member within the college/university setting.
7. Utilize the Boyer aspects of scholarship in planning to meet promotion and tenure criteria in 3 and 5 years.
8. Predict the impact of healthcare reform on the role of staff development educator in a healthcare organization.
9. Predict the impact of healthcare reform on the role of nursing faculty in a college/university.

Module 1. Overview of Higher Education

I. Historical perspective.
II. Mission.
III. Organizational structure, governance, funding.
IV. Measuring organizational effectiveness and cultural competence
  A. Internal measures
    1. Self-study
  B. External measures
    1. Accreditation
    2. Use of tools to measure individual and organizational competence.
V. Issues affecting contemporary higher education
  A. Diversity and cultural competence
  B. Diverse students
    1. Cultural
    2. Ethnic
    3. Gender
    4. Sexual orientation
    5. Disability
  C. Cost.

Module 2. Faculty Role in Higher Education

I. Teaching.
II. Service.
III. Scholarship
  A. Research
  B. Publication
  C. Presentation.
IV. Boyer aspects of scholarship
  A. Teaching
  B. Application
  C. Integration
  D. Discovery.

Module 3. Nursing Education Within the College/University Setting

I. Historical perspectives.
II. Technical versus professional education.
III. Liberal arts as a foundation for nursing practice.
IV. Role of nursing faculty compared to role of non-nursing faculty.
V. Socialization of nursing faculty.

Module 4. Faculty Orientation and Mentoring

I. Academic freedom.
II. Performance evaluation.
III. Promotion and tenure.
IV. Due process.
V. Professional conduct.

Module 5. Issues Related to Nursing Students: How Do We Integrate TCN?

I. Academic integrity.
II. Professional conduct of students.
III. Students' rights.
IV. Evaluation of students.
V. Disability.
VI. Confidentiality.
VII. Due process.

Module 6. Integrating TCN Concepts in Staff Development

I. Roles of nurse professional development specialist
  A. Educator
  B. Manager
  C. Consultant
  D. Researcher.
II. Educator role
  A. Staff orientation and professional development
  B. Mandatory education
  C. Unit-specific education
  D. Credentialing
    1. Certification
    2. Magnet recognition
  E. Preparing policies and procedures.
III. Issues Affecting Staff Development Educators
  A. Impact of financial cutbacks
  B. Preparing nurses to meet new challenges
  C. Competency assessment.

Index

Tell Me Your Story

1
We are from the same source.
Separate only in shape
Speech or form.

2
Yet something stirs
at the recognition of each other.
While the language is different
The story is the same:
a story of pain
or joy…abundance or lack
…of illness or health.

3
Tell me the story.
In your way: your lifeways, folk healing.
I would listen
While reflecting on mine.

4
Together we can fill the gaps.
And soon perhaps
None will remain.

Drew Yates Sagar